Topical Reviews in
Anaesthesia

Topical Reviews in

Anaesthesia

Volume 1

EDITED BY

J. Norman MB, ChB, PhD, FFARCS

Professor, Department of Anaesthetics
Southampton General Hospital, Tremona Road
Southampton

AND

J. G. Whitwam MB, ChB, PhD, MRCP, FFARCS

Reader in Clinical Anaesthesia, Department of Anaesthetics
Hammersmith Hospital, Du Cane Road, London

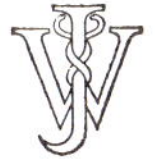

Bristol
John Wright & Sons Ltd
1980

Published by John Wright & Sons Ltd., 42–44 Triangle West, Bristol BS8 1EX.

British Library Cataloguing in Publication Data

Topical reviews in anaesthesia.
Vol. 1
1. Anaesthesia
I. Norman, J. II. Whitwam, J. G.
617′.96 RD81

ISBN 0 7236 0539 4

Printed in Great Britain by John Wright & Sons Ltd.,
at The Stonebridge Press, Bristol BS4 5NU

Preface

It can be argued that any new journal is unwelcome in an already overburdened market. However, it is the very number and diversity of sources of information that provide the justification for this new series of reviews, since the theory and practice of anaesthesia encompass the application of knowledge from a large variety of clinical and scientific disciplines. Any one individual may find it difficult to keep abreast of the literature, still less to weigh the balance of evidence for any particular point of view. It was felt that, with removal from the constraints in length imposed by existing anaesthetic journals publishing original material, it would be possible to review the 'present state of the art' using a multidisciplinary approach.

There are some subjects in which, after several years of research and the publication of a wealth of literature, it would appear appropriate to take stock of the situation. In some areas of clinical work in recent years there has been either a change of emphasis or the development of a view by consensus which has led to a standardization of approach which may be apparent only to someone well versed in all aspects of the particular subject. These considerations are paramount in selecting topics for review. However, the reviews will encompass not only the more scientific basis of anaesthesia, but it is proposed that two or more articles in each number will be relevant to the clinical aspects of the specialty. It seemed appropriate to start the series with a discussion of the evidence for the current views on the mechanisms of anaesthesia. A non-didactic approach has been adopted for clinical reviews so that whenever possible the evidence is presented for any statements which are made or views expressed, and the reasons are given for the principles underlying any particular clinical approach.

Five articles were commissioned for this first number, but one of these, on neuromuscular function, was so comprehensive as to justify its publication as a separate monograph*. It is hoped that the four papers presented here will be of interest to clinicians, will help teachers to formulate concepts and at the same time provide an adequate bibliography to be of use to a potential research worker.

Reviews of this type are intended to enable a reader to become *'au fait'* with the subject in a way that would otherwise be time consuming and difficult, and hence they should provide a service that is not readily available in the existing literature.

J. N.
J. G. W.

*Bowman W. C. (1980) *Pharmacology of Neuromuscular Function: With Special Reference to Anaesthetic Practice.* Bristol, John Wright & Sons Ltd.

Contributors

B. G. Covino PhD, MD
Professor of Anaesthesia, Harvard Medical School and Chairman, Department of Anesthesiology, Affiliated Hospitals Center, Boston, Massachusetts, USA

J. M. Manners MB, ChB, DobstRCOG, FFARCS
Consultant Anaesthetist, Department of Anaesthetics, Southampton General Hospital, Southampton

Felicity Reynolds MD, FFARCS
Senior Lecturer and Head of Anaesthetic Academic Unit, St Thomas's Hospital Medical School, London

C. D. Richards BSc, PhD
Senior Lecturer in Physiology, Royal Free Hospital School of Medicine, London

Contents

Foreword

Since the time of John Snow, anaesthetists have been trying to make anaesthesia less of an art and more of a science. However, to become expert in the specialty requires spending many years in practice and study, and it is very difficult within the same time to acquire enough scientific knowledge to be able to read basic scientific literature with understanding, although this understanding is essential for the progress of the specialty. The *Topical Reviews in Anaesthesia* represent an attempt to help in this process and are the result of careful collaboration between anaesthetists and scientists, so that these texts should not be difficult for the average practising anaesthetist to understand. One should not be deterred by the fact that one's scientific knowledge might be somewhat rusty; the scientific starting point in all the reviews is no more advanced than that to be expected of any good practising anaesthetist.

All the basic scientists with whom I have personally worked have had clear ideas of the eventual use to which their scientific discoveries might be put, and in *Topical Reviews* it is obvious that they understand the necessity to explain themselves so that they do not appear as incomprehensible 'boffins'. The *Reviews* are therefore not only informative, but I predict that most anaesthetists will actually enjoy reading them.

J. G. Robson C.B.E.
Director and Professor of Anaesthetics,
Royal Postgraduate Medical School, London

C. D. Richards

1 The Mechanisms of General Anaesthesia

INTRODUCTION

This review is concerned with the actions of general anaesthetics on the central nervous system and their relation to the production of the anaesthetic state. It is not an account of the received opinion of the mechanism of anaesthesia, as no such opinion exists, rather it reflects the reviewer's interests and prejudices. To present a coherent picture of such a vast field is difficult especially as the experimental evidence derives from techniques ranging from physical chemistry to psychology. I have therefore been selective in my choice of literature although I believe that none of the important work and ideas of the field has been omitted.

What is anaesthesia? The *Shorter Oxford Dictionary* defines anaesthesia as 'the loss of feeling or sensation; insensibility'. Implicit in this definition is the concept of perception, the conscious appreciation of sensation and the involvement of the higher nervous functions characteristic of the brain. In the search for the nervous mechanisms that are the basis of the anaesthetic state, it is helpful to have some understanding of the physiological processes that underlie sensation. This forms the first section of the review, and as the purpose of anaesthesia is to control pain, this section is heavily biased towards the somatosensory system as it is this system that transmits the sensations of pain. The subsequent sections are concerned with specific questions about the mechanisms of anaesthesia. How are anaesthetics taken up by, and distributed in the brain? Do anaesthetics cause a specific pharmacological lesion in the brain that is responsible for anaesthesia? If not, what effects do they have that may contribute to the anaesthetic state? What are the changes in nerve cell physiology that underlie the functional deficits caused by anaesthetics? Finally, what is the molecular basis of anaesthetic action?

SENSORY PROCESSING

Somatosensory Pathways

Sensation begins with the excitation of a specific end-organ in the skin, joints, muscle or viscera. These end-organs are generally regarded as specific to particular modalities such as touch, deep pressure or local temperature. They are of four types: free nerve endings, encapsulated nerve terminals (e.g. Ruffini corpuscles), lamellated nerve terminals (e.g. Pacinian corpuscles) and nerve terminals associated with specialized epithelial cells (Merkel cells). Of these types, two are of particular interest to the anaesthetist: free nerve endings which appear to be the end-organs for nociception [203, 265] and the Pacinian corpuscles which sense deep pressure [100]. In general, there is no clear-cut correspondence between the conduction velocity of peripheral nerve fibres and the modality of sensation, but it appears that the slower conducting A δ myelinated fibres (4–30 ms^{-1}) and the unmyelinated C fibres (0·4–2 ms^{-1}) transmit sensation of pain in man other than pinprick [45, 108, 307]. The afferent nerves pass into the spinal cord via the dorsal horn and ascend the neuraxis by three pathways: the dorsal columns, the spinocervical tract and the spinothalamic tract.

The ascending dorsal column fibres consist of branches of primary afferents which are rapidly conducting and transmit sensations of touch, vibration and muscle stretch. These fibres make their first synapse in the dorsal column nuclei – the cuneate and gracile nuclei. These nuclei have a somatotopic arrangement of the projections from the body surface and it is here that the first stage of sensory integration takes place in this pathway [97, 196]. The second order fibres emanating from these two nuclei cross over and pass forward to the ventrobasal thalamus where they synapse [49, 209]. The third order sensory thalamic neurones then relay this information to the primary somatosensory cortex [124].

The spinocervical tract ascends in the dorsal funiculus of the spinal cord. Unlike the ascending dorsal column sensory fibres, it consists of second order sensory fibres whose cell bodies lie in laminae III–V of the dorsal horn [30, 286]. These fibres can be excited by skin pressure, hair movement and various noxious stimuli such as C fibre stimulation and noxious heat or cold [34]. These second order afferents terminate in the lateral cervical nucleus [177, 212], the cells of which give rise to third order sensory nerve fibres that pass to the contralateral medial lemniscus and thence to the ventrobasal thalamus [146]. The thalamic cells then project to the somatosensory cortical receiving areas [124].

The spinothalamic tract ascends in the ventrolateral quadrant of the spinal cord and appears to originate in laminae I, IV–VIII in the monkey spinal cord [180, 275, 298]. The cells in lamina I have been reported to respond selectively to noxious stimuli [44, 199]. The ascending tract has three components: one that projects to the medullary reticular formation, the spinobulbar pathway; another that projects to the reticular formation, the 'palaeospinothalamic pathway'; and the third converges with the medial lemniscus to terminate in the thalamus [9]. This third pathway is well developed in primates and conveys the sensations of touch, itch, pain and temperature [298].

The ventrobasal thalamus receives information from each of the three main sensory pathways. This places it at the centre of the sensory projections from the periphery and the posteriolateral thalamic nuclei possess detailed maps of the contralateral body surface. These nuclei project to the somatosensory areas of the cortex [124] and receive in turn a substantial projection from it [209, 230]. Indeed, this descending cortical projection exerts a profound tonic inhibition on the cells of the ventrobasal thalamus [10, 14]. From the primary cortical receiving areas the response to a sensory input disseminates throughout the cortex where it is integrated with information from other pathways before the appropriate motor actions are taken.

Modulation of Sensory Processes

Normal transmission along the classical sensory pathways has a high margin of safety through each synaptic relay. Yet we know from our everyday experience that we are aware of only a few of the stimuli that daily assault our senses. It follows, therefore, that the response of the nervous system to peripheral stimulation is modified by other factors such as the level of arousal or the presence of other stimuli. Apart from the indirect regulation of the amount of light reaching the eye by the iris, and the volume of sound transmitted to the cochlea by the tensor tympani, the modulation of sensory perception does not take place in the periphery but within the central nervous system itself, at a spinal or supraspinal level. This modulation takes several forms: for example there is convergence of sensory information in the dorsal column nuclei so that stimulation of one specific receptor causes the discharge of a specific cell in the nuclei but inhibits the discharge of neighbouring cells – 'surround inhibition' [97, 98]. Similarly, strong noxious stimuli, which elicit responses that do not travel in the ascending dorsal columns but in the spinocervical and spinothalamic pathways, are able to inhibit the passage of sensory information through the dorsal column nuclei and facilitate the transmission of sensory information through the ventrobasal thalamus [15]. The facilitation of thalamic transmission can cause desynchronization of the cortical electroencephalogram (EEG) – the so-called arousal response (*see below*). In addition to the modulatory influence of the ascending pathways there are descending influences from the cortex on the thalamus [118], the brain stem reticular formation [87, 109, 274] and the dorsal column nuclei [65, 243]. Thus the cortex can exert a direct excitatory influence on the activity of cells in the dorsal column nuclei and an indirect inhibitory influence via the midbrain reticular formation. The spinocervical nuclei also receive descending control from the cortex [31].

The term brain stem reticular formation has been used to indicate a diffuse structure in the lower regions of the brain that has a modulatory influence on cortical function [88]. Angel [11] has pointed out that there are differences of opinion about the exact composition of the brain stem, though it may be taken to include the medulla oblongata, pons and mesencephalon, and that the original concept of diffuse cellular network has had to be modified because the reticular formation has subsequently been shown to consist of several moderately clearly defined cellular regions. Additionally, there are components in the thalamus that may be considered to be part of the reticular formation – those thalamic nuclei that receive a direct projection from the reticular formation such as the reticular thalamic nuclei, as well as those regions that have cells of similar structure to those of the brain stem reticular formation, the intralaminar thalamic nuclei. The role of these nuclei in evoking electrical activity in the cortex was studied by Dempsey and Morrison [68], who showed that low frequency stimulation of the intralaminar thalamic nuclei elicited high voltage negative waves in the cortex which showed a characteristic waxing and waning pattern similar to that seen in the EEG during the alpha rhythm. Later Moruzzi and Magoun [181] found that high frequency electrical stimulation in the brain stem and intrathalamic nuclei gave rise to electrocortical desynchronization, i.e. brought about a change in the electrocorticogram from low frequency high voltage waves to high frequency low voltage waves (*Fig. 1.1*). This change was later shown to be

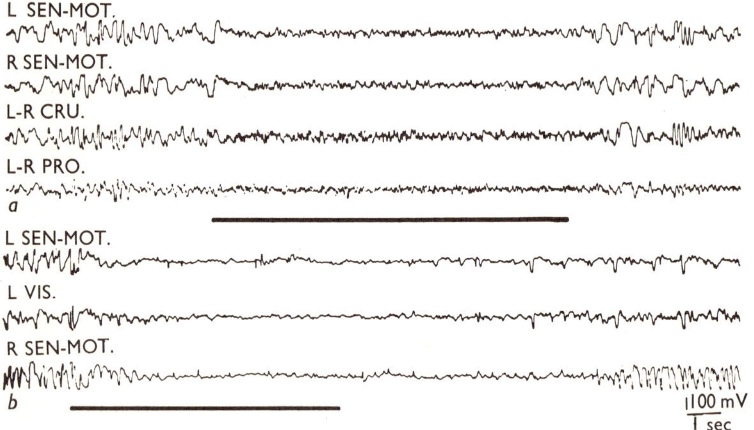

Fig. 1.1. The desynchronization of the electrocorticogram (ECoG) by stimulation of the reticular formation. *a,* From an encéphale isolé preparation. Initially the ECoG has a pattern of low frequency, high voltage waves. Stimulation of the reticular formation (black bar) causes the emergence of a high frequency, low voltage pattern. *b,* From an intact cat anaesthetized with chloralose. The abbreviations on the left indicate the positions of the recording leads. (*From Moruzzi and Magoun [181].*)

accompanied by signs of behavioural arousal [86]. These observations led to the general acceptance of the view that the arousal reaction could be attributed to excitation of an ascending component of the reticular formation and that the activity of the cortex (and consequently conscious experience) was controlled by the brain stem. Such a view is oversimplified for the following reasons among others (*see also* Angel [11]): first, low frequency stimulation of the intralaminar thalamic nuclei gives rise to synchronized cortical waves, while high frequency stimulation of the same structures gives rise to the desynchronized waves [68, 181]. Second, it assumes an equivalence between EEG pattern and behavioural state that is not justified: for example, it is possible to dissociate the behavioural state of an animal from its EEG pattern [157, 297] by treatment with

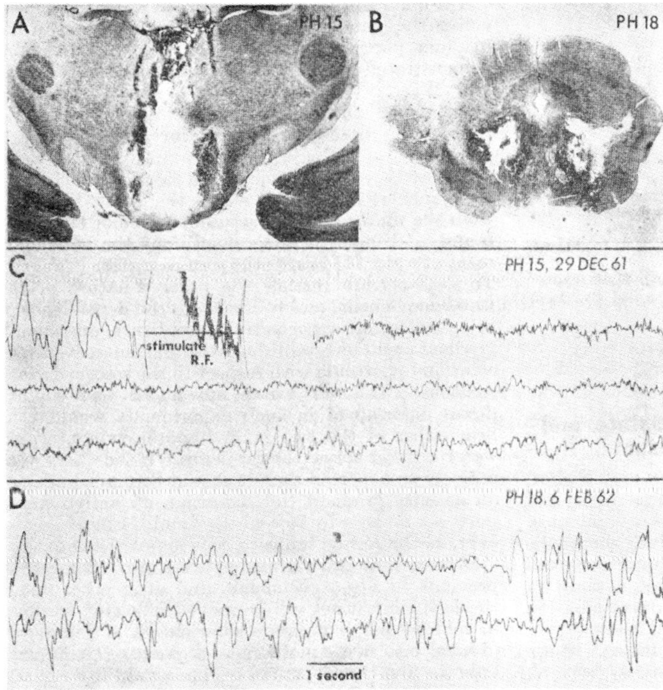

Fig. 1.2. The effect of lesions in the brain stem and hypothalamus on the electrocorticogram (ECoG). A, C, From cat PH 15. A shows the lesion in the hypothalamus. This cat was in permanent coma after the lesion. The ECoG shows normal desynchronization following stimulation of the reticular formation but no behavioural arousal. B, D, From cat PH 18. B shows the lesion in the reticular formation. The ECoG was recorded during visual tracking by the awake animal. The same ECoG pattern was also present before and after the tracking session. The two ECoG tracings are continuous. (*From Feldman and Waller [78].*)

atropine where the EEG is synchronized (similar to that seen during sleep) although the animal is behaviourally awake. Third, Feldman and Waller [78] showed that large lesions could be made in the ascending reticular formation which produced animals with a permanently synchronized EEG but which were behaviourally awake. They also showed that lesions in the hypothalamus could produce comatose animals with a permanently desynchronized EEG (*Fig. 1.2*). Clearly therefore, while the brain stem reticular formation has important modulatory influences on sensory processes and cortical activity (viz. the arousal reaction), it is quite erroneous to regard it as the site of consciousness, i.e. perceptual experience, as the following section will make clear.

The Role of the Cortex in Sensory Experience

Here we must consider the difficult question of consciousness and its localization in the brain, which lies at the heart of any discussion of the mechanisms of general anaesthesia. Without going further into philosophical discussions about the meaning of words we may accept the simple definition proposed by Cobb [50] that consciousness is an awareness of environment and of self. This definition implies perceptual experience, that is to say that not only can we respond to a stimulus but that we are aware of what we are doing. Thus reflex actions, however complex, are unconscious in the sense that they may, and indeed often do, occur before we are aware of them and they can occur without our being aware of them, e.g. during general anaesthesia or sleep. Clearly consciousness is not an all-or-none phenomenon, but a graded state. Our problem is therefore that of estimating awareness – a difficult task. We may ask a man whether he is aware of events occurring around him, but we cannot quantify how aware he is. In animals we are reduced to inferring consciousness from behavioural responses.

Although we have to consider where consciousness may be located in the brain, this is a hazardous pursuit. Indeed, Walshe [288] has commented that precise definition of consciousness is impossible as 'we are from time to time differently conscious' and that discussion of the localization of consciousness is 'anatomising an abstraction'. Nonetheless, the question is important and will not go away just because it is difficult. Early neurologists considered the cortex as the site of consciousness because it was the outgrowth of cortex that distinguished the brain of man from that of other animals. Later observers noted that large areas of cortex could be removed under local anaesthesia without loss of consciousness but that tumours of the brain stem and diencephalon frequently caused coma. Following the work of Moruzzi and Magoun [181] on the brain stem (*see above*), these observations became over-interpreted and the view developed that consciousness was localized in the brain stem. Thus Feldberg [77], writing in 1959 about the experiments of Goltz on decorticate dogs, remarked that while the animals possessed a consciousness vastly different from that of normal dogs, their condition was that of idiocy not unconsciousness. However Cairns [37], after reviewing the evidence for the role of the brain stem in the maintenance of consciousness, wrote 'I must emphasise again that unconsciousness accompanying organic lesions of the brain stem and thalamus is largely a disorder of crude consciousness. . . . There is nothing in this view to controvert the older view that the cerebral cortex is *essential* for the higher levels of consciousness' (my italics). More recent evidence suggests that consciousness in the sense of perceptual awareness, is in fact a cortical phenomenon.

Consider first the condition of decorticate animals and men. Decorticate animals or hydrocephalic children may live for considerable periods of time. Cairns reports one hydrocephalic child who survived for 20 years. Thus the cerebral cortex is not essential to life. Such patients sleep and wake, react to hunger and thirst, to loud sounds, to crude visual stimuli; they may be able to discriminate unpleasant and pleasant tastes and they have some crude motor control over their limbs. Similar results have been reported for decorticate dogs [77]. In all these instances the cortex is either totally absent or virtually destroyed while the thalamus and brain stem are intact. Writing on human anencephalic or hydrocephalic children, Cairns [37] comments 'However one may regard it, there is in these monsters a somatic activity amounting to a kind of wakefulness or consciousness which takes place without participation of the cerebral cortex.' There is some truth in this view. However, we cannot know whether these monsters have 'awareness of self and environment' as Cobb's definition of consciousness requires. Moreover, their behaviour is devoid of the characteristics of their normal brethren. They are not imbeciles like severely handicapped mongols but automata without the essential ingredient that would make them human.

It is well known that ablation of the specific sensory cortex causes a failure of perception even though the peripheral sensory apparatus may be intact. Thus ablation of the visual cortex in man causes a loss of sight. Partial ablation would give blindness in the corresponding part of the visual field even though the eye and lower visual centres in the superior colliculus remained intact. Recent experiments with patients who have such lesions [201, 227, 240] have thrown new light on the problem of consciousness. As expected, they all report that they cannot see objects placed in the part of the visual field corresponding to their scotoma, i.e. they are not aware of such objects. Yet they have some residual sensation. Powerful stimuli may be perceived as bright lights without clear form, and careful psychological testing has shown that such patients can discriminate monocular from binocular stimuli and that they are better at discriminating the position of dark bars in visual space than normal subjects [227]. They can control their eye movements sufficiently to fixate in the region of an object flashed into their visual field even though they cannot 'see' the object [201]. Similar differences between normal monkeys and those with lesions in the visual cortex have been described [117, 295].

Other evidence of the role of the cortex in consciousness comes from the work of Sperry on patients with disconnected cerebral hemispheres [261, 262]. Such a situation arose as a result of treatment of severe epilepsy by section of the corpus callosum, the anterior commissure and the hippocampal commissure. Apparently this drastic surgery did not result in major disturbances of personality in these patients, but Sperry has shown that they behave as though there was 'an apparent doubling in most of the realms of conscious awareness. Instead of the normally unified single stream of consciousness, these patients behave in many ways as if they have two independent streams of conscious awareness, one in each hemisphere, each of which is cut off from and out of contact with the mental experiences of the other. In other words each hemisphere seems to have its own separate and private sensations; its own perceptions; its own concepts; and its own impulses to act, with related volitional cognitive and learning experiences' [262]. The experimental evidence for this view was obtained by a variety of tests of which I shall briefly discuss only the stereognostic ones. Subjects sat at a table containing simple everyday objects hidden from view by a screen. They were asked to pick one object with one hand and describe it. Objects retrieved with the right hand were correctly identified as expected because the right hand projects to the left, dominant, hemisphere which contains the speech centres. However, if a subject was asked what he held in his left hand, his left hemisphere did not know and was reduced to guessing. If however, the minor right hemisphere was allowed to express itself by asking the subject to retrieve the same object from a bag containing other objects with the left hand, then this was done accurately. From a variety of tests like this, Sperry concluded that each hemisphere of the brain in these patients could comprehend and solve such problems, but that the minor hemisphere was handicapped by having no control over speech so that careful tests were necessary to show its competence. Wider testing showed significant differences in the capabilities of the two hemispheres (*Fig. 1.3*), but did not suggest that the minor hemisphere was in any sense unconscious. In fact, despite the separateness of the experiences of the two hemispheres, Sperry found that emotional responses could be transmitted from the right hemisphere to the left even though the left hemisphere was unaware of the triggering stimulus.

It seems justifiable to conclude from this evidence that the cortex is the site of sensory perception and conscious experience. However, it is also apparent that certain deep structures including the ascending reticular formation, thalamus, hypothalamus and limbic system strongly influence the activity of the cortex. Lesions in the brain stem, hypothalamus and thalamus can result in permanent coma despite the presence of an intact cortex. Conversely, animals with an intact brain stem and thalamus but without a cortex are automata. Normal cerebral activity requires both an intact cortex and intact lower structures. A simple analogy may help to express this interdependence: the system is like a lighting circuit with one bright light (consciousness) and several very dim ones (higher reflex actions) controlled by a switch (somewhere in the lower brain structures). If the switch is damaged, the circuit fails and nothing will be illuminated. However, if the main light is broken or removed, operation of the switch will result only in dim illumination. Only with an intact switch and an intact light will the whole scene be illuminated.

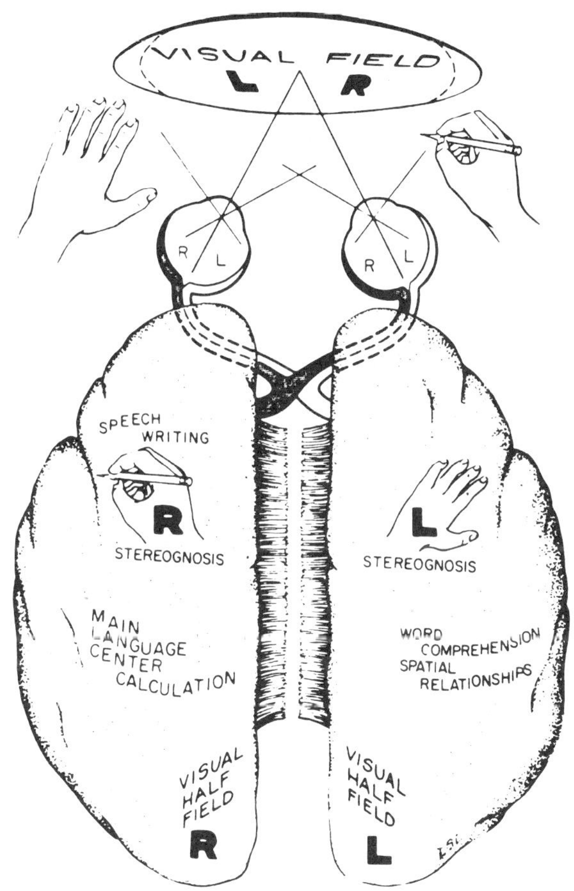

Fig. 1.3. The localization of basic cerebral functions in the major and minor hemispheres revealed by behavioural tests after cutting the corpus callosum and anterior commissure. (*From Sperry [261]*.)

THE ACTIONS OF ANAESTHETICS ON THE CENTRAL NERVOUS SYSTEM

From what has already been discussed, it is apparent that general anaesthesia must result from the actions of anaesthetics on one or more of the following structures: brain stem, hypothalamus, thalamus and cerebral cortex. The question is whether there is any evidence to suggest that the function of one of these structures is affected by anaesthetics before the function of any other. If such evidence were to be found, it would then be possible to infer that this structure was a primary target for the action of general anaesthetics and that anaesthesia was the result of a specific pharmacological lesion in the brain at that site. In contrast, impairment of function at all four sites would imply a more general, diffuse, action on the brain. The evidence bearing on this question has been obtained by both indirect and direct experimental approaches.

The evidence obtained by indirect methods – studies of anaesthetic distribution in the brain and the effects of anaesthetics on cerebral metabolism will be considered first, and will be followed by an account of the evidence obtained from the more direct electrophysiological studies of anaesthetic action on nervous activity.

Uptake and Distribution of Anaesthetics

Anaesthetics are, generally speaking, rather lipid-soluble substances and their uptake into the brain is dictated not by regional differences of permeability but by local cerebral blood flow [161]. Grey matter has a higher blood flow than white matter and the regions with the highest blood flow are the inferior colliculus, sensory areas of the cerebral cortex and the geniculate bodies. The reticular formation has only about one-half the blood flow of the primary sensory cortex (Table 1.1) [145, 211].

Table 1.1. The Effects of Thiopentone on Regional Blood Flow in the Brain of the Cat

	Normal blood flow ($ml.g^{-1}$ min^{-1})	*Percent decrease with thiopentone*
Sensorimotor cortex	1·38 ± 0·12	53
Auditory cortex	1·30 ± 0·05	45
Visual cortex	1·25 ± 0·06	38
Lateral geniculate	1·21 ± 0·08	35
Hypothalamus	0·84 ± 0·05	35
Thalamus	1·03 ± 0·05	31
Cerebellar nuclei	0·87 ± 0·07	29
Association cortex	0·88 ± 0·04	22
Inferior colliculus	1·80 ± 0·12	22
Reticular formation	0·59 ± 0·05	NS
Cerebral white matter	0·23 ± 0·02	NS

Data from Landau et al. [145] and Reivich et al. [211].

Thus agents like thiopentone that have a high blood–brain partition coefficient distribute preferentially in the cerebral grey matter, the highest levels being attained during the initial stages of anaesthesia. In contrast, phenobarbitone is taken up slowly and though there is an initial preferential distribution in the cerebral grey matter, the highest levels of anaesthetic in grey matter are attained slowly and there is little distinction between the different regions of the brain or even between grey and white matter [38] (*Fig. 1.4*). From the scanty evidence available it appears, therefore, that anaesthetics distribute preferentially to grey matter but

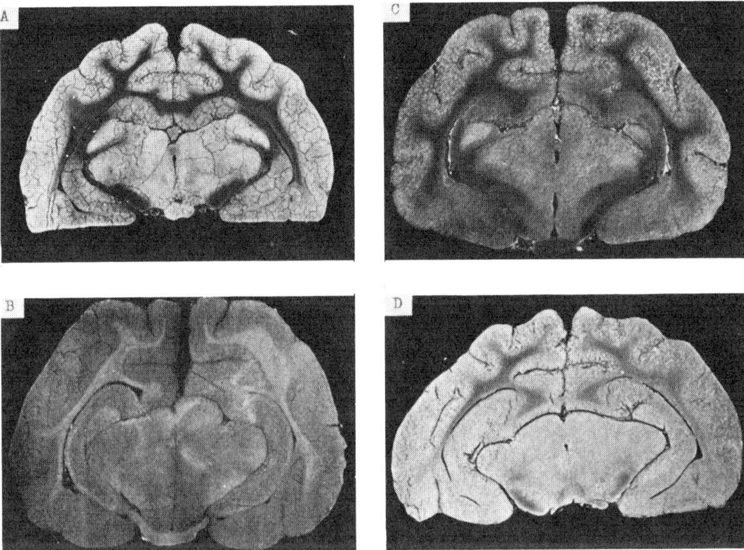

Fig. 1.4. Autoradiographs showing the distribution of radio-labelled thiopentone (A, B) and phenobarbitone (C, D). A, 3 min after injection of ^{35}S thiopentone. B, 10 min after injection. C, 5 min after injection of ^{14}C phenobarbitone. D, 30 min after injection. Note rapid initial uptake of ^{35}S thiopentone into grey matter and its equally rapid loss. Phenobarbitone shows slower uptake into grey matter. (*From Cassano et al. [38].*)

there is no evidence of preferential accumulation of anaesthetics in the grey matter of particular regions of the brain [51, 52].

Effect of Anaesthetics on Cerebral Metabolic Activity

Early studies indicated that the administration of anaesthetics caused a depression of the cerebral metabolic rate. Later experiments on the action of thiopentone on regional blood flow showed that the greatest reductions in blood flow occurred in the sensory–motor cortex, auditory cortex, visual cortex and lateral geniculate body [145]. Despite its normal high value, the blood flow of the inferior colliculus showed a relatively small change during anaesthesia and there was no significant change in a number of other structures including the reticular formation and the cerebral white matter. It has generally been assumed that these changes in metabolic rate reflect a reduced metabolic demand rather than a direct depressant action of anaesthetics on cellular respiration and that the reduction of the metabolic demand reflects a decrease in nervous activity [255]. Recent work with the newly developed 2-deoxyglucose technique of mapping local glucose uptake [257] has confirmed the essential correctness of this view. There is a close correspondence between local cerebral blood flow, local glucose uptake and local nerve activity [210, 256].

Using the 2-deoxyglucose technique, Sokoloff et al. [257] found a generalized depression of local glucose uptake throughout the brains of rats anaesthetized with thiopentone when compared to that of normal, awake rats (Table 1.2). In agreement with the earlier results on cerebral

Table 1.2. The Action of Thiopentone on Local Cerebral Glucose Uptake

	Local cerebral glucose uptake (μmol. 100 g^{-1} min^{-1})		
	Control	*Anaesthetized*	*Percentage decrease*
Visual cortex	111 ± 5	64 ± 3	–42
Auditory cortex	157 ± 5	81 ± 3	–48
Parietal cortex	107 ± 3	65 ± 2	–39
Sensorimotor cortex	118 ± 3	67 ± 2	–43
Lateral geniculate body	92 ± 2	53 ± 3	–42
Ventral thalamus	98 ± 3	55 ± 1	–44
Hypothalamus	63 ± 3	43 ± 2	–32
Inferior colliculus	198 ± 7	131 ± 8	–34
Pontine grey matter	69 ± 3	46 ± 3	–33
Corpus callosum	42 ± 2	30 ± 2	–29

Data from Sokoloff et al. [257].

blood flow, the greatest reductions occurred in the sensory areas of the cortex, the thalamus and the geniculate bodies. Similar results have been reported on the effects of γ-butyrolactone on local cerebral glucose metabolism in the rat [302].

However, when the effects of a wider range of anaesthetics on cerebral metabolic activity are considered, the picture is much less clear-cut. Broadly speaking, anaesthesia is accompanied by a decrease in cerebral metabolic rate but this effect is not uniform amongst all anaesthetics and is not simply dose related, as a glance at Table 1.3 will show. Both cyclopropane [5] and ether [253] appear to have a biphasic effect on cerebral oxygen uptake, an initial depressant effect followed by a rise to near normal values as the dose administered is increased. Ketamine produces a decrease in cerebral metabolic rate that is not statistically significant [267]. Only with Ethrane (enflurane) [253], halothane [159] and methoxyflurane [269] has a clear dose-related depression of oxygen uptake been established.

Local cortical glucose consumption also shows variation between anaesthetic agents but the evidence is scanty. Shapiro et al. [248] have mapped local cortical glucose consumption in normal awake monkeys, monkeys anaesthetized with halothane or pentobarbitone or sedated with phencyclidine. The pattern is markedly different for each agent, the most

Table 1.3. The Effects of Some Anaesthetics on Cerebral Oxygen Consumption

Anaesthetic	*Dose*	*Cerebral oxygen uptake (ml. 100 g^{-1} min^{-1})*	*Percentage change*	*Species*	*Ref.*
Cyclopropane	0	3·2 ± 0·3	–	Man	5
	13%	2·27 ± 0·26	–29%		
	37%	2·24 ± 0·26	–30%		
	0	2·82 ± 0·12	–	Man	5
	5%	1·67 ± 0·31	–41%		
	20%	2·50 ± 0·35	–12%		
Diethyl ether	0	3·0	0	Man	253
	2·4%	2·0	–34%		
	4·5%	2·7	–11%		
Ethrane	0	3·0		Man	253
	0·85%	2·28	–25%		
	2·0%	2·0	–33%		
	3·0%	1·53	–50%		
Halothane*	0	6·6 ± 1·4	–	Dog	159
	0·5%	5·7 ± 1·6	–14%		
	2·0%	4·0 ± 1·1	–39%		
Hydroxydione	0	3 1 ± 0 1		Man	99
	–	1·7 ± 0·2	–45%		
Ketamine	0	2·82 ± 0·15	–	Man	267
	3 mg/kg	2·48 ± 0·1	–12% $P > 0·1$		
Methoxyflurane*	0·1%	5·67 ± 0·24	–	Dog	269
	0·25%	5·11 ± 0·22	–10%		
	0·44%	4·37 ± 0·26	–33%		
Thiopentone	0	3·3	–	Man	
	–	2·1	–36%		113
	25 mg/l blood	1·5	–55%		198

*Experiments with halothane and methoxyflurane were carried out in dogs anaesthetized with 70 per cent N_2O, 30 per cent O_2 and are values for cerebral cortex, not whole brain.

striking difference being a large increase in local glucose consumption over most of the cortex (except the preoccipital and occipital cortex) in the presence of phencyclidine and a moderate increase in the glucose consumption of the temporal lobe in animals anaesthetized with pentobarbitone (*Fig. 1.5*). A detailed analysis of the action of halothane on local glucose consumption throughout the brain revealed significant decreases only in the occipital cortex, periaqueductal grey matter, reticular formation and inferior colliculus.

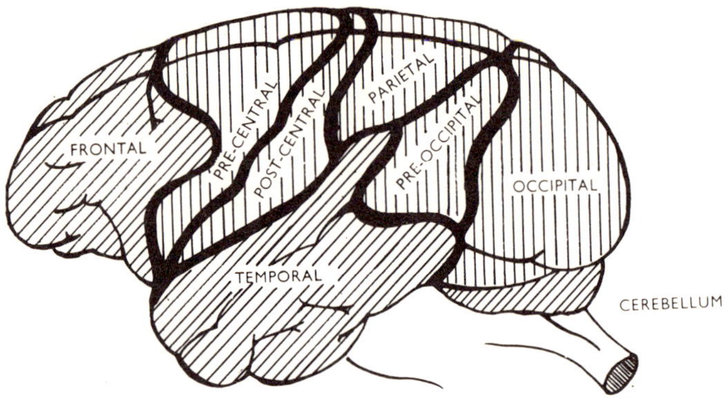

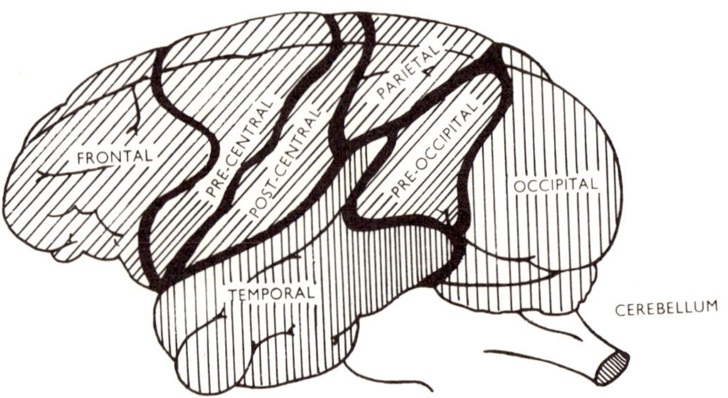

Fig. 1.5. Composite maps of the superficial cortical local cerebral metabolic rate determined by the deoxyglucose method for awake monkeys and for monkeys anaesthetized by halothane, pentobarbitone, and phencyclidine. (*From Shapiro et al. [248].*)

PENTOBARBITAL

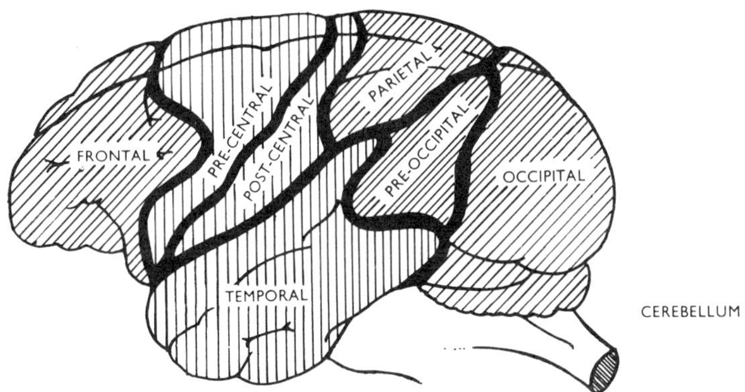

PHENCYCLIDINE

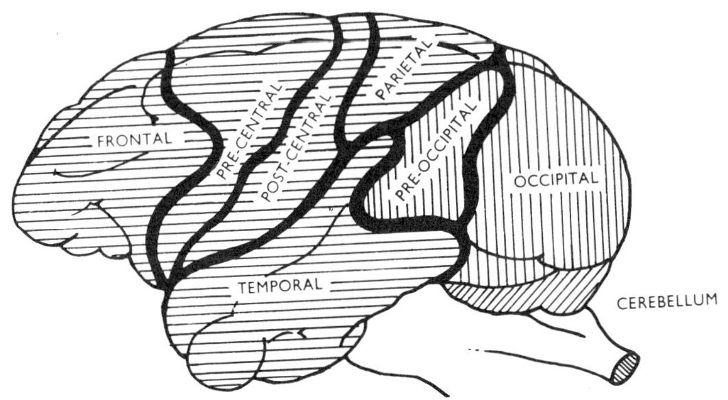

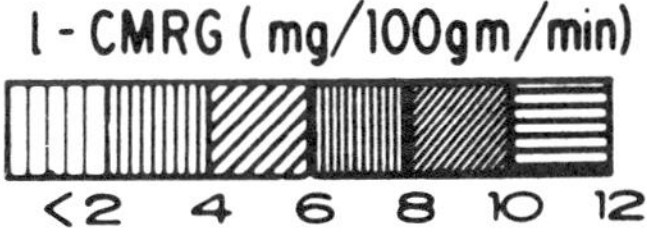

As it has been established that local cerebral glucose uptake is correlated with local nerve activity [210, 256], these results imply that anaesthetics do not cause a uniform depression of activity throughout the nervous system nor is the pattern of change common to all anaesthetics. However, it must be remembered that these methods are largely indirect and Landau [145] has remarked that they are 'rather like trying to measure what a factory does by measuring the intake of water and the output of sewage. . . only secondary inferences can be made regarding function.' Nonetheless, the same organ is being studied in the presence of different perturbing agents. If they all acted in a common way, we may reasonably expect to see a common pattern of perturbation emerging. The fact that this is not so suggests that there are likely to be considerable differences in the way different anaesthetics produce anaesthesia.

Actions on the Spinal Cord and Ascending Sensory Systems

It is clear that the actions of anaesthetics on the spinal cord are not directly implicated in the production of general anaesthesia: spinal block is not accompanied by unconsciousness. However, the modulation of sensory transmission by anaesthetics at a spinal level will necessarily affect the response of the higher centres to peripheral stimuli. Furthermore, anaesthetics are employed not only for the suppression of pain but also for the suppression of motor movement during surgery, much of which will be due to simple withdrawal reflexes.

It is an old observation that motor responses to painful stimulation are obtunded by general anaesthetics. Indeed, the action of anaesthetics on reflex activity was one of the observations that led Sherrington [249] to the concept of the synapse. Recent work has been directed towards the mechanisms underlying this depression. The effect of anaesthetics on monosynaptic and polysynaptic reflex pathways can be studied by observing the response of ventral root fibres to stimulation of the appropriate dorsal root and measuring the change in the amplitude of the ventral root response when an anaesthetic is applied. The recorded potential consists of a brief initial, short latency response (the monosynaptic response) and is followed by another of long duration which has many irregularities (the polysynaptic response). A wide variety of anaesthetics depress these responses [125, 228, 260] (*see Fig. 1.6*). In general it has been assumed that transmission through a polysynaptic pathway must be more vulnerable to the action of anaesthetics than that through a monosynaptic pathway [303]. However, several studies indicate that this is not true of spinal pathways where the evoked potential of the monosynaptic stretch reflex is more readily depressed than that of polysynaptic pathways [127]. Within a given pathway the vulnerability of sequential steps will depend not on the number of synapses but on the security of synaptic transmission at each step.

Detailed consideration of the mechanisms of action of anaesthetics on

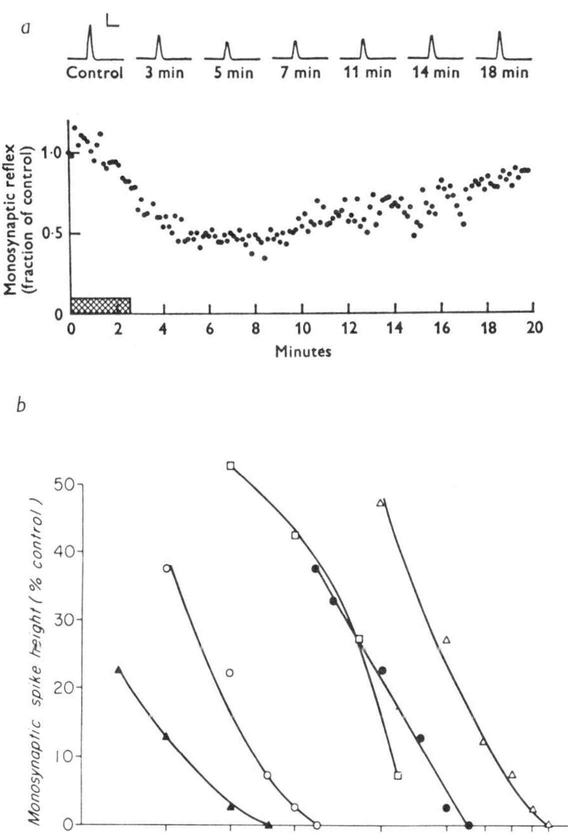

Fig. 1.6. Depression of the monosynaptic spinal reflex discharge recorded from ventral roots by various anaesthetics. *a,* Time-course of the depression of the monosynaptic reflex discharge of triceps surae motoneurones by thiopentone (10 mg/kg i.v., hatched area on abscissa). Top, sample responses recorded at the times indicated. *b,* The effects of various volatile anaesthetics on the height of the monosynaptic spike recorded from a lumbosacral ventral root following stimulation of the corresponding dorsal root. (○) halothane, (●) ether, (△) cyclopropane, (▲) methoxyflurane, (□) fluroxene. (*a, From Weakly [292]. b, From de Jong et al. [125].*)

synaptic transmission will be deferred to a later section (*see* p. 30). Broadly, however, we may expect synaptic transmission to be depressed as a result of (*a*) a decrease in excitatory synaptic transmission; (*b*) an increase in tonic postsynaptic inhibition arising from local or descending (i.e. supraspinal) pathways; (*c*) an increase in tonic presynaptic inhibition. Local *phasic* inhibitory mechanisms cannot be involved in the suppression of monosynaptic responses because of their short latency. It is unlikely that an increase in tonic descending inhibitory action is responsible for the depression of spinal reflexes brought about by anaesthetics, as Frank and Ohta [79, 80] have shown that the inhibitory effect of the reticulospinal pathway on reflex activity is abolished by a wide variety of anaesthetics including chloralose, nitrous oxide, paraldehyde, pentobarbitone, procaine and tribromoethanol (*see Fig. 1.7* for example). Intracellular recording from motoneurones has revealed no consistent hyperpolarization of the membrane potential during the application of anaesthetics [260, 292], so that an increase in tonic postsynaptic inhibitory activity seems unlikely, especially as Weakly [292] found that barbiturates did not depress the amplitude of miniature excitatory postsynaptic potentials (EPSPs) when the reflex response was depressed. However, Nicoll [189] has shown that barbiturates can induce a hyperpolarization of the postsynaptic membrane of frog spinal motoneurones similar to that observed after application of the putative inhibitory transmitter, γ-aminobutyric acid (GABA). Similarly, an increase in the tone of presynaptic inhibitory fibres is a possibility difficult to exclude. Nevertheless, the simplest explanation for the depression of spinal reflexes is that anaesthetics act directly on excitatory synaptic transmission. This hypothesis is also consistent with the observation that anaesthetics do not block impulse conduction in the afferent fibres but decrease the intracellularly recorded EPSP of motoneurones [260, 292].

In principle, anaesthetics could affect all of the components in the ascending sensory systems. However, as we shall see, the synaptic processes that occur in the dorsal horn, ventrobasal thalamus and the cortex are the most vulnerable to anaesthetic action. Furthermore, anaesthetics exert a profound depressant action on the non-specific sensory pathways of the reticular formation.

There appear to be no detailed experiments on the modulation of receptor function by anaesthetics, but de Jong and Nace [126] have reported that the response of cutaneous receptors to touch or to hair movements was not affected by ether, halothane, methoxyflurane or nitrous oxide. Moreover, the conduction of impulses along the peripheral nerve fibres from the receptors to the dorsal horn was unaffected – this conclusion was apparently true for Aα, Aδ and C fibres. In agreement with this Thornton et al. [272] found that halothane : nitrous oxide anaesthesia did not affect the excitability of the ulnar nerve of man. However, Rosner et al. [236] later reported that ether, nitrous oxide and cyclopropane *increased* the conduction velocity of ulnar nerve fibres while Ethrane had no such effect. The mechanism underlying this observation is obscure but most of the experimental variables were well controlled. As a rule, *in vitro* studies show that general anaesthetics have no effect on nerve conduction at normal clinical doses (i.e. at the doses that are achieved during the maintenance phase of anaesthesia). However, at higher concentrations

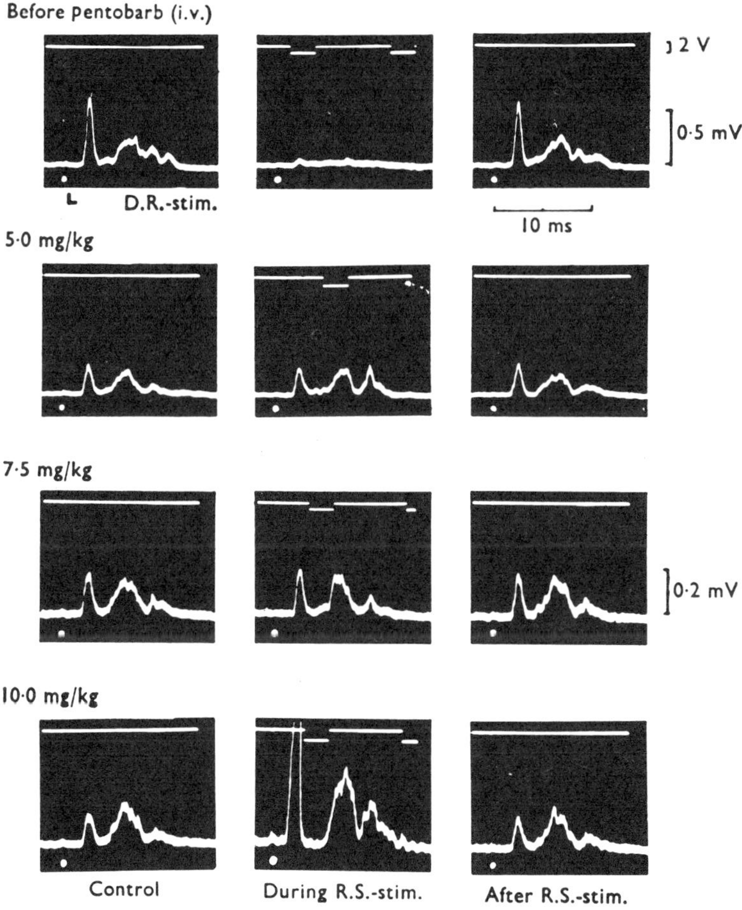

Fig. 1.7. The effect of pentobarbitone on the reflex potentials recorded from a ventral root before, during and after stimulation of the reticular formation. Dorsal root stimulation (white dots) produced monosynaptic and polysynaptic potentials. Before the anaesthetic was administered, stimulation of the reticular formation suppressed the responses to dorsal root stimulation. Administration of pentobarbitone progressively blocked this inhibition. Note the greater vulnerability of the initial monosynaptic response to depression by pentobarbitone when compared to the later polysynaptic wave and the change in the voltage calibration for the lower two rows. (*From Frank and Ohta [79].*)

all general anaesthetics are capable of blocking impulse conduction in nerves [244]. Nonetheless, it is evident that the analgesic and anaesthetic actions of general anaesthetics are not attributable to blockade of peripheral nerve conduction. In this major respect their action differs from that of local anaesthetics.

The activity of cells in the dorsal horn is depressed by a wide variety of anaesthetics. Thus Wall [287], in his pioneering studies, found that anaesthetic doses of pentobarbitone depressed the spontaneous activity of cells in laminae IV, V and VI and that the activity evoked by peripheral stimulation of C fibres was also depressed. Similar results have later been reported for lamina IV neurones by de Jong and Wagman [128], who found that the cutaneous receptive fields of touch-sensitive neurones in lamina IV of the dorsal horn of the monkey became smaller in extent

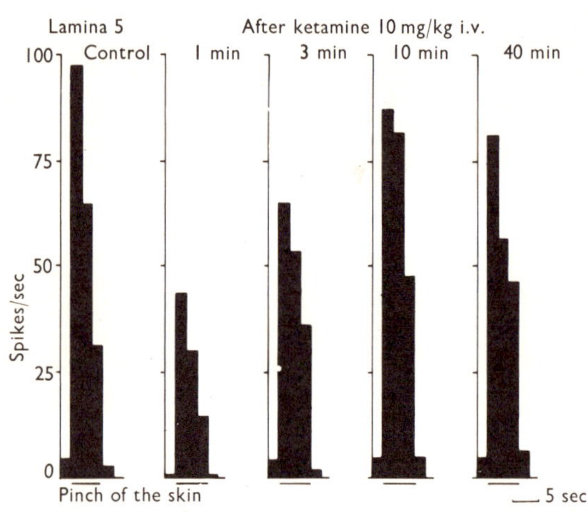

Fig. 1.8. The effect of ketamine on the activity of a lamina V cell responding to a pinch of the skin. The depression is short lived and reversible. (*From Conseiller et al. [56].*)

during the administration of halothane. The spontaneous activity of cells in other laminae is depressed during anaesthesia induced by a variety of agents including ether, halothane and thiopentone [136]; the cells in laminae IV, V and VI show the greatest depression [107]. Kitahata et al. have observed a selective depression of activity of cells in laminae I and V by ketamine [137] and lamina V by nitrous oxide. Conseiller et al. [56] have reported similar findings for laminae IV and V cells with ketamine (*Fig. 1.8*). Such observations have been considered by various authors to be the basis of the analgesic or even anaesthetic actions of anaesthetics [126]. Clearly, such effects must contribute to the analgesic and anaesthetic actions of general anaesthetics but the extent of this contribution is difficult to assess. Heavner and de Jong [107] have pointed out that although ether, halothane and thiopentone all affect the activity of cells in lamina V in a similar way, ether is a good analgesic whereas halothane and thiopentone are notoriously poor.

While the effects of anaesthetics on sensory processing in the spino-cervical and spinothalamic systems have not been studied, the effects on the dorsal column pathway have received considerable attention. In general the transmission of impulses from the forelimb (excited either by electrical stimulation or by natural stimuli) through the cuneate nucleus is remarkably stable [16, 66, 140]. Anaesthetics, apparently, do not appreciably upset this transmission at doses normally used for surgery. However, Galindo [93] reported that synaptic transmission through the cuneate nucleus was depressed by halothane and pentobarbitone. The reason for this discrepancy is not clear but may reflect the differences of technique. Thus, Dawson et al. [66] stimulated the forepaw and recorded responses in the cuneate nucleus and specific sensory cortex in rats anaesthetized with trichloroethylene. Angel and Unwin [16] used natural peripheral stimuli in rats anaesthetized with urethane. Both groups found that increasing anaesthetic depth did not change the sensitivity of the cuneate cells to peripheral stimulation. However, Galindo recorded the response of cuneate cells to natural peripheral stimuli, to stimulation of the peripheral nerve and to stimulation of the dorsal columns. In all cases anaesthetics depressed synaptic transmission through the cuneate nucleus. His animals were decerebrated and so were free of any descending cortical or thalamic influences. Angel [11] also notes that cells in the cuneate nucleus which were not monosynaptically activated, and those that showed an initial monosynaptic response followed by a longer latency response, did show a decrease in responsiveness with increasing depth of anaesthesia. Similar changes in excitability have been reported for cells in the rostral third of the cat gracile nucleus [97, 98]. Thus, we may conclude that sensory information passing through the dorsal column nuclei will be little changed by increasing anaesthetic depth but, in certain circumstances, it may be blocked at this level.

Action of Anaesthetics on Thalamic Transmission

From the dorsal column nuclei, sensory information is passed to the ventrobasal thalamus and thence to the cortex. Information traversing this pathway is affected both by spontaneous changes in excitability coincident with synchronous cortical activity and by anaesthetics. King et al. [134] found that the electrical response to stimulation of the medial lemniscus recorded from the internal capsule showed small increases in latency when the electrocorticogram showed synchronous electrical activity. They attributed this increase in latency to a decrease in the electrical tone arising from the midbrain reticular formation. They observed a similar increase in latency when small doses of pentobarbitone or thiopentone (10 mg/kg) were administered and concluded that low doses of barbiturates caused a reduction in reticular activity and this in turn led to depressed transmission through the thalamus. They noted that higher doses of barbiturates (20–30 mg/kg) had proportionately greater effects on the response recorded from the internal capsule and concluded that, at higher concentrations, barbiturates directly affected transmission through the ventrobasal thalamus. Similarly, Dawson et al. [66] noted that the cortical response to electrical stimulation was dependent upon the depth of anaesthesia maintained by trichloroethylene and postulated that this effect was due to a direct action of trichloroethylene on the ventrobasal thalamus. Later work has confirmed the correctness of this view. Angel and Unwin [16] have shown that urethane depresses the activity of cells in the ventrobasal thalamus which responds to a stimulus to the cuneate nucleus with monosynaptic latencies. According to Angel [11], the decrease in transmission can be attributed to a direct action on the synapses of the ventrobasal thalamus. Anaesthetic depth had no effect on the cortical response to stimulation of the thalamocortical afferents and he concluded that the excitability of the cortical cells is unchanged by anaesthetics. Nonetheless, he cautions that these results 'cannot be interpreted as meaning thalamic transmission of sensory information is of prime importance for the anaesthetic state but this particular site of synaptic transfer is more susceptible to anaesthetic agents than either that in the dorsal column nuclei or primary somatic sensory cortex excited monosynaptically by dorsal column or thalamocortical afferents respectively.'

Actions on Sensory Cortex

Reduced cortical responses to sensory stimulation have been reported by many workers. However, different anaesthetics appear to produce different effects on the cortical responses evoked by various stimuli. We have already seen that the response of the somatosensory cortex of the rat to stimulation of the contralateral forepaw is depressed by two anaesthetics (urethane and trichloroethylene) and similar changes, namely a decrease in amplitude and an increase in latency, have been observed with other anaesthetics [13]. However, in man a uniform change is not evident. Somatosensory-evoked responses (SERs) recorded from the cortex using extracranial scalp electrodes and percutaneous stimulation of the ulnar nerve (i.e. an analogous situation to the experiments on rats described above) consist of two components, an early short latency potential of small amplitude and short duration followed by a larger amplitude response of long duration. Clark and Rosner [48] refer to the early and late components of the SER as 'specific' and 'non-specific'. The specific responses correspond to those recorded directly from the cortex by conventional electrophysiological techniques; they are largest at places overlying the contralateral post-Rolandic sensory cortex and reflect nerve activity generated in that region. They thus represent the direct cortical response to stimulation of specific somatosensory pathways. Non-specific parts of the average somatic-evoked responses in man are diffusely and bilaterally distributed, occur at greater latencies than the specific component and are thought to reflect cortical activity driven from the

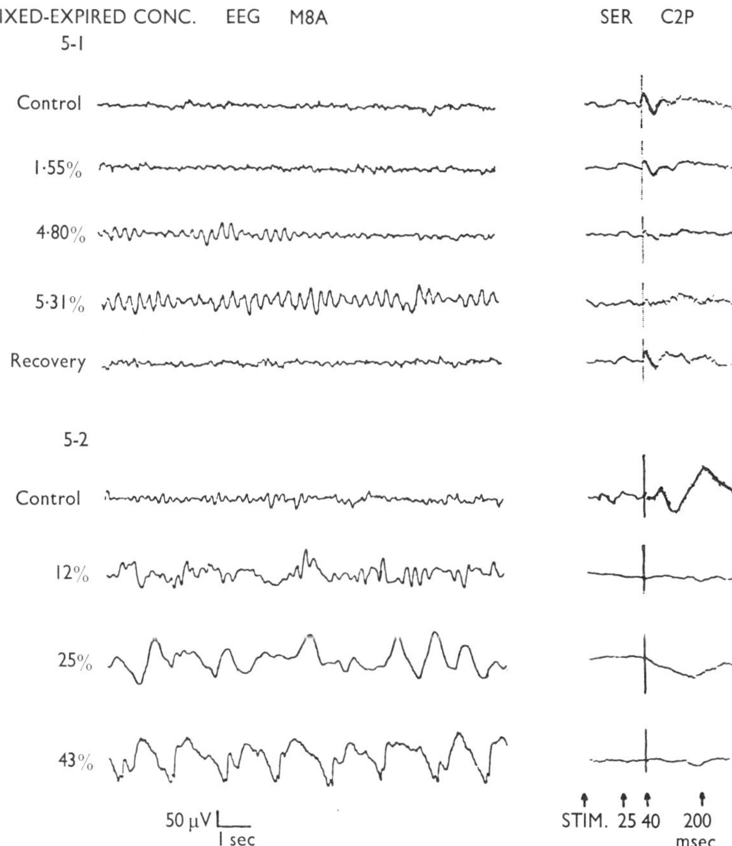

Fig. 1.9. The effect of cyclopropane on the electroencephalogram (EEG) and somatic-evoked responses (SER) of a conscious (5–1) and an unconscious (5–2) man. EEG: monopolar, frontal. SER: averaged monopolar recordings at the post-Rolandic scalp in response to stimulation of the contralateral radial nerve. Note dual time-base, fast to the left of the vertical bar, slow to the right. The subject 5–1 loses the response of the SER in 5·3 per cent cyclopropane and has a synchronized EEG but does not lose consciousness. (*From Clark and Rosner [48]*.)

mesencephalic reticular formation. At subanaesthetic concentrations, cyclopropane decreased or abolished both the specific and non-specific components of the SERs [114] (*Fig. 1.9*). In contrast, subanaesthetic concentrations of ether, Ethrane, methoxyflurane and nitrous oxide had little effect on the specific component but depressed the non-specific activity [114]. Higher doses affected both components but Ethrane produced a specific evoked response of abnormally long latency and amplitude as anaesthesia was deepened [47]. Barbiturates have been reported to depress the non-specific components of the SERs, whilst leaving the specific component intact [1].

Visual-evoked potentials and auditory-evoked potentials are also modulated by anaesthetics in different ways [70–72]. Thus barbiturates and ether depress non-specific visual-evoked potentials at lower doses than those required to depress the specific component, and nitrous oxide and halothane show a similar selectivity for the non-specific components. However, auditory-evoked potentials are apparently depressed by halothane [64, 135] and ether [179] but are augmented by chloralose [300].

Reticular Formation

Stimulation of the reticular formation in lightly anaesthetized or unanaesthetized drowsy animals causes an alerting or arousal reaction in the electrocorticogram in which slow synchronous electrical waves of low frequency and high amplitude are supplanted by rapid electrical waves of high frequency and low amplitude [181] (*see* p. 4). This reaction is accompanied by signs of behavioural arousal, even in lightly anaesthetized animals [86]. Furthermore, lesions in the brain stem may result in coma (p. 6). These striking observations suggested that the reticular formation may have a role in the genesis of anaesthesia. French et al. [89] set out to test this hypothesis by simultaneously recording evoked potentials from the specific sensory pathways (medial lemniscus or sensory cortex) and the central brain stem in response to auditory stimuli or stimulation of the sciatic nerve. They found that administration of ether or pentobarbitone blocked activity recorded from the classical sensory pathway. They also showed that this effect did not require the presence of an intact cerebral cortex and concluded that it was a direct result of anaesthetic action on the reticular formation. This led them to postulate that this action of anaesthetics 'participates in an explanation of the anaesthetic state'. Other workers have extended these original observations by recording evoked activity in the thalamus and reticular formation. They have found that nitrous oxide, ethylene or cyclopropane reduced the evoked responses recorded in the reticular formation more than those recorded in the thalamus [63]. A similar result has been reported for halothane [64].

Arduini and Arduini [18] have shown that the arousal response to reticular stimulation and olfactory stimulation is blocked by low doses of pentobarbitone (*Fig. 1.10*). King [133] investigated the mechanism of this effect, and showed that while barbiturates blocked the arousal response, they augmented the recruitment response of the cortex to stimulation of the non-specific thalamic nuclei. She also found that mephenesin and benzothiazoles had no effect on the arousal response but blocked the recruitment response. She concluded that 'Since recruitment responses were shown to be interrupted by stimulation of the reticular activating system, barbiturates may be considered to increase recruiting activity by blocking the tonic activity of the reticular formation which normally limits the distribution and reduces the amplitude of responses evoked from the diffuse thalamic projection system.' This statement implies that the actions of barbiturates are primarily on the reticular formation, but it does not take into account the actions of barbiturates on the normal intracortical tonic activity which may also influence recruiting activity.

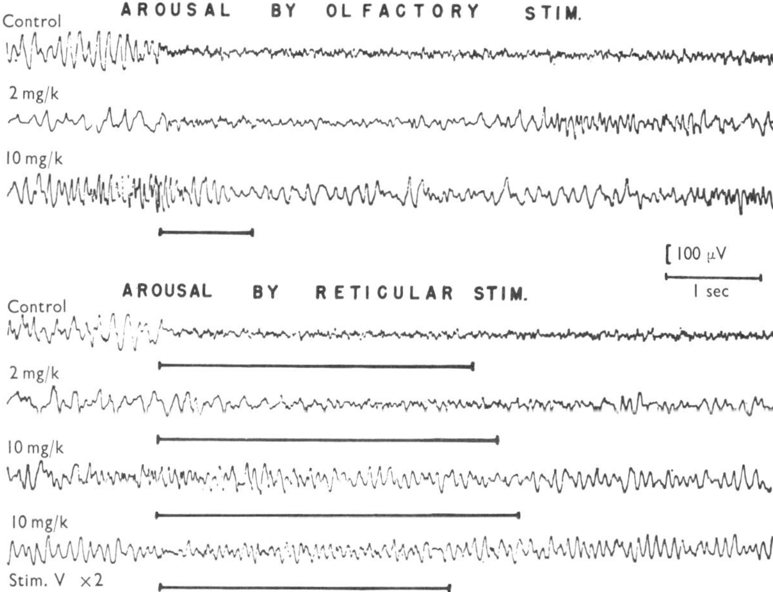

Fig. 1.10. The effect of pentobarbitone (Nembutal) on electroencephalogram (EEG) arousal in response to olfactory and reticular stimulation in a rabbit. The black bars indicate the period of stimulation in each case. (*From Arduini and Arduini [18].*)

Thus interpreted, these experiments carry the hypothesis of French et al. [89] one step further, in that both the anaesthetic action and the EEG action of the barbiturates are attributed to a depressant action on the reticular formation. This is the basis of the simple hypothesis that anaesthetics act primarily by depressing the ascending activity of the reticular formation to impair normal cortical activity.

Implicit in this view of anaesthetic action is the assumption that all anaesthetics are central nervous system depressants and that they have a common mode of action. Furthermore, it also assumes that the reticular formation is a single entity exerting a tonic effect upon the cortex and that the state of the EEG can be equated with the level of consciousness. These assumptions are all questionable.

While the mode of action of anaesthetics is still a controversial field and the neurological mechanisms are by no means thoroughly worked out, it is becoming increasingly clear that anaesthetics do not have essentially identical effects on the nervous system. The barbiturates have a depressant action on the central nervous system and this is reflected not only in behavioural changes but also in the depression of the cerebral metabolic rate (p. 11). In contrast, agents like phencyclidine and ketamine which produce a state of anaesthesia very different from that produced by barbiturates cause little reduction in the cerebral metabolic rate (Table 1.3, p. 13) and some increase in the local cerebral glucose uptake (*Fig. 1.5,* p. 14). There are also differences in the action of anaesthetics on the gross electrical activity of the brain [235]. Thus, while barbiturates block the arousal reaction, they augment the recruitment response and synchronize EEG. Ether, however, blocks the arousal reaction and the recruitment response [133], yet it too produces a synchronized EEG, albeit somewhat different in character from that produced by the barbiturates. Alpha-chloralose [300] increases the response of the reticular formation to auditory stimuli, yet it produces a state of profound anaesthesia in which the preparation is unusually responsive to auditory stimuli. However, auditory stimuli do not arouse or awaken the animal. Winters has attempted to provide a unifying hypothesis in which he proposes that there is a continuum of neurological activity in which anaesthetics may affect the activity of the nervous system by either depressing it below the normal awake state or by elevating it above normal to produce a cataleptic anaesthesia. In this system he proposes [300] that the actions of all anaesthetics on the reticular formation are not uniform but that they are essential to anaesthetic activity. 'The reticular activating system is influenced by all anaesthetics; some inhibit its action and some hyperexcite the system resulting in a functional disorganisation. Some agents traverse both excitation and depression (diethyl ether). Others induce only stage II catalepsia, e.g. nitrous oxide, ketamine, γ-hydroxybutyrate, α-chloralose, phencyclidine, trichloroethylene and enflurane. Others produce no stage II but progress directly from stage I to stage III, e.g. halothane and barbiturates.' This is a more realistic approach to the action of anaesthetics on the reticular formation than the earlier view as Magni et al. [160] have shown that perfusion of the caudal brain stem via the vertebral arteries with barbiturates desynchronizes the EEG, while perfusion of the more anterior part via the carotid arteries synchronizes the EEG (i.e. even by such gross techniques the reticular formation can be divided into a caudal desynchronizing region and an anterior synchronizing region). The difficulty with Winters' hypothesis is that it equates EEG pattern with gross neurological activity rather than synchronous nerve activity. Thus although 'cataleptic' anaesthetic agents like phencyclidine and ketamine either increase or do not significantly change cerebral metabolic rate, other 'cataleptic' agents such as Ethrane [253] and γ-hydroxybutyrate [302] produce a monotonic depression of cerebral metabolic rate that is related to the dose administered.

A recent version of the hypothesis that anaesthetics act primarily by influencing the activity of the reticular system is due to Angel [12]. He has pointed out that the reticular formation exerts both a facilitatory and an inhibitory influence on the transfer of sensory information through the ventrobasal thalamus. He and his colleagues have recorded from neurones in the thalamic reticular nucleus and found that they could be grouped into two classes on the basis of their firing rate and its alteration during anaesthesia. Type A cells had a low irregular resting discharge rate that increased in frequency during anaesthesia. Type B cells had a high discharge rate that decreased during anaesthesia. Since Angel had already shown that anaesthetics block somatosensory transmission in the ventrobasal thalamus, he proposed that anaesthetics 'functionally denervate' the cerebral cortex by increasing reticular inhibition and decreasing reticular facilitation of ventrobasal thalamic transmission via the actions on these two classes of neurone. As a hypothesis it has two serious weaknesses. Firstly, the assumption that type A cells have an inhibitory action and that type B cells have a facilitatory action on thalamic transmission is unproved. Secondly, the assumption that decreases in thalamic responsiveness to sensory stimulation are exclusively due to the influence of the reticular formation is improbable. There is also a strong descending influence of the cortex on the thalamus (p. 3).

There is ample evidence from the foregoing paragraphs that the activity of the reticular formation and its influences on cortical activity are affected by general anaesthetics. The crucial question is whether the loss of ascending non-specific sensory activity is directly responsible for the loss of consciousness. The evidence in favour of this hypothesis is based on the selective depression of sensory-evoked potentials in the reticular formation and on the changes in the EEG caused by stimulating either the reticular formation or a sensory modality. However, psychophysical experiments with cyclopropane have shown that this anaesthetic can block both the specific and non-specific components of the sensory-evoked potential before the subjects lose the ability to perceive a stimulus [46]. This suggests that neither the diffuse influence of the reticular formation nor a large sensory-evoked potential are essential to perception. We have already seen that it is possible to dissociate the appearance of the EEG from the behavioural state either by drugs or by lesions in the ascending reticular formation (p. 5). Indeed, Feldman and Waller [78] found that gross lesions in the brain stem produced animals which had a permanently synchronized EEG but which showed normal behavioural patterns. Furthermore, Bremer [28] has reported that sensory stimulation will only give rise to an arousal reaction in the EEG if the sensory cortex for that modality remains intact. These observations suggest that the actions of anaesthetics on the activity of the reticular formation are not *essential* for the production of the anaesthetic state.

Anaesthetic Action on Intracortical Transmission

So far we have considered the action of anaesthetics only on those cortical responses that are directly related to an afferent barrage. However, somatosensory information arriving at the cortex is integrated with information arising from the other special senses and is influenced by the prevailing emotions. It is the totality of these activities that determines what action will be taken in response to a specific stimulus (*see* p. 3). These higher functions of the nervous system are largely effected by the cerebral cortex and the actions of anaesthetics on these processes are therefore likely to be of considerable importance in the anaesthetic state.

The first direct evidence of a specifically cortical action of anaesthetics was provided by Burns [36]. He studied the action of anaesthetics on the evoked electrical activity of neurologically isolated slabs of cerebral cortex. These isolated slabs were prepared by exposing the cerebral cortex of a cat under anaesthesia. A long gyrus was selected for the preparation and its underlying subcortical white matter was severed by undercutting the gyrus at a depth of 7 mm. The lateral connexions from the gyrus to neighbouring areas of the cortex were then cut leaving only the pia intact to preserve the blood supply. At this stage the animal was decerebrated and the anaesthetic was withdrawn. Thus prepared, the cortical slab was functionally denervated but still possessed millions of viable cortical neurones with their local connexions largely intact. Unlike normal cerebral cortex, these slabs were electrically silent unless stimulated. Strong stimuli to the cortical surface elicited a complex long-lasting response that could be recorded from the cortical surface. Burns showed that this consisted of two components: an initial negative response that was a conducted response in the superficial nerve fibres of the cortex and a long-lasting positive component that was due to the electrical activity of cells within the cortex. Anaesthetics administered systemically in sufficient dose to anaesthetize a normal cat had no effect on the early negative response due to the direct conduction of impulses in the superficial fibres, but greatly depressed the longer latency responses which were attributable to the discharge of the cortical cells. Smaller doses of anaesthetic produced proportionately smaller effects. Since the conducted response was unaffected by these doses of anaesthetic, the decrease in the late response could be attributed to an action on the interconnexion between the cortical cells, i.e. to an action on synaptic transmission within the cortex itself. Burns himself thought that the most likely explanation for the depressant action of the anaesthetics was a decrease in excitatory synaptic activity, but an increase in intracortical inhibitory activity could have contributed to the depression. Since this early work other evidence has accumulated to show a direct action of anaesthetics on cortical cells. A wide range of anaesthetics including ether, halothane, trichloroethylene, barbiturates and steroids have been shown to depress excitatory synaptic transmission in *in vitro* preparations of olfactory cortex at doses comparable to those required for the maintenance of general anaesthesia [215] (*Fig. 1.11*). Similar results have been found with *in vitro* preparations of

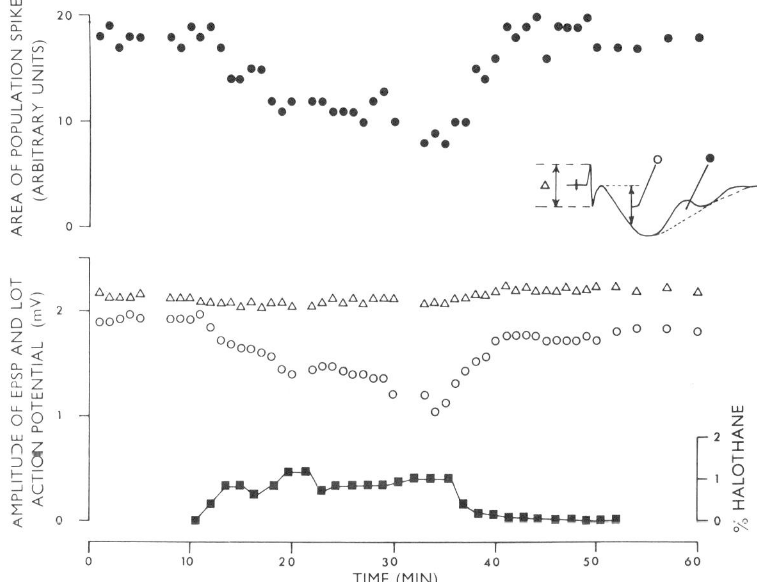

Fig. 1.11. The effect of halothane on synaptic transmission in the olfactory cortex. Inset shows a schematic drawing of the evoked potentials; initially there is a sharp biphasic wave which reflects conduction of impulses in the afferent axons (△). This is followed by a negative wave which is an excitatory synaptic wave (EPSP) (○). On the EPSP is superimposed a positive peak (●) whose area is proportional to the number of cells firing in response to the EPSP. Note that halothane (0·8–1 per cent) depressed the EPSP and population spike but spared the initial conducted response. (*From Richards [214]*.)

hippocampus [226]. Nicoll et al. [190] have shown that barbiturates increase the duration of inhibitory postsynaptic potentials in the hippocampus. These results demonstrate that general anaesthetics are capable of profoundly influencing synaptic transmission in the cerebral cortex at doses corresponding to those required for anaesthesia although they do not, of course, establish that anaesthetic actions on the cortex are *required* for general anaesthesia.

Summary

General anaesthetics affect neural function at all levels of the neuraxis from the spinal cord to the cerebral cortex. All of these effects will in some measure contribute to the anaesthetic state although those on the brain stem, thalamus and cerebral cortex will be of prime importance as these structures have been implicated in the maintenance of the conscious state. The hypothesis that anaesthetics act primarily on the ascending reticular function was shown to be oversimplified. Various manoeuvres will result in a dissociation between the activity of the reticular formation and that of the cerebral cortex. Furthermore, the arousal response to a specific stimulus requires that the sensory cortex for that modality be intact.

The actions of general anaesthetics on neural transmission are not due to the blockade of impulse conduction in the major afferent pathways of the nervous system or to a block of peripheral nerve conduction. However, regions of synaptic contact are susceptible to the actions of anaesthetics. Various mechanisms could account for this blockade – increased firing threshold, increased inhibitory tone or a direct depressant action on excitatory synaptic transmission. Evidence was advanced in support of the last of these possibilities. A more detailed discussion of all three possibilities follows.

ACTION OF ANAESTHETICS ON SYNAPTIC TRANSMISSION

Mechanisms of Synaptic Transmission

We have seen that nerves entering the central nervous system from peripheral receptors make a series of synaptic connexions as they ascend to the brain. This same organizational feature is found throughout the nervous system and is fundamental to its integrative processes. The synapse is a point of contiguity between two nerve cells where one, the presynaptic cell, is in a position to modify the activity of the other, the postsynaptic cell. Synaptic transmission is of two types, excitatory and inhibitory; inhibitory synaptic transmission can be further divided into two subclasses, presynaptic inhibition and postsynaptic inhibition.

All synaptic processes are essentially the same; they begin with the conduction of a nerve impulse along the axon of the presynaptic cell to its nerve terminals where it causes the release of a small amount of a chemical substance (a 'transmitter') into the synaptic cleft. The transmitter diffuses across the cleft to the surface of the postsynaptic cell where it interacts with receptor proteins to which it binds selectively. The receptor changes its conformation (shape) once the transmitter is bound and in some way the permeability of the postsynaptic membrane to certain of the extracellular ions increases. It is the nature of this change in ionic permeability (or conductance) that determines the character of a synapse (i.e. whether it is excitatory or inhibitory). Excitatory synaptic transmission is associated with an increase in conductance to sodium and potassium ions which causes a local fall in membrane potential (the excitatory postsynaptic potential or EPSP) which spreads along the surface of the cell by a passive process called electrotonic conduction. If the fall in membrane potential is of sufficient magnitude at the cell body to reach the threshold depolarization for cell discharge, the cell will fire. Inhibitory postsynaptic transmission is associated with an increased postsynaptic conductance to chloride ions. This tends to raise the membrane potential (hyperpolarization) and gives rise to the inhibitory postsynaptic potential (IPSP) which inhibits cell discharge because a greater depolarization is required to reach the threshold for spike initiation.

In any physiological situation, the activity of many synapses on the dendrites of a single neurone interact to produce a sum potential that determines the prevailing level of membrane potential at the cell body. The importance of an individual synapse in the modulation of a cell's excitability is a function of its distance from the cell body. Synapses remote on the distant branches of the dendritic tree will have less influence on cell activity than those next to the cell body. (For a more detailed discussion of the physiology of synapses *see* references 73, 129, 142.)

The mechanisms underlying presynaptic inhibition are rather less well understood. The evidence for its existence stems from an observation of Frank and Fuortes [82] that stimulation of group Ia muscle afferents from a particular muscle diminished the excitatory postsynaptic activity in the motoneurones of its antagonistic muscles. There was no detectable change in the membrane permeability or membrane potential of the affected cells and so this phenomenon was termed 'remote inhibition'. Later work has suggested, but not proved, that presynaptic inhibition results from a depolarization of the inhibitory fibres on the primary afferent terminals (for references *see* Angel [11]). This depolarizing action is considered to diminish the amplitude of the action potential and consequently the amount of transmitter it causes to be released.

It is generally assumed that, as anaesthetics have a depressant effect on behaviour, their effects on synaptic transmission in the central nervous system will be essentially depressant. This assumption is broadly true, but anaesthetics such as ketamine cause little neuronal depression if their effects on cerebral metabolism are a guide, while others like ether during stage II anaesthesia and α-chloralose enhance the significance of auditory stimuli. These observations suggest that anaesthetics will not have a uniform depressant action on synaptic transmission throughout the central nervous system, a certain degree of selectivity is to be expected. Furthermore, depression of synaptic transmission should not be taken to imply a complete blockade comparable to that produced by curare at the neuromuscular junction during paralysis, merely a reduction in the effective transfer of information.

In principle, anaesthetics could depress synaptic transmission at a particular relay by decreasing the efficacy of excitatory synapses, by increasing the efficacy of inhibitory synapses, by raising the threshold depolarization of the postsynaptic cell required for its discharge or by any combination of these effects. It cannot be assumed that there is a specific action upon excitation simply because a general anaesthetic causes a reduction in synaptic transmission through a particular synaptic pathway in an intact animal. Only under the most favourable circumstances is it possible to attribute the effect of an anaesthetic to a specific action on excitation or to some other synaptic process. Detailed study of the *mechanisms* by which anaesthetics affect synaptic transmission is therefore restricted to those pathways in which indirect influences can either be controlled or eliminated.

Anaesthetic Action on Excitatory Synaptic Transmission

Modern attempts to elucidate the mode of action of anaesthetics on synaptic transmission may be said to date from the work of Larrabee and Posternak [148] who showed that chloroform, chloretone, ether and pentobarbitone depressed excitatory synaptic transmission through mammalian sympathetic ganglia at lower concentrations than those required to depress the compound action potential of the afferent axons (*Fig. 1.12*). These experiments were conducted *in vitro* and so the effects reflected a direct depressant action on excitatory synapses. Subsequently, it has been shown that ether and the barbiturates depress monosynaptic reflexes in the spinal cord and this depression is paralleled by a depression of motoneurone EPSPs [260, 292]. Anaesthetics have also been found to depress extracellularly recorded EPSP field potentials in preparations of the olfactory cortex [213, 214, 221] and hippocampus [226] maintained *in vitro.* In all of these studies the depression of excitatory synaptic transmission could be demonstrated with concentrations comparable to those required for anaesthesia in the intact animal. However, Nicoll [188] has found that the unusual dendrodendritic excitatory synapses between the mitral cells and the granule cells of the olfactory bulb are resistant to depression of anaesthetics until high concentrations are reached.

As anaesthetics depress excitatory synaptic transmission both *in vitro,* in preparations of the nervous system that have neither spontaneous activity nor intact inhibitory pathways, and *in vivo* where short-latency monosynaptic spinal reflexes are depressed, a direct action of anaesthetics on excitatory synapses has been established. For further analysis it is convenient to divide excitatory synaptic transmission into four components: (*a*) conduction of impulses along afferent axons and their branches to the nerve terminals; (*b*) the release of transmitter from the nerve terminals into the synaptic cleft; (*c*) the binding of transmitter to the receptor sites on the postsynaptic membrane and its associated ionic conductance change; (*d*) the initiation of a nerve impulse in the postsynaptic neurone.

Effects of Anaesthetics on Presynaptic Nerves

Sherrington [249], in his classic book, attributed the action of anaesthetics to a depressant effect on synaptic transmission because he found that reflex activity in the spinal cord was abolished by low concentrations of

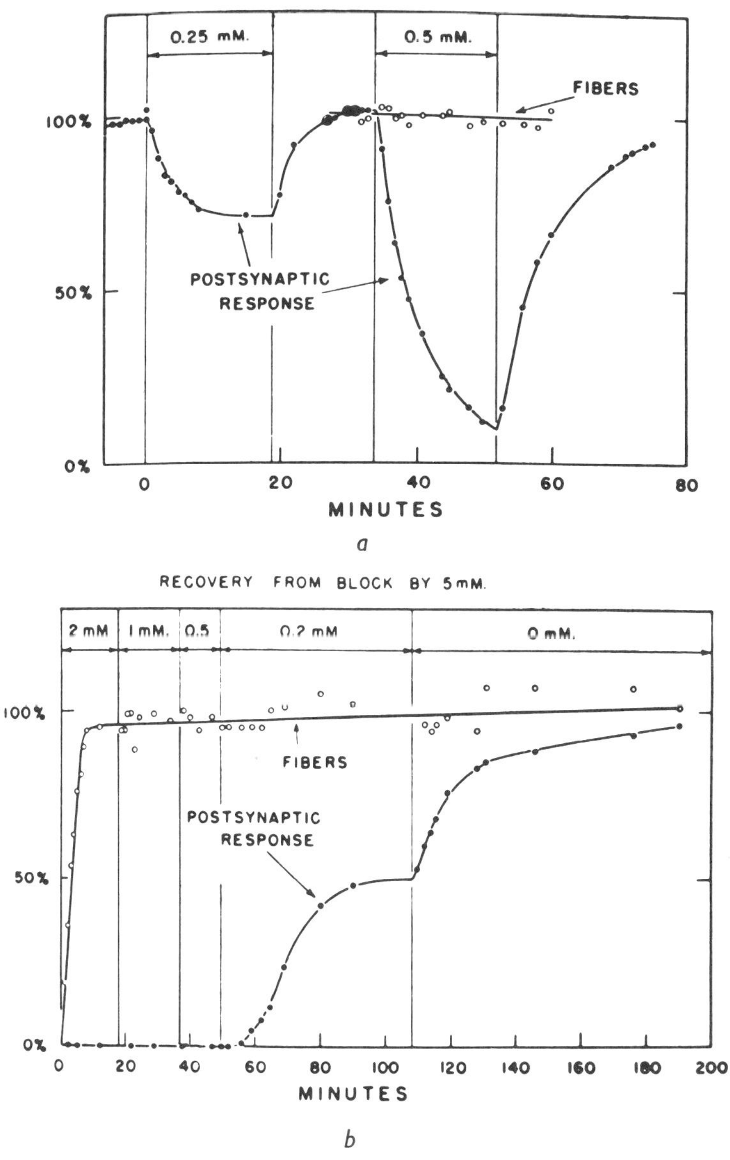

Fig. 1.12. The action of pentobarbitone on synaptic transmission in sympathetic ganglia. *a*, Selective depression of the postsynaptic response (•). *b*, Recovery from total block by 5 mM pentobarbitone. Note the rapid recovery of the presynaptic conducted response and the slower recovery of the synaptic component. All response amplitudes are expressed as a percentage of initial control values. (*From Larrabee and Posternak [148].*)

chloroform while nerve impulse conduction in motor axons was preserved. Since that time it has been virtually axiomatic that general anaesthetics exert a selective depressant action on central synapses whilst leaving nerve conduction unimpaired. That this view was only partially correct was shown by Larrabee and Posternak [148] in their early work on sympathetic ganglia. They found that clinically useful general anaesthetics including chloroform, ether and pentobarbitone all had a selective depressant action on synaptic transmission as the early work had suggested. However, they also found that the short-chain alcohols and urethane had no selective action on synapses, synaptic transmission showing a depression parallel to that of the compound action potential of the afferent nerve fibres. Yet these substances are able to produce anaesthesia. They considered that the susceptibility of synaptic transmission to the action of anaesthetics could reflect a low safety factor for impulse conduction in the terminal branches of the afferent axons. This idea was later revived by Frank and Sanders [81] and by Seeman [244, 263] who attributed all the actions of general anaesthetics on synaptic transmission to a blockade of nerve impulses in afferent axons and thereby attributed general anaesthesia to this mechanism.

This idea is based on two observations. First, substances which are local anaesthetics, such as procaine, can produce a level of general anaesthesia corresponding to stage II and this anaesthetic action is synergistic with that of general anaesthetics such as the barbiturates [81]. Second, there is evidence that the susceptibility of peripheral axons to blockade by both general and local anaesthetics increases as their diameters decrease [94, 164, 186]. Thus small axons are more readily blocked by anaesthetics than are large ones. These authors therefore suggested that the apparently selective depression of synaptic transmission by general anaesthetics resulted from a depression of conduction in the fine terminal branches of the afferent axons [263]. This idea is attractive because both local and general anaesthesia can be explained on the basis of a single cellular lesion – a failure of nerve conduction.

It is certainly true that general anaesthetics can block nerve conduction if sufficiently high concentrations are applied to a nerve. However, if all synaptic depression is to be explained on the basis of a depression of nerve conduction, evidence is required to show that the blockade of synaptic transmission in the central nervous system itself can be attributed to a depression of nerve conduction in the afferent nerve fibres. The evidence against this view derives from experiments on the action of anaesthetics on impulse conduction in the lateral olfactory tract (LOT). This tract is a prominent band of white matter coursing along the anterior ventrolateral surface of the brain. Its fibres arise chiefly from the mitral and tufted cells of the olfactory bulb, have a diameter of 1–2 μm and conduct at about 8 $msec^{-1}$ [202, 218]. The colateral fibre branches that are distributed over the surface of the cortex have a conduction velocity of 1·5–3 $msec^{-1}$ from which we may estimate their diameter to be 0·3–0·5 μm [291]. These fine branches make extensive synaptic connexions in the cortex and the anatomical arrangement is favourable for recording both the compound action potential of the LOT fibres, that of their colaterals and the synaptic activity of the postsynaptic cells [213, 214]. It was found that concentrations of anaesthetics sufficient to depress synaptic transmission by 50 per cent or more (equivalent to an amount of anaesthetic likely to be found only during very deep anaesthesia) had no effect on nerve conduction in the LOT or in the fine colateral fibres (*Fig. 1.13*). Similar results were

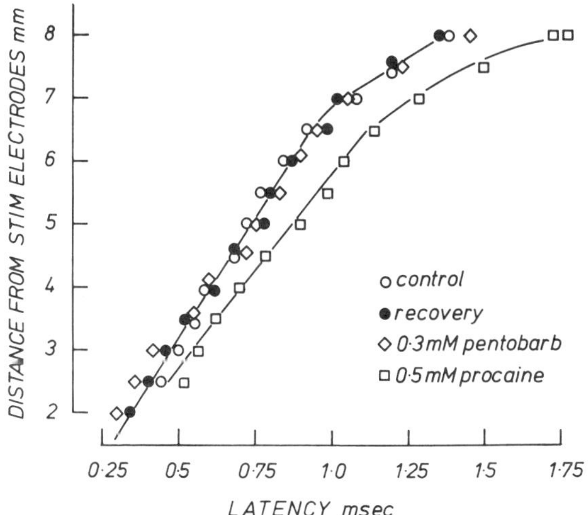

Fig. 1.13. A comparison of the effect of procaine and pentobarbitone on impulse conduction in the lateral olfactory tract. The latency to the initial peak of the action potential is plotted as a function of the distance between the recording and stimulating electrodes. Note the change in slope at 7 mm corresponding to the end of the visible part of the olfactory tract. 0·3 mM pentobarbitone and 0·5 mM procaine both depress the synaptic waves by 50 per cent but while pentobarbitone has no significant effect on conduction in the tract, procaine slows conduction appreciably.

obtained when the action of anaesthetics on the perforant path fibres of the hippocampus were studied. These fibres have a diameter of 0·6–0·8 μm and make *en passage* synapses with the granule cells (i.e. there are no terminal arborizations) [184]. Finally, if the action of a general anaesthetic that has a 'selective' depressant action on synaptic transmission, such as pentobarbitone, is compared with an agent that specifically blocks the sodium channel of nerves, such as tetrodotoxin, certain differences become apparent. Concentrations of pentobarbitone sufficient to block synaptic transmission by 50 per cent (about 0·3 mM) have no very obvious effect on the nerve impulse conduction in the LOT, whereas equivalent concentrations of tetrodotoxin or procaine slow nerve conduction appreciably (*Fig. 1.13*) and raise the threshold for excitation (i.e. decrease the excitability of the nerve fibres).

In conclusion, most general anaesthetics depress excitatory synaptic transmission at concentrations lower than those required to depress nerve conduction in the afferent axons or their terminal branches. As the EPSPs themselves are depressed, this result suggests that it is the process of chemical transmission itself that is affected by anaesthetics. The exceptions to this general rule include the lower alcohols, urethane and the short-acting intravenous agent, propanidid. These agents have effects on synaptic transmission very similar to those of local anaesthetics.

Action of Anaesthetics on Chemical Transmission

Chemical transmission consists of two processes – the release of transmitter and the binding of released transmitter to the postsynaptic membrane. These two processes are difficult to study in the brain itself as few neurotransmitters have been identified and assigned to specific pathways. Consequently, most of the available evidence is based on experiments with substances whose transmitter role has not been firmly established.

Action of Anaesthetics on Transmitter Release

The most satisfactory evidence that anaesthetics can decrease the amount of transmitter released by nerve impulses comes from the experiments of Matthews and Quilliam [163] on acetylcholine (Ach) release from the superior cervical ganglion. They showed that several central nervous system depressants including amylobarbitone decreased the amount of Ach released by stimulation of the preganglionic fibres (*Fig. 1.14*). Electrophysiological evidence in favour of a reduction in the release of a central nervous system transmitter by anaesthetics has been provided by Weakly [292] in his elegant experiments on the action of barbiturates on the stretch reflex of triceps surae motoneurones. Weakly showed that low doses of barbiturates depressed the motoneurone EPSPs in response to stimulation of single Ia afferent fibres, but the amplitude of the individual miniature EPSPs was unaffected. Since it is believed that the EPSP is made up of a number of miniature EPSPs ('quanta') all released together, Weakly concluded that the EPSP was depressed because the number of quanta released by the Ia nerve terminals was reduced (i.e. there was a decreased secretion of transmitter when the anaesthetics were administered).

Experiments on the frog neuromuscular junction suggest that barbiturates can *increase* the quantal content of the end-plate potential (i.e. the amount of transmitter released), the depression of neuromuscular transmission being attributed to a large decrease in the sensitivity of the postsynaptic membrane to Ach [204, 247, 271, 296] (*see below*). This effect of barbiturates occurs at high concentrations of pentobarbitone (0·5–1·0 mM) and its relevance to anaesthesia is not clear [247].

The nature of the transmitter at the synapses between the Ia afferents and the motoneurone is unknown so a direct verification of Weakly's experiment cannot be achieved. However, neurochemical studies on slices of hippocampus have shown that the Ca^{2+}-dependent K^+-evoked release of the putative inhibitory transmitter, GABA, is depressed by low concentrations of barbiturates [121]. Similarly, it has been shown that barbiturates reduce the K^+-evoked release of Ach from slices of cerebral cortex [229]. This reduction in release of neurotransmitters has also been shown to occur in isolated nerve terminals (synaptosomes) [104].

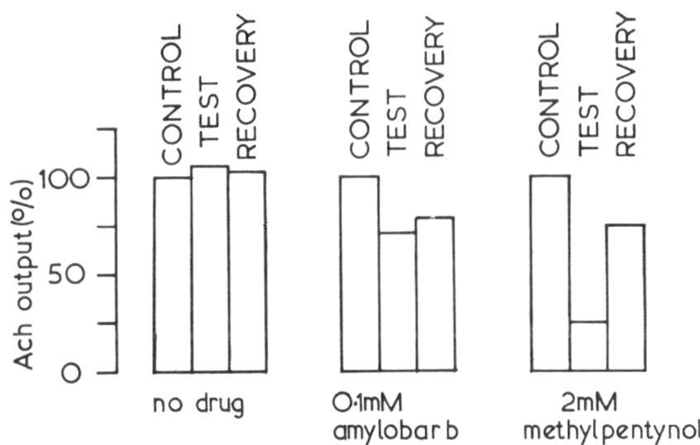

Fig. 1.14. The influence of amylobarbitone and methylpentynol on acetylcholine (Ach) output from sympathetic ganglia. Three periods of stimulation were used and the amount of Ach released during each was expressed as a percentage of that released in the first period. The drug was added only for the second (test) period of stimulation. The depression of Ach by both drugs is statistically significant. (*From data of Matthews and Quilliam [163].*)

If the evidence that anaesthetics reduce the secretion of neurotransmitters from afferent nerve terminals is accepted, we need to establish how this is brought about. It is improbable that anaesthetics exert an inhibitory action on the synthesis of neurotransmitters or on their storage in the nerve terminals. During anaesthesia the levels of Ach in the brain are actually increased [60], although this increase is not uniform throughout the brain [178, 187]. Similar results have been reported for the levels of dopamine, noradrenaline [232] and serotonin [231] during anaesthesia with cyclopropane and halothane. The brain levels of GABA are unchanged during anaesthesia with Althesin (a mixture of two steroid anaesthetics, alphaxalone and alphadalone acetate) or ketamine, although they are decreased by halothane [22]. The levels of glutamate (a putative excitatory transmitter) were unchanged by halothane but depressed by Althesin and ketamine. The significance of these changes is difficult to assess as both glutamate and GABA are intimately involved in general cerebral metabolism. However, it is clear that there is no general depression of the levels of transmitter substances during anaesthesia.

The electrophysiological evidence is also inconsistent with a direct inhibitory action of anaesthetics on presynaptic synthesis or storage of transmitter. Rapid stimulation of afferent nerves gives rise to a potentiation of the EPSPs (frequency potentiation) which is undiminished in the presence of anaesthetics. Similarly, post-tetanic potentiation of EPSPs (after a rapid train of afferent volleys) is readily observed in the presence of anaesthetics. These observations further suggest that the presynaptic stores of transmitter are readily available for release by nerve impulses [213, 214, 226, 258, 259].

Although a decrease in the height of the action potential arising from a local anaesthetic action on the afferent nerve fibres could lead to a reduction in the amount of transmitter released [130, 268], such a mechanism is unlikely to account for the selective depression of synaptic transmission discussed in the previous section (p. 34). Nevertheless, the depression of EPSPs by non-selective drugs such as procaine, urethane and the short-chain primary alcohols is almost certainly due in part to this mechanism.

It appears that the reduction in transmitter release caused by general anaesthetics is due to a direct action on the neurosecretory process itself, possibly by interfering with the influx of calcium into the presynaptic nerve terminal [24].

Action of Anaesthetics on Receptors

Most studies of the effects of anaesthetics on the sensitivity of nerve cells to putative transmitters have been conducted *in vivo,* often in decerebrate or spinal animals. However, the detailed connectivities and synaptic physiology of these cells are usually unknown. The interpretation of such experiments in terms of a specific change in the sensitivity of receptors to a particular putative transmitter is therefore rather difficult. The cells frequently have spontaneous activity and the pattern of behaviour during exposure to an anaesthetic is likely to be influenced by the action of the anaesthetic on other neurones to which they are synaptically connected. In an attempt to overcome the confusion caused by these problems I shall deal first with those studies that have used *in vitro* preparations of brain and spinal cord and then attempt to reconcile the results with those obtained by more conventional electrophysiological methods.

The olfactory cortex is especially useful for such studies as it can be maintained *in vitro* under suitable incubation conditions for many hours. It has no spontaneous activity but can be excited by stimulation of the LOT which synaptically activates cells of the cortex [222, 223]. The synaptic waves thus evoked are depressed by concentrations of anaesthetic comparable to those required for general anaesthesia [213, 214, 221]. Finally, there is some circumstantial evidence to implicate glutamate as the excitatory transmitter, between the LOT and the cells in the olfactory cortex [27, 216]. The sensitivity of cells in the olfactory cortex to iontophoretically applied glutamate was depressed by a variety of anaesthetics. (Iontophoresis is a technique for applying small quantities of a drug from a glass micropipette to single nerve cells by brief electrical pulses.) These anaesthetics were ether, methoxyflurane, trichloroethylene, pentobarbitone and alphaxalone [224, 225]. The concentrations required for the depression to occur were comparable to those required to depress synaptic transmission in the olfactory cortex (*Fig. 1.15a*). However, the

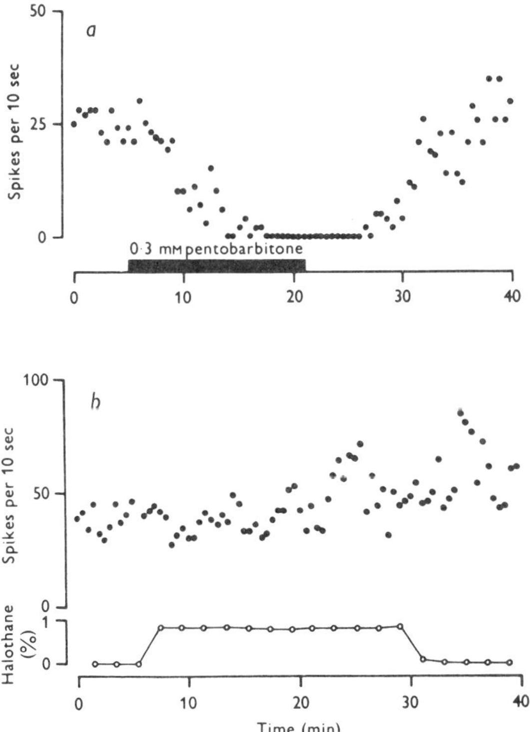

Fig. 1.15. The action of anaesthetics on the sensitivity of two cells in *in vitro* preparations of the prepiriform cortex to iontophoretically applied L-glutamate. *a*, The effect of 0·3 mM pentobarbitone on the responses of a cell 270 μm deep in the prepiriform cortex. The cell was excited by a 20 nA, 10 sec pulse of glutamate every 30 sec throughout the experiment. The number of impulses elicited by each pulse of glutamate is plotted against time from an arbitrary zero. 0·3 mM pentobarbitone completely suppressed the cell's response to the pulses of glutamate. The effect was reversible. *b*, The effect of 0·8 per cent halothane on the responses of a cell 290 μm deep in the prepiriform cortex. This cell was excited by 35 nA, 10 sec pulses of glutamate every 30 sec. There was little, if any, depressant effect of halothane.

The experiments from which *a* and *b* are taken, were conducted in saline solutions containing 10 mM magnesium to block the normal evoked synaptic activity. The halothane was applied to the preparation in the gas phase [214]. (*From Richards and Smaje [224].*)

sixth agent tested, halothane, had no depressant action on the sensitivity of the receptors to glutamate until its concentration was considerably in excess of that required to depress synaptic transmission (*Fig. 1.15b*). Similar results were obtained when the experiments were repeated after synaptic transmission had been blocked by high Mg^{2+} concentrations in the bathing medium to exclude the possibility of indirect synaptic influences. Thus these results reflected direct actions of anaesthetics on the glutamate sensitivity of the cells studied. If the effects on the glutamate sensitivity reflect changes in the sensitivity of the postsynaptic receptors themselves, the synaptic depression caused by ether, methoxyflurane, trichloroethylene, pentobarbitone and alphaxalone would be the result of a decrease in the sensitivity of the postsynaptic receptors to the transmitter, while that caused by halothane would be principally due to a decrease in the amount of transmitter released from the nerve terminals [225]. A similar conclusion has been reached by Zorychta et al. for the action of halothane on synapses between Ia afferents and motoneurones in the spinal cord [306]. However, recent experiments with sympathetic ganglia have shown that halothane depresses both the potentials evoked by stimulation of the preganglionic nerve and the action of nicotinic agonists. These results suggest that halothane may reduce the sensitivity of the nicotinic receptors on the postsynaptic membrane to Ach [43].

The glutamate receptors of the neocortex show similar results to those of the olfactory cortex when studied under similar *in vitro* conditions [225]. Barker and Ransom [21, 207] have found that mouse spinal neurones grown in tissue culture also have a reduced sensitivity to glutamate when pentobarbitone is applied. Studies *in vivo* have given results that are broadly consistent with those just described. Crawford and Curtis [59], Crawford [58] and Galindo [93] have all reported that the sensitivity of neurones to glutamate is reduced by barbiturates, while it is little affected by halothane. There is nothing in all this evidence to suggest that the actions of anaesthetics (other than halothane) on synaptic transmission are exclusively due to an effect on the postsynaptic membrane. Indeed it is probable that both pre- and postsynaptic actions of anaesthetics contribute to depression of synaptic transmission.

Acetylcholine receptors in the brain are predominantly muscarinic [138] and so tend to produce slow, long-lasting effects when they are activated, unlike the nicotinic receptors of the sympathetic ganglia and neuromuscular junction. Nevertheless, muscarinic receptors are thought to mediate slow synaptic excitation and inhibition both in sympathetic ganglia [294] and in the brain [141]. Several anaesthetics including methohexitone, halothane and methoxyflurane have been reported to abolish muscarinic excitation of cortical neurones *in vivo* [39]. These observations are of especial interest as the arousal response of the cortex to reticular formation stimulation was thought to be mediated by a cholinergic process [90]. However, recent experiments *in vitro* with

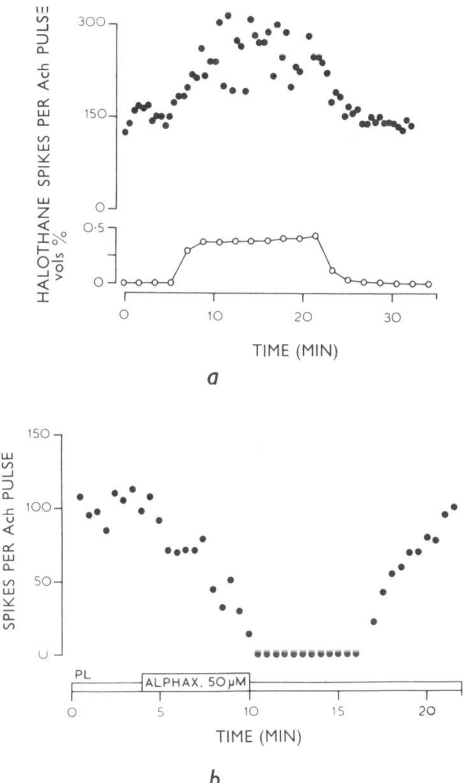

Fig. 1.16. The action of halothane and alphaxalone on the sensitivity of neurones in the olfactory cortex to iontophoretically applied acetylcholine (Ach). *a* and *b* were constructed from records taken from separate experiments. In *a* the cell was excited by a 70 mA pulse of Ach for 15 sec every 30 sec. Halothane was applied to the preparation in the gas phase (*see Fig. 1.15*). In *b* the cell was excited by a pulse of 75 nA Ach for 10 sec every 30 sec. The alphaxalone was administered as a steroid component of phospholipid vesicles. A control suspension of phospholipid without alphaxalone was superfused before and after the administration of the drug (PL). (*From Smaje [252].*)

preparations of olfactory cortex and neocortex have failed to confirm these findings. Smaje [252] found that, of six anaesthetics tested, only alphaxalone depressed the muscarinic responses to Ach while volatile anaesthetics actually enhanced them (*Fig. 1.16*). Pentobarbitone had no consistent depressant effect. These results obtained by Smaje were broadly similar to those reported 6 years earlier by Crawford [58] in his studies on decerebrate cats. Smaje also showed that these effects could be observed in preparations in which synaptic transmission had been blocked by decreasing the Ca^{2+} and raising the Mg^{2+} of the bathing fluid. Therefore the results reflect effects of anaesthetics on the muscarinic sensitivity of the postsynaptic membrane.

The effects of anaesthetics on the receptors of neurones to other putative excitatory transmitters have not yet received attention. However, there is a large amount of data on the action of anaesthetics on the nicotinic receptor of the neuromuscular junction. This receptor is unlikely to be typical of central nervous system receptors, if only because the evidence just discussed shows sharply differing effects on the two types of central nervous system receptor which have been studied. Nonetheless, the receptors of the neuromuscular junction are more amenable to detailed study, and detailed studies are necessary to throw light on the precise mechanisms by which anaesthetics perturb receptor function. A number of anaesthetics including the barbiturates and local anaesthetics decrease the amplitude of miniature end-plate potentials (MEPPs) [91, 205, 239, 273]. Since the prevailing view is that each MEPP reflects a predetermined amount of transmitter being released from the presynaptic nerve terminal [129], a decrease in the amplitude of the MEPPs presumably reflects a decrease in the sensitivity of the postsynaptic membrane to the transmitter (Ach). In contrast, ethanol increases both the amplitude and duration of MEPPs and the associated permeability changes (miniature end-plate currents or MEPCs) [92, 205]. Other alcohols (propanol, butanol and pentanol) also increased the duration of the MEPCs [92]. General anaesthetics including chloroform, ether, halothane and enflurane all decreased MEPCs [273].

Using a new technique developed by Verveen and Derksen [283] in Leiden and by Anderson and Stevens [8] in Seattle, Quastel and Linder [205] have analysed the pattern of the noise induced in the postsynaptic membrane by application of acetylcholine [131] and how it changes when anaesthetics are administered. They have shown that the increase in the duration of the MEPCs that is caused by alcohols is due to an increase in the time that the individual channels remain open (their relaxation time, or lifetime, is increased). Thus the permeability changes of the postsynaptic membrane to small ions last longer. This effect, together with a change in the sensitivity of the postsynaptic receptors to Ach could explain the dual actions of the alcohols on the MEPCs. Conversely, volatile anaesthetics apparently decrease the lifetime of the change that occurs in response to a given amount of Ach. Thus the effect of an anaesthetic may vary from receptor to receptor and the same receptor may show different effects with different anaesthetics. These results have profound implications for theories of anaesthesia as we shall see.

Anaesthetic Action on the Electrical Properties of the Postsynaptic Membrane

Anaesthetics may have effects on the electrical properties and excitability of the postsynaptic neurone in addition to their direct actions on chemical transmission. First, they could increase the resting conductance of the postsynaptic membrane by making it more permeable ('leaky') to the small ions of the extracellular fluid (e.g. Na^+, K^+ and Cl^-). This would have the effect of decreasing the passive spread of the EPSPs from the active synaptic regions and so would decrease the excitatory tone at the cell body. Second, anaesthetics could decrease the excitability of the postsynaptic neurone by raising the threshold depolarization required for cell discharge. A combination of both effects is also possible.

These possibilities have been tested in the olfactory cortex [213, 214, 221] and hippocampus [226] by a careful analysis of the synaptic field potentials. In each region, the synaptic field potentials consist of two components, an initial wave which is negative near the synapses and which reflects the strength of the synaptic depolarization, and one or more positive peaks; the area of the first of these peaks is a measure of the number of neurones discharging in response to the initial synaptic volley. By careful measurement, a relationship between the amplitude of the initial synaptic wave (the population EPSP) and the number of cells firing can be established. If anaesthetics either raised the threshold for cell discharge or if they decreased the electrotonic propagation of the synaptic potentials, then this relationship would be shifted so that a larger EPSP would be required to fire the same number of cortical cells. Such a change can be seen when the levels of Ca^{2+} and Mg^{2+} are raised (*Fig. 1.17a*). However, this relationship is not affected by anaesthetics (*Fig. 1.17b-d*). They simply reduced the size of the synaptic potential for a given stimulus strength, i.e. the effects on excitatory transmission in these areas of the cortex could be attributed solely to an action on chemical transmission.

Intracellular recordings from spinal motoneurones by Somjen and Gill [260] were broadly consistent with this view. They found that although ether and thiopentone increased the firing threshold of some motoneurones, they decreased that of others. Their results were obtained from spinal cats given high doses of thiopentone (30 mg/kg), but the concentration of ether administered was not specified. Adequate control of blood pressure and blood gases (Pa,o_2, Pa,co_2) was not evident. Weakly [292], however, found lower doses of pentobarbitone and thiopentone (5–10 mg/kg) had no effect on either the electrical threshold or the conductance of the motoneurone membrane.

The data discussed so far is relevant only to agents which have a selective depressant action on chemical transmission. It is probable that agents which depress synaptic transmission by virtue of their actions on nerve conduction would elevate the firing threshold of neurones as this effect accompanies their blockade of nerve impulse conduction. Preliminary experiments with tetrodotoxin, procaine and propanidid and the synaptic field potentials of the olfactory cortex suggest that this is so.

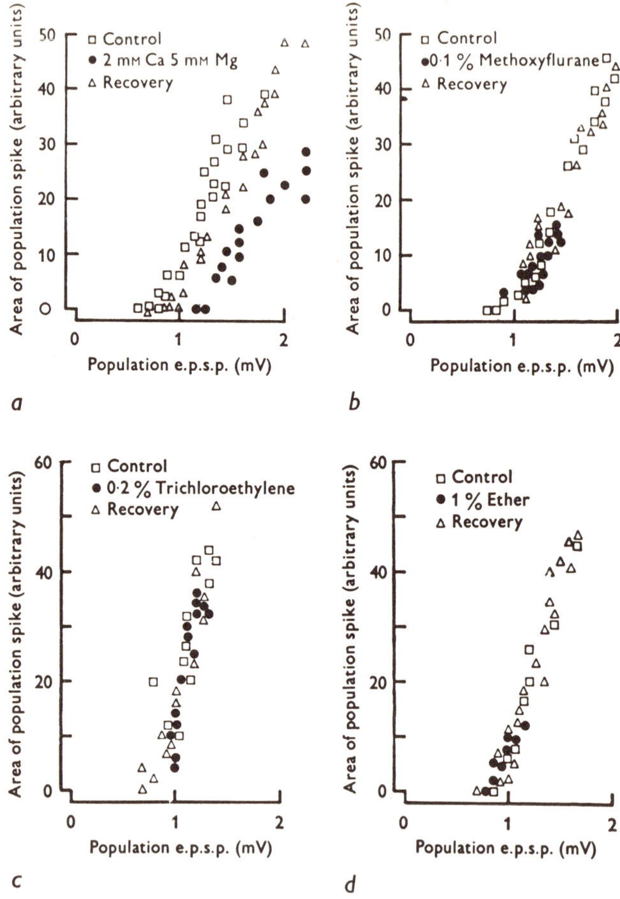

Fig. 1.17. The effects of anaesthetics on the relationship between the population EPSP and the discharge of granule cells in the hippocampus. *a,* Increasing the levels of calcium and magnesium causes a rightward shift in the curve indicating that these ions had increased the threshold for cell discharge. *b–d,* Methoxyflurane, trichloroethylene and ether did not cause such a shift, indicating that the depressant effects of these anaesthetics on synaptic transmission was not due to a decrease in the excitability of the granule cells. (*From Richards and White [226].*)

Summary

Anaesthetics can be divided into two broad classes on the basis of their effects on excitatory synaptic transmission. The first class includes local anaesthetics, the primary alcohols, propanidid and urethane, all agents which have no selective depressant action on chemical transmission. Such agents appear to act primarily by a blockade of nerve impulse conduction which causes a consequential depression of the EPSPs and an elevation of the electrical threshold both in the afferent nerve fibres and in the postsynaptic cells. The second class includes volatile anaesthetics such as ether and halothane, the barbiturates and steroids, all of which depress chemical transmission before they affect nerve impulse conduction. Agents of this class appear to have no effect on the firing threshold of neurones at normal anaesthetic doses. These two classes are distinct, but there are areas of overlap; thus the alcohols and local anaesthetics have a direct action on the postsynaptic receptors of the neuromuscular junction and the selectivity of agents of the second class is relative and varies both with the anaesthetic and the dose applied.

Action of Anaesthetics on Inhibitory Transmission

Analysis of the action of anaesthetics on inhibitory synaptic transmission is difficult because inhibitory pathways operate via excitatory interneurones. Direct stimulation of the inhibitory nerve fibres themselves is seldom possible. It is therefore difficult to attribute the effects of anaesthetics on inhibitory synaptic processes to a direct action on inhibitory synapses rather than to some subtle change in the properties of an excitatory interneurone. Modulation of the influence of some other pathways on the inhibitory process in question is also possible.

In contrast to the general depressant effects of anaesthetics on excitatory synaptic transmission, presynaptic inhibition is enhanced by both chloralose and pentobarbitone (*Fig. 1.18*), although it is depressed by ether, paral-

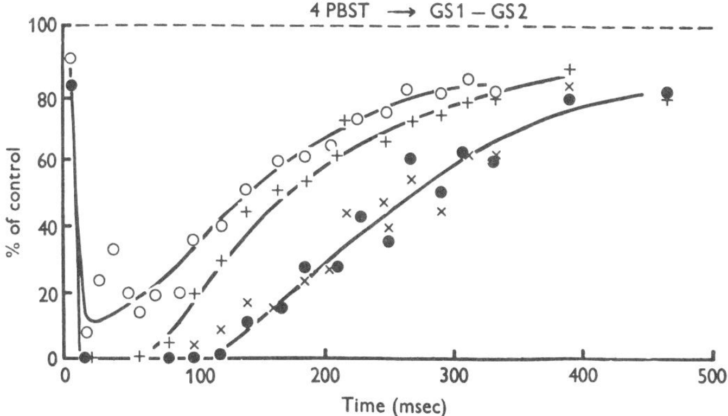

Fig. 1.18. The effect of pentobarbitone on the presynaptic inhibition of a monosynaptic reflex. Two volleys to the gastrocnemius (GS) nerve were given at intervals of 1–500 msec and the height of the monosynaptic response recorded from the first sacral ventral root was recorded. The first volley evoked no response but facilitated the response to the second volley. If the volleys to the GS are preceded by a short train of shocks to the posterior-biceps semitendinous nerve the response to the GS shocks are depressed for over 200 msec. If pentobarbitone is administered (20 mg/kg, •) the depression is intensified and prolonged, after 3 h the effect of pentobarbitone had partly worn off (+) but a second injection of pentobarbitone (×) again intensified the inhibition. (*From Eccles et al. [75].*)

dehyde, urethane and chloral hydrate [75, 241]. Similarly, postsynaptic recurrent inhibition in spinal motoneurones [149] and CA1 hippocampal pyramidal cells [190] is increased by barbiturates. Postsynaptic recurrent inhibition in the olfactory bulb is increased by a number of anaesthetics including the barbiturates, halothane and urethane, but it is depressed by ethanol (*Fig. 1.19*) [188, 264]. The reticulospinal inhibitory pathway is readily blocked by anaesthetics [79, 80] and Weakly et al. [293] could find no evidence of an increase in direct postsynaptic inhibition in motoneurones following the administration of barbiturates.

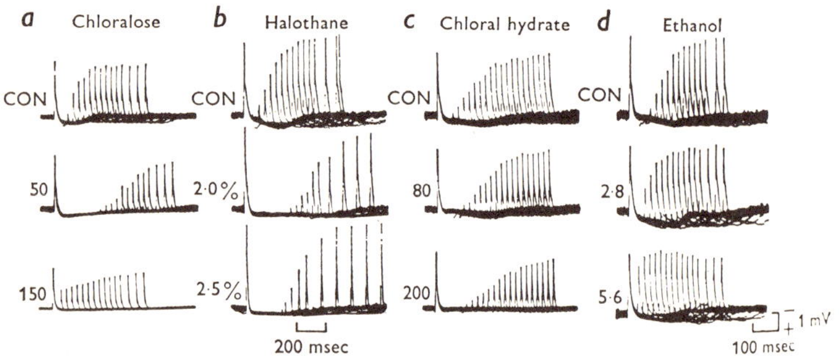

Fig. 1.19. The effect of anaesthetics on the inhibition of olfactory bulb mitral cells by granule cells. The tcp record is the control for each series. The dose of chloralose and that of chloral hydrate are given as mg/kg, that of halothane as per cent inhaled in a halothane–oxygen mixture and the dose of ethanol as g/kg. The calibration at the lower right-hand corner applies to all records except the lowest of column *b* where the sweep speed is halved. Note that the anaesthetics except for ethanol initially intensify and prolong the inhibition of the mitral cell response to antidromic stimulation of the lateral olfactory tract. Increasing the dose of chloralose threefold leads to a block of the inhibitory effect. Increasing the dose of ethanol progressively decreases the inhibition. (*From Nicoll [188].*)

The block of inhibitory synaptic transmission in certain pathways by anaesthetics [76, 79, 80, 293] may readily be explained by mechanisms similar to those involved in the block of excitatory synaptic transmission. The block itself could result from a direct depressant action on the inhibitory synapses themselves or on excitatory interneurones or both.

It is more difficult to explain how the activity of some inhibitory synapses is augmented by anaesthetics. One possibility is that the activity of excitatory interneurones or of the inhibitory cell itself is increased in some way by the action of anaesthetics. These cells characteristically discharge at high frequencies, after their excitation (examples of this pattern of behaviour can be seen with both Renshaw cells in the spinal cord [74] and basket cells in the hippocampus [6, 7]). If these trains became prolonged, then the inhibition they would exert on the postsynaptic cells would be increased. There is some evidence that this happens as the activity of Renshaw cells to ventral root stimulation is increased by ethanol [169] and their sensitivity to iontophoretically applied Ach (their normal excitatory transmitter) is also slightly increased by chloralose [23]. An alternative possibility is that the enhancement is the result of a direct action on chemical transmission at the inhibitory synapse itself. (It is difficult to see how a block of afferent nerve conduction could account for such a phenomenon.) Although there is evidence that the barbiturates can increase the amount of transmitter released from the presynaptic nerve terminals at the neuromuscular junction [204, 247, 271, 296] (p. 36), there is no comparable evidence to suggest that they increase the release of inhibitory transmitters. Indeed the available evidence suggests that barbiturates depress the release of the putative inhibitory transmitter GABA both from slices of hippocampus [121] and from synaptosomes [104]. If, however, the released transmitter remained in the synaptic cleft for a longer period because the mechanisms for its removal had been inhibited, its effect would be prolonged. This idea was suggested by Cutler and his colleagues [62], but later work has refuted the idea, neither the high affinity nor the low affinity uptake of GABA by small brain slices is inhibited by barbiturates at concentrations normally required for anaesthesis [121]. The remaining possibility is that barbiturates (and possibly other anaesthetics) increase the effect the transmitter has on the postsynaptic membrane. Nicoll [189] has shown that pentobarbitone increases the effect of GABA on frog motoneurones and itself produces a GABA-like effect. Similarly, pentobarbitone enhances the hyperpolarizing action of GABA on spinal neurones grown in culture [208], but does not enhance that of another inhibitory amino acid, glycine (*Fig. 1.20*). This effect presumably reflects an increase in the lifetime of the activated ionic channels as the affinity (cf. the action of alcohols on the MEPCs) of the receptor for GABA is not increased by barbiturates. The action of GABA on cat spinal neurones is apparently enhanced by barbiturates although that of glycine is not [158]. One further hypothesis, as yet unsubstantiated, that may explain the enhancement of inhibition by barbiturates is that when they reduce the release of transmitter they also prolong the time over which the transmitter is released. This would not account for the increase in the intensity of the inhibition which would have to be attributed to a postsynaptic effect, but it could contribute to the increase in its duration.

Summary

Anaesthetics appear to have direct actions on both excitatory and inhibitory synaptic transmission. In general it appears that excitatory synaptic transmission is depressed by anaesthetics while inhibitory synaptic transmission may be either depressed or enhanced depending upon the pathways involved. These differential effects of anaesthetics have considerable implications for the action of anaesthetics on the nervous system as a whole.

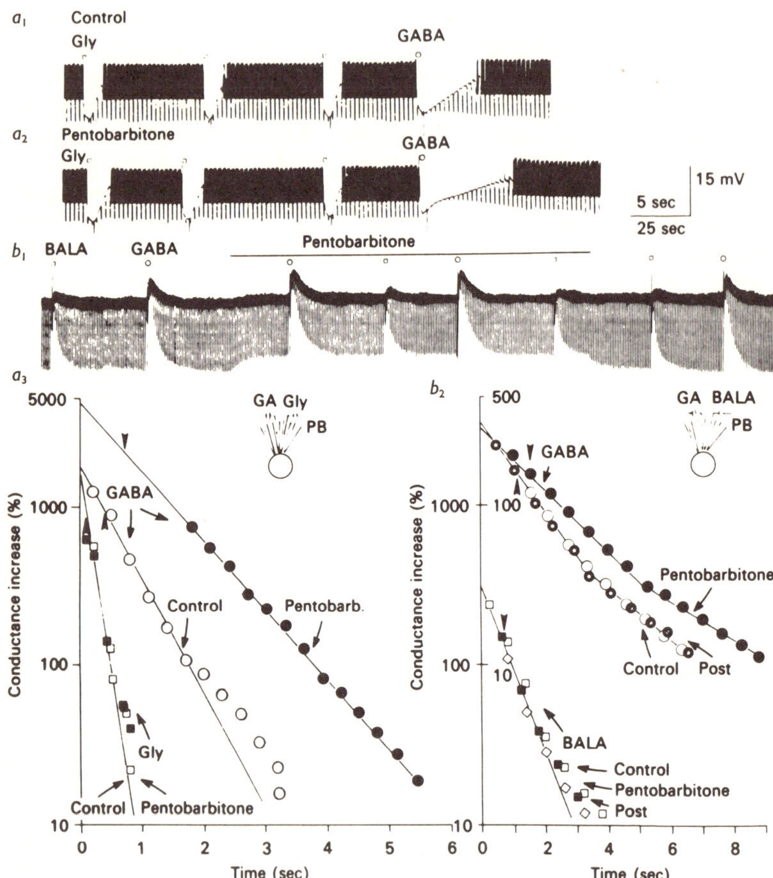

Fig. 1.20. The selective enhancement of the action of γ-aminobutyric acid (GABA) by pentobarbitone on a cerebellar–brainstem neurone maintained in tissue culture (*a*). A smaller effect is seen with a spinal neurone (*b*). a_1, a_2 show specimen records of the effects of glycine and GABA on the membrane resistance monitored by constant current hyperpolarizing pulses and its modulation by 0·1 mM pentobarbitone. a_3 is a plot of the time-course of the conductance increase for various conditions. b_1 and b_2 show similar records for a spinal neurone responding to pulses of β-alanine (□) and GABA (○). (*From Barker and Ransom [21].*)

THEORIES OF ANAESTHESIA

Anaesthetics as a group share no distinguishing chemical features. Substances range from inert inorganic gases such as nitrous oxide through simple organic compounds such as hydrocarbons (both halogenated and non-halogenated), alcohols and ketones to complex organic molecules such as barbiturates and steroids; all have satisfactory anaesthetic properties.

Inert substances like xenon and the alkanes (methane, ethane etc.) are effective anaesthetics, while highly reactive chemical substances are unsuitable as their effects are toxic and irreversible. Thus, whatever the mechanism of anaesthesia, it does not require a specific chemical reaction to occur in the neurones of the brain. Indeed, the absolute requirement for a freely reversible depression of central nervous system function suggests that the mechanism involves physiochemical processes that do not require the formation of covalent chemical bonds.

It has been assumed as an initial working hypothesis that all anaesthetics work in essentially the same way (the unitary hypothesis of anaesthesia). Because of the extraordinarily wide range of substances that possess anaesthetic properties, much experimental effort has concentrated on regularities observed in correlations of the physical properties of anaesthetics with their anaesthetic potency (e.g. lipid solubility [168], hydrate dissociation pressure [176, 195], van der Waals constants [304], molar refractivity [195], molecular polarization [194]). The most satisfactory of these is the remarkably good correlation between the potency of anaesthetic gases and vapours and their solubility in olive oil. This correlation holds over a 30 000-fold concentration range [171] (*Fig. 1.21*). Non-volatile anaesthetics have recently been included in this correlation [83]. This empirical approach has been further refined by correlating the solubility of anaesthetics in solvents of different polarity with their anaesthetic potency. This detailed analysis suggested that anaesthetics dissolve in a hydrophobic region in the body which has some polar and some non-polar characteristics (i.e. properties intermediate between a pure hydrocarbon such as hexane (non-polar) and the lower alcohols or water (highly polar) [171]).

The question then is: where in the neurones are the regions that have these solvent properties? Cells consist of a watery phase (the cytoplasm) containing large amounts of soluble protein and a lipid phase (the membranes) also containing protein. Relative to anaesthetic molecules, protein molecules are large, so it is conceivable that anaesthetics may act by binding to hydrophobic regions of cytoplasmic proteins to inhibit their function and so cause metabolic alterations that lead to anaesthesia. However, although several soluble proteins [116, 143, 301] can bind anaesthetics, there is no evidence to suggest that anaesthetics materially affect their physiological function at the concentrations attained during anaesthesia. Furthermore, anaesthetic effects can be demonstrated in artificial membranes [182] and in nerves whose axoplasm has been removed and replaced by artificial solutions [84, 85, 185]. Consequently, it is now widely accepted that anaesthetics act primarily by a direct interaction with nerve membranes. Krnjević has pointed out that the plasma membrane is only a small part of the total membranes of a cell and that there is no *a priori* reason for assuming that this membrane rather than those of the cell mitochondria, say, is the primary site of action of anaesthetics on the

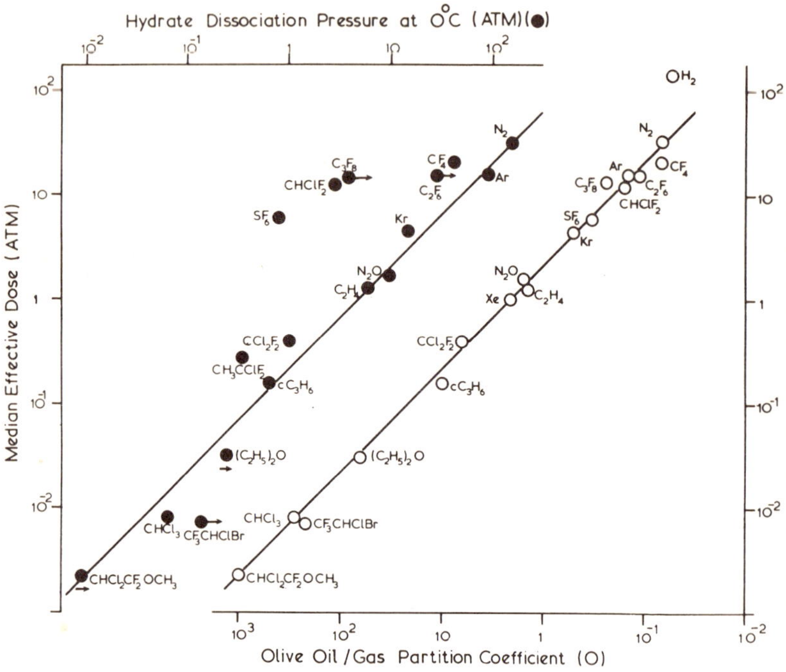

Fig. 1.21. The correlation between the anaesthetic potency of various anaesthetics and their olive oil/gas partition coefficients (right graph, ○) or their hydrate dissociation pressures (left graph, ●). The anaesthetic potency was defined as the pressure of anaesthetic required to abolish the righting reflex of 50 per cent of a group of mice. (*From Miller et al. [171].*)

membrane system of a cell [139]. Equally, it should be recognized that it is through the medium of the plasma membrane that a nerve cell interacts with its fellows so that it is always true that anaesthetic actions *per se* must be mediated through modifications of the function of the plasma membrane. Whether the actions of anaesthetics are due to direct actions on the plasma membrane or to indirect actions mediated via some generalized metabolic disturbançe must now be considered.

It has been known for many years that anaesthetics depress cellular respiration [284]. Moreover, we have seen earlier (p. 11) that cerebral metabolism is depressed during general anaesthesia maintained by a wide variety of anaesthetic agents. These observations have led to the view that anaesthesia is caused by depression of cerebral oxidative metabolism, i.e. to a form of chemical asphyxia. Biochemical studies have established that anaesthetics inhibit oxidative metabolism by a block of electron transport in the mitochondrial membranes [40, 101, 175]. However, the concentrations required to inhibit mitochondrial function by 50 per cent are greatly in excess of the amount required for anaesthesia (about two to six times greater than the minimum alveolar concentration required for surgical anaesthesia for a variety of inhalational agents [53]). That anaesthetics can inhibit oxygen uptake and electron transport is not in doubt. The question at issue is this: do they produce their anaesthetic effects by their action on cellular respiration? This view has been vigorously championed by Quastel in particular [206], but close examination reveals serious weaknesses in the hypothesis. As I have already indicated, the concentrations of anaesthetics needed to interfere with the respiration of intact tissue slices or isolated mitochondria are high compared to those required to produce anaesthesia. The correlation between anaesthetic potency *in vivo* and that

Table 1.4. The Effect of Anaesthesia on the Levels of ATP and Creatine Phosphate in Whole Brain*

Treatment	*Creatine phosphate*	*ATP*	*ADP*	*Total high energy phosphate*	*Ref.*
Control	3·63 ± 0·09	2·95 ± 0·04	0·03 ± 0·01	10·07	96
220 mg/kg phenobarbitone	5·08 ± 0·18	3·12 ± 0·07	0·26 ± 0·05	11·95	
135 mg/kg amylobarbitone	4·87 ± 0·07	3·20 ± 0·08	0·20 ± 0·01	11·66	
4·5 per cent ether	4·42 ± 0·09	3·19 ± 0·06	0·22 ± 0·04	11·19	
Control	3·21 ± 0·05	2·21 ± 0·05	0·43 ± 0·02	–	67
1·5 per cent halothane	3·75 ± 0·11	2·19 ± 0·07	0·43 ± 0·02	–	
Ketamine	3·32 ± 0·16	2·13 ± 0·04	0·48 ± 0·01	–	

*All values are expressed as μM/g wet wt.

required to inhibit mitochondrial respiration *in vitro* is poor (e.g. *in vitro* amylobarbitone > thiopentone and halothane > methoxyflurane; *in vivo* thiopentone > amylobarbitone and methoxyflurane > halothane). Other substances that inhibit cell respiration such as cyanide or azide do not cause anaesthesia, nor do they block synaptic transmission which is sensitive to anaesthetic agents [147]. The administration of sublethal doses of cyanide is accompanied by convulsions and an increase in brain lactate; a lethal dose of cyanide reduces cytochrome oxidase activity by about one-half, causes substantial decreases in the level of 'high energy' compounds such as creatine phosphate and adenosine triphosphate (ATP) and increases cerebral lactate [4, 192]. All of these data point towards cerebral anoxia. In contrast, during anaesthesia maintained with a variety of anaesthetics no evidence of cerebral anoxia could be found [67, 96, 191, 200]. Indeed in all cases there was a slight increase in the brain levels of 'high energy' compounds (Table 1.4) and a decrease in brain lactate. It seems that the decrease in cerebral metabolic rate that occurs during general anaesthesia is a result of a decrease in nervous activity and is not its cause.

Krnjević has proposed an ingenious variation of this hypothesis. He discovered that certain metabolic inhibitors such as 2,4-dinitrophenol had a hyperpolarizing action on cortical neurones which could be attributed to an increase in the permeability of the membrane to potassium [95]. He therefore argued that if anaesthetics depressed mitochondrial activity they would no longer accumulate Ca^{2+} efficiently and this would lead to an increase in intracellular Ca^{2+}. Injecting Ca^{2+} into nerve cells is associated with an increase in membrane permeability to potassium and a decrease in excitability [165]. Thus an accumulation of intracellular calcium could account for the depression of synaptic transmission seen throughout the nervous system. He further suggested that this hypothesis could explain the depression of muscarinic excitation of cortical cells because muscarinic excitation is mediated by a *decrease* in cell permeability to potassium, and concluded 'Since a possible involvement of cortical cholinergic pathways in cortical arousal has long been suspected, this hypothesis could explain a special vulnerability to anaesthetics of neural processes underlying consciousness' [139].

However, there is no evidence that anaesthetics impair the ability of mitochondria to accumulate Ca^{2+} unless oxidative metabolism and ATP production are also affected [102]. We have already seen that cerebral ATP levels are not depressed during anaesthesia. Furthermore, the available evidence suggests that anaesthetics do not affect the electrical excitability of cortical cells as this hypothesis predicts (p. 40). Finally, it appears that the muscarinic responses of cortical cells are not invariably depressed by anaesthetics as the hypothesis predicts. Smaje [252] has shown that certain anaesthetics actually enhance the muscarinic response to Ach of cells in the olfactory cortex and Crawford [58] found little evidence of a block of muscarinic excitation. To conclude, there is no evidence that the changes in synaptic efficacy that occur during anaesthesia are secondary to metabolic changes occurring within the cell. The effects are best explained by direct interactions between anaesthetics and the various components of the neuronal membranes that subserve synaptic transmission.

Current Views of Membrane Structure

Before proceeding further it is necessary to have some knowledge of current ideas of membrane structure. It is now generally agreed that mammalian membranes consist of a bilayer of phospholipid molecules in which proteins are embedded. The phospholipid molecules are aligned so that the polar head groups (containing the phosphate and basic radicals) are oriented outward towards the aqueous environment and the long fatty acid hydrocarbon chains form a hydrophobic phase at the centre of the bilayer. The membrane proteins are embedded in the lipid bilayer or penetrate through it (*Fig. 1.22*) [251]. Studies of the physical properties of membranes by sophisticated techniques such as nuclear magnetic resonance (NMR) and electron-spin resonance (ESR) have shown that the mobility of the methylene groups of the phospholipid hydrocarbon chains increases with the distance from the polar head group regions so that the head group region and the immediately subjacent methylene groups form a gel-like region (i.e. are relatively stiff), while the core of the bilayer has

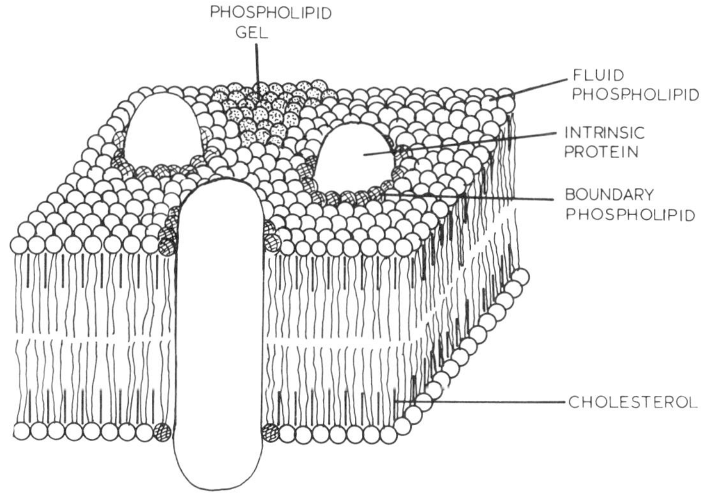

Fig. 1.22. A diagrammatic representation of the structure of a mammalian plasma membrane. The membrane shown consists of a single penetrant protein surrounded by a layer of bound phospholipid which is embedded in a fluid matrix of phospholipid and cholesterol. A region of phospholipid gel is also shown (stippled) to indicate the possible lateral phase separation of membrane lipid although it is improbable that it would exist at normal body temperature (*see text*). (*From Richards [217].*)

the characteristics of a liquid hydrocarbon. The exact fluidity of a membrane depends upon its precise phospholipid composition, the presence or absence of cholesterol (which tends to stiffen the membrane) and the temperature [33, 144, 162]. There is evidence to suggest that a number of intrinsic membrane-bound enzymes require the presence of a ring of lipid molecules to stabilize them in their active form. Metcalfe and his group [110, 289, 290] have investigated the properties of this annular lipid and its role in the regulation of the calcium transport protein of the sarcoplasmic reticulum. They found that the activity of the enzyme–lipid complex depended upon the composition of the phospholipid associated with the protein. Dioleyl lecithin, a phospholipid that has a low melting point (gel–liquid phase transition temperature) permitted higher enzymic activity at low temperatures (24–30 °C) than dipalmitoyl lecithin which has a high melting point. They found that adding 50 mM benzyl alcohol to the incubation medium increased the enzymic activity, an effect they attributed to the fluidizing effect of the alcohol upon the lipid (*see below*). Conversely, adding cholesterol in sufficient amounts to cause it to displace some of the protein-bound phospholipid resulted in inhibition of enzymic activity.

The Action of Anaesthetics on Membrane Structure

Given that anaesthetics produce their characteristic effects by direct interaction with the plasma membrane, with what constituents of the membrane do they interact? Two main alternatives present themselves: anaesthetics could dissolve in the membrane lipid, modify its physical properties and so indirectly affect the function of the membrane proteins associated with synaptic transmission (or action potential propagation) or they could bind directly to the membrane proteins to perturb their function.

Historically, emphasis has been given to the striking correlation between the potency of anaesthetics and their lipid solubility. It is, therefore, hardly surprising that the cell lipids have been for long regarded as the most probable site of anaesthetic action. Clear formulation of this concept is found in the lipid solubility rule of Meyer [168]: anaesthesia commences when any chemically indifferent substance has attained a certain molar concentration in the lipids of the cell; the value of this critical concentration depends on the animal species under study but not on the chemical nature of the anaesthetic. Meyer himself appreciated that this is not strictly a theory of anaesthesia but what he called 'an experimentally observed regularity that any theory of anaesthesia must take into account'. Some years later Mullins [183] pointed out that when anaesthetics dissolve in membrane lipids (or any other solvent for that matter) they occupy an amount of space that depends both upon their concentration and the size of the individual anaesthetic molecules. He therefore proposed the critical volume hypothesis, which postulates that anaesthesia occurs when a critical volume fraction of anaesthetic is achieved in the cell membranes and further suggested that the membrane expansion caused by anaesthetics would lead to occlusion of pores in the membrane which would, in turn, prevent the passage of ions. This was a landmark, as it was the first attempt to provide a mechanistic explanation of anaesthetic action.

Recent experiments by Miller et al. have attempted to test these two hypotheses. Initial attempts to distinguish between them by solubility arguments were inconclusive, although they did reaffirm the importance of the correlation between lipid solubility and anaesthetic potency [171]. In their later work they concentrated on the effects of pressure on the potency of anaesthetic gases and showed that the variation of potency of four anaesthetic gases (nitrous oxide, nitrogen, carbon tetrafluoride and sulphur hexafluoride) at different pressures was more consistent with the critical volume hypothesis than with the simple lipid solubility rule [172]. They calculated that the active site would expand by 0·2–0·6 per cent (v/v) during anaesthesia. Their calculation assumed that the active site had solvent properties and a compressibility similar to benzene or carbon disulphide, both of which are relatively compressible. (If the site of anaesthetic action were to be less compressible than these solvents its expansion during anaesthesia would also be less.) The critical volume hypothesis, unlike the lipid solubility rule, could also accommodate the early observation that the effects of anaesthetics on tadpoles and bacteria could be reversed by high hydrostatic pressure [122, 123]. Later work has shown that anaesthesia induced in mice [156, 173, 299], newts [156] and tadpoles [103] by a wide variety of agents can be reversed by pressure. This pressure data provides clear evidence that the site of action increases its volume when anaesthetics are bound, but does not by itself allow any inference to be made about the nature of the site itself, i.e. whether it is lipid or protein.

Evidence that cell membranes expand during anaesthesia has been provided by Roth and Seeman [237, 238, 246]. A wide variety of anaesthetics protect red cells from hypotonic haemolysis and this protective action can be attributed to an anaesthetic-induced expansion of the red cell membrane. Calculations suggested that in the presence of concentrations of anaesthetic sufficient to cause general anaesthesia, the surface area of the red cell membrane expands by about 0·4 per cent and concentrations of anaesthetic sufficient to cause nerve block (i.e. local anaesthesia) expand the area of the red cell membrane by about 2 per cent. Similar membrane area expansion has been shown for monolayers of dipalmitoyl lecithin exposed to partial pressures of halogenated anaesthetics similar to those required for general anaesthesia [281]. Lately, there has been some evidence that alkanes and benzyl alcohol may increase the thickness of artificial phospholipid membranes (black lipid membranes) [19, 20, 105, 106].

Simple solubility models of anaesthetic action are rather unhelpful when the problem of how anaesthetics perturb membrane function is considered. So the various ways in which anaesthetics modify the physical properties of membrane lipids have been considered as potential mechanisms of anaesthesia. Specifically these are the fluidity of membrane lipids, their physical phase (i.e. whether they are in the crystalline or liquid state) and the thickness of the bilayer.

Membrane Fluidity

About 10 years ago Metcalfe et al. [167] were studying the binding of benzyl alcohol to erythrocyte membranes by NMR spectroscopy and found that the rotation of the alcohol molecules was restricted when they were present at low concentrations in the membrane, but the degree of restriction diminished as the concentration of the alcohol in the membrane increased. To explain this phenomenon they suggested that the alcohol increased the disorder of the membrane making it more fluid. Colley and Metcalfe [54] following on from this work showed that a series of *n*-aryl alcohols of varying chain length had a fluidizing action and concluded that 'Whatever the primary region of localisation in the bilayer, the effect of alcohols in fluidizing the structure is sensed by the whole of the lipid molecule in its steric interactions with neighbouring lipids.' These results have profound implications because a localized increase in fluidity caused by an anaesthetic should be transmitted via lipid–lipid interactions to specific functional proteins such as receptors. Furthermore, we have already seen that the fluidity of the bilayer phospholipids influences the function of certain membrane proteins. Later work using ESR methods has extended these observations and shown that a wide variety of anaesthetics fluidize membrane lipids [115, 150, 278]. Trudell et al. [279] have even shown that increasing pressure antagonizes the fluidizing effect of anaesthetics.

In view of the apparently universal ability of anaesthetics to fluidize membrane lipids, it is not surprising that the fluidizing action of anaesthetics came to be regarded as the probable mechanism of anaesthesia (*Fig. 1.23*). This idea was reinforced by the work of Lawrence and Gill

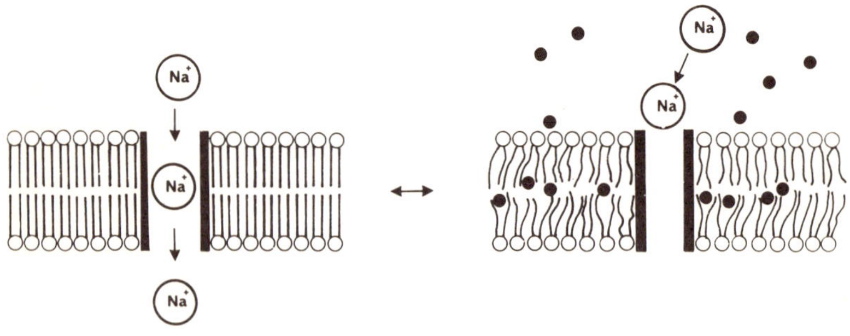

Fig. 1.23. A schematic representation of the membrane fluidity hypothesis of anaesthetic action. On the left the membrane is represented as a series of oriented phospholipid molecules in which an ion channel is embedded. Adding anaesthetic (•) disorders the phospholipid hydrocarbon chains rendering them more fluid and this change is sensed by the ion channel which undergoes a conformational change that impairs its function.

[151] who found that non-anaesthetic lipid-soluble substances, e.g. *n*-hexadecanol, tetradecane and certain cannabinoids (derivatives of cannabis extracts) did not fluidize membranes. However, this view is not universally accepted. Boggs et al. [26] have pointed out that the amount of anaesthetic in the membrane lipid during general anaesthesia is small (about 5 mM per mole of lipid) and at such low concentrations there are no detectable

changes in the fluidity of phospholipids (*Fig. 1.24*). Furthermore, even with concentrations of anaesthetic sufficient to cause local anaesthesia (i.e. nerve block) the changes in fluidity are small. Most of this work has been performed on artificial phospholipid–cholesterol membranes which, unlike normal membranes, do not contain proteins. When natural synaptosomal membranes have been studied, it has been found that concentrations of halothane and barbiturates comparable to those found during anaesthesia do not increase membrane fluidity but decrease it [233, 234].

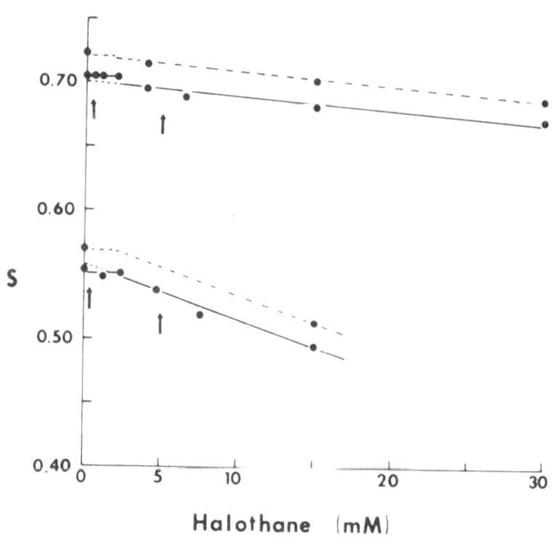

Fig. 1.24. The effect of halothane at 1 atmosphere (———) and 130 atmospheres (– – – –) pressure on the order parameter (S) of 8 doxylalamitate (upper curves) and 12 doxylstearate (lower curves) in phosphatidylcholine–cholesterol vesicles. The arrows indicate the concentrations of halothane required for general anaesthesia (left) and nerve block (right). Note that while increasing halothane decreases the order parameter (fluidizes the lipid) little change in S is seen at the concentrations relevant for anaesthesia. The effect of pressure is not specific to the action of halothane but reflects a generalized decrease in fluidity as the pressure is increased. (*From Boggs et al. [25].*)

The *n*-alkanols (ethanol, propanol etc.) show an increasing capacity to fluidize membranes as the chain length increases up to hexanol; thereafter the fluidizing action decreases until at decanol it is no longer present [220]. Alkanols with a chain length greater than ten carbon atoms decrease membrane fluidity (at least up to C14). Yet alkanols up to dodecanol (C12) (i.e. alkanols having both fluidizing and rigidifying actions) can anaesthetize tadpoles [29] and block nerve impulse conduction [220]. Furthermore, the actions of butanol and dodecanol on nerve conduction are synergistic not antagonistic as the fluidity hypothesis would predict [220]. Thus, there is no correlation between the fluidizing action of alkanols and their anaesthetic activity so that the fluidizing action of anaesthetics cannot be a *general* mechanism of anaesthetic action.

Lipid Phase Transition Theories

Consider a pure phospholipid such as dimyristoyl lecithin (DML) which has fully saturated hydrocarbon chains. At a low temperature, say 0 °C, it exists in a gel state with both head groups and hydrocarbon chains oriented in an orderly manner. As the temperature is raised there is little change in the motional freedom of the molecules until a critical temperature is reached at which the hydrocarbon chains melt (23 °C in the case of DML). This is the phase transition temperature (T_t). Above T_t the hydrocarbon chains show little increase in their fluidity as the temperature rises [41, 193]. Mixtures of two phospholipids show two T_ts corresponding to those of the constituents of the mixture. Thus the component with the higher T_t remains in a condition of lateral phase separation after the other has melted [250]. Melting of phospholipid monolayers is associated with an increase in their surface area [280].

There is now ample evidence to show that anaesthetics of all kinds, e.g. alcohols [111, 119, 220], amines [120, 282], barbiturates [153] and steroids [55] lower the T_t of various phospholipids just as salt lowers the melting point of ice (*Fig. 1.25*). Furthermore, amounts of anaesthetic sufficient to cause nerve block decrease T_t by 3–5 °C [152, 153].

On the basis of this information Trudell [277] has suggested that anaesthetics may work by decreasing the T_t of phospholipids which exist in the membrane in a condition of lateral phase separation. In detail he proposes that anaesthetics partition into the membrane and melt some of the phospholipids which exist in the gel state. This leads to an increase in the lateral pressure exerted by the membrane lipid on specific functional membrane proteins, which in turn inhibits their function and culminates in anaesthesia.

An alternative hypothesis based on this idea has been proposed by Lee [152] for the action of anaesthetics on nerve conduction. He has postulated that the sodium channel of nerve is maintained in an optional conformation by an annulus of rigid lipid molecules (similar to a gel state) and that anaesthetics fluidize this lipid, so causing the channel to relax into an inactive conformation. Clearly, this model could be extended to include other membrane proteins such as receptors or ion channels (*Fig. 1.26*).

These hypotheses are rather implausible. First, although there is evidence that there are lateral segregations of membrane lipids in bacteria, there is no evidence that upsetting this segregation results in functional deficits [193, 270]. Second, the phospholipids of mammalian membrane do not have saturated hydrocarbon chains but are partially unsaturated and such

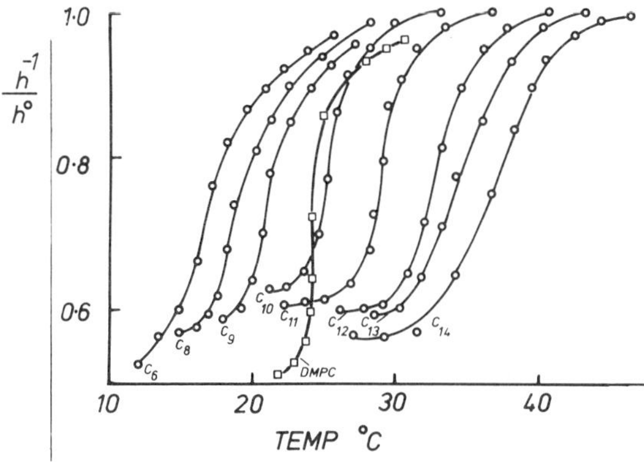

Fig. 1.25. The effect of a series of alcohols on the phase transition temperature of dimyristoyl phosphatidylcholine DMPC (□). The ordinate h^{-1}/h^0 is an arbitrary measure of membrane fluidity. Low values of h^{-1}/h^0 represent a gel-like state, high values a fluid state. Alcohols with a chain length of less than 10 carbons decrease the phase transition temperature. Decanol has little effect, while undercanol (C11), dodecanol (C12), tridecanol (C13), and tetradecanol (C14) all elevate the phase transition temperature. (*From Richards et al. [220].*)

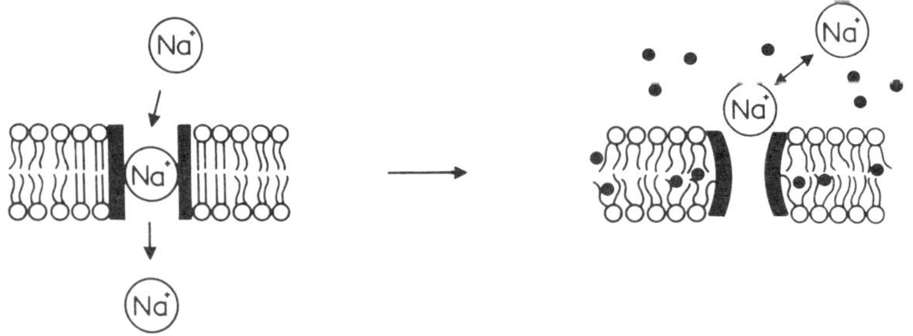

Fig. 1.26. A diagrammatic representation of the lipid phase transition hypothesis of anaesthetic action. Lee postulates that the sodium channel (black bars) is held in its optimal conformation by a ring of rigid lipid molecules (shown here by the straight chains) and that this lipid–protein complex is embedded in a matrix of fluid phospholipids. The addition of anaesthetics (•) fluidizes the boundary lipid and causes the protein conformation to collapse, so impairing its function.

lipids do not show sharp phase transitions but a progressive increase in fluidity as the temperature is raised. Third, mammalian nerve membranes contain large amounts of cholesterol (roughly one cholesterol molecule for every two phospholipid molecules) which suppresses phase transitions in lipid membranes [33, 144]. Fourth, short-chain alkanols fluidize membrane phospholipids and lower their T_t, while long-chain alkanols decrease the fluidity of phospholipids and raise their T_t (*Fig. 1.27*). However, both long- and short-chain alkanols are anaesthetics and their actions are synergistic not antagonistic as these hypotheses would suggest [220]. Finally, the effects of temperature on the potency of anaesthetics are not consistent with these models. If these hypotheses are correct, lowering the temperature should decrease the effectiveness of anaesthetics, both because the temperature difference between ambient and T_t will widen and because lowering the temperature decreases the amount of anaesthetic taken up by the membrane lipid. In fact, the potency of various volatile anaesthetics increases as the temperature is

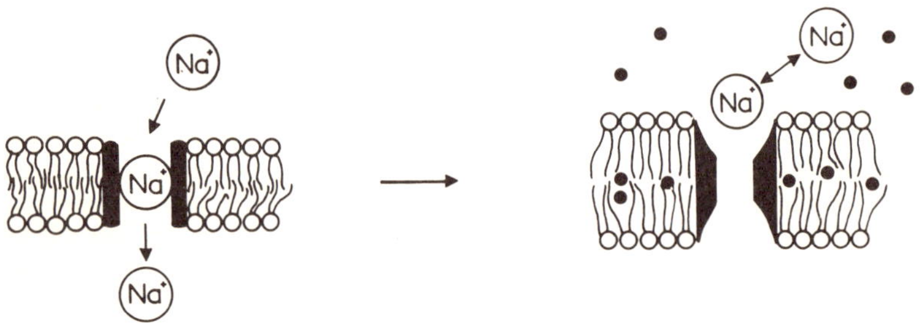

Fig. 1.27. The dynamic–tension model of anaesthetic action. Here the membrane is thought to consist of two layers of phospholipid whose hydrocarbon chains interdigitate. The lipid–protein interactions are thought to be very strong. Addition of anaesthetic molecules (•) increases the thickness of the bilayer by causing the separation of the hydrocarbon chains. This stretches the outer face of the protein, distorts its conformation and so inhibits its function.

lowered [42]. Furthermore, the local anaesthetic action of benzyl alcohol increases as the temperature is lowered while that of butanol is not greatly altered, which suggests that cooling by itself does not make nerve conduction more vulnerable to perturbation by anaesthetics [166, 220]. These temperature studies have wider implications for theories of anaesthesia to which I shall return.

Membrane Expansion

Seeman and Roth [246] have calculated that the surface area of red cells expands by 0·4 per cent in the presence of concentrations of anaesthetic sufficient to cause general anaesthesia and by 2–3 per cent in the presence of concentrations sufficient to block nerve impulse conduction. They assumed that the membrane expansion was uniform and noted that if this was true the membrane expansion was some ten times the actual volume occupied by the anaesthetic molecules in the membrane. Seeman attributed this expansion to the fluidizing action of anaesthetics on membrane lipids and to conformational changes in membrane proteins. He hypothesized that this disordered lipid membrane disrupted the normal function of membrane proteins (enzymes, ion channels and receptors) and resulted in anaesthesia [244].

The idea of membrane volume expansion has been revived by recent work on black lipid membranes. Two groups independently proposed that anaesthetics increase membrane thickness by separating the hydrocarbon tails belonging to each surface of the bilayer [19, 20, 105, 106] (*Fig. 1.27*). The resulting distortion of the normal lipid–protein interactions was considered to affect the operation of ion channels and other membrane functions and so cause anaesthesia. These studies were based on measurements of the electrical capacity of the lipid bilayers and Haydon et al. [106] have reported similar changes in the electrical capacity of the giant axon of the squid.

Although these ideas are plausible they produce serious quantitative problems. It seems incontrovertible that anaesthetics increase the surface area of membranes by about 2 per cent at concentrations required for local anaesthesia. The capacitance changes suggest that the thickness increases by 15–30 per cent, i.e. there must be a total volume increase of 30–60 per cent for an amount of anaesthetic occupying only 0·3 per cent of the initial membrane volume! Furthermore, Seeman [245] later studied the effect of ethanol on the volume of artificial lipid membranes (liposomes) by precision densitometry and found that the volume of the membranes increased exactly by the amount of space occupied by the anaesthetic in the membrane. He drew the conclusion that the observed expansion of natural membranes must be the result of conformational changes in the membrane proteins. However, this would imply that the proteins would have to increase their volume by more than 3 per cent during local anaesthesia – an improbably large value, as proteins have a volume change of only 2–3 per cent between their native state and their fully unfolded state [305]. This discrepancy can be resolved if it is conceded that the area of the membranes increases at the expense of their thickness (i.e. if the thickness *decreases* by a small amount it is possible to reconcile the data on the red cell membranes with that of the densitometry [217, 276]). What of the capacitance measurements? There are difficulties with this technique because the thickness changes are inferred from indirect measurements. Furthermore, the membranes are formed in the presence of a hydrocarbon solvent and it may be that more of this solvent is retained in the membrane when anaesthetics are applied [19]. Other explanations of the data are also possible. In any event, direct measurement by X-ray and neutron diffraction techniques have shown no significant change in membrane thickness in the presence of various volatile and gaseous anaesthetics [83]. At present, therefore, there is no clear evidence that anaesthetics actually increase membrane thickness as these hypotheses propose.

The Effect of Temperature on Anaesthetic Action

The various hypotheses of anaesthetic action that are based on interactions between membrane lipids and anaesthetics, all suggest that increasing temperature and anaesthetics alter the physical properties of the membrane lipids in the same manner. Clearly, if anaesthetics are supposed to alter some relatively gross physical property such as membrane fluidity or a critically balanced phase separation then other means of producing that change should produce the same effect. Furthermore, such hypotheses predict that the potency of anaesthetics should increase with increasing temperature, partly because the changes caused by anaesthetics are similar to those of increasing temperature, and partly because the partition coefficient of anaesthetics increases with temperature. However, as temperature itself profoundly influences physiological performance the extent of this synergism is difficult to predict. All that can be stated with confidence is that less anaesthetic should be required to anaesthetize an animal or block nerve conduction as the temperature rises.

Experiments with intact mammals have been attempted but are of little value as hypothermia produces torpor. Consequently, any change in anaesthetic potency with temperature would be difficult to interpret unambiguously. To overcome this problem Cherkin and Catchpool [42] acclimatized goldfish to different temperatures. After acclimatization to a particular environmental temperature, the concentration of anaesthetic needed to anaesthetize the goldfish at that temperature was determined. This procedure was followed at other temperatures and the change in the relative potency of anaesthetics with temperature was determined. Cherkin and Catchpool found that there was a monotonic increase in anaesthetic potency as the temperature decreased (*see Fig. 1.28*). This result strongly suggested that those theories of anaesthesia based on lipid solubility were incorrect.

More recently, Metcalfe and Richards [166] determined the potency of benzyl alcohol and butanol as nerve blocking agents at different temperatures. They showed that cooling a nerve by 10–15 °C had little effect other than to decrease conduction velocity. The potency of butanol was little changed over this temperature range but that of benzyl alcohol markedly increased. Since they also showed that the partition coefficient for these alcohols between the aqueous phase and the membrane varied in the same direction and by a proportionate amount, the results could not simply be explained on a simple lipid solubility model [220] (e.g. fluidity, membrane thickness).

To conclude, the effects of temperature on anaesthetic potency are not consistent with the lipid solubility of anaesthetic action. Anaesthetic potency does not always correlate with lipid solubility.

Membrane Proteins as the Site of Anaesthetic Action

The effects of temperature on anaesthetic potency are not consistent with

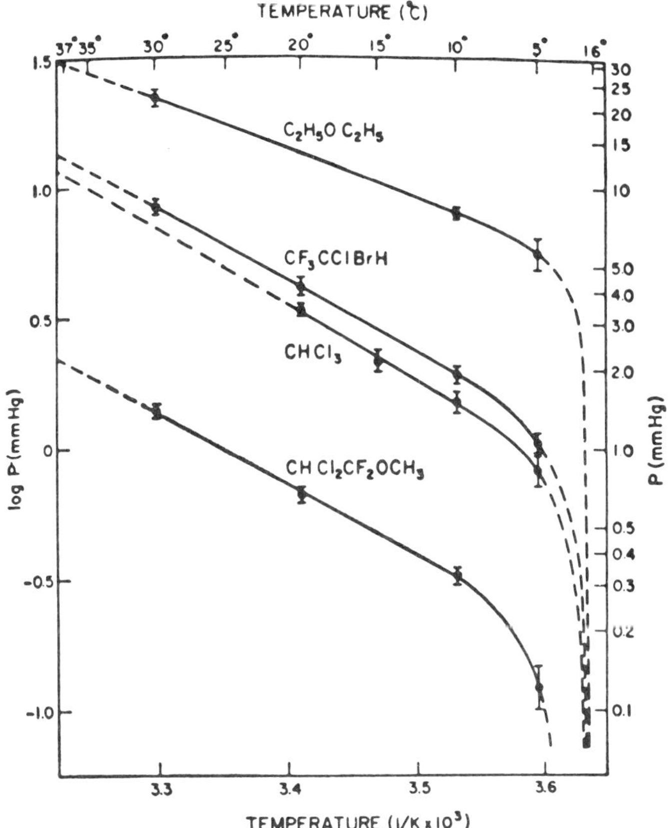

Fig. 1.28. The relationship between body temperature and the partial pressure of various volatile anaesthetics required to anaesthetize 50 per cent of a sample of goldfish. Each point represents 50–190 fish; the vertical bars indicate the 95 per cent confidence limits. (*From Cherkin and Catchpool [42]*.)

the idea that the primary site of anaesthetic action is membrane lipid. However, the strong correlation between anaesthetic potency and solubility in olive oil suggests that the site of action has a hydrophobic nature. Since anaesthetics have little effect on the function of cytoplasmic proteins, the remaining possibility is that anaesthetics work by direct perturbation of membrane proteins. Various other pieces of evidence are consistent with this idea.

First, the simple solubility models predict that optical isomers of anaesthetics (which differ in shape but not in chemical constitution) should have identical anaesthetic properties. Although this is true for the isomers of halothane [132], it is not true for other optically active anaesthetics [35, 285]. Thus the optical isomers of hexobarbitone have a twofold difference in anaesthetic potency for equal brain levels. Certain amine local anaesthetics (RAC 109) show a two- to eightfold difference in potency on different nerves [3]. Steroid anaesthetics show intricate structure–activity relations and in a few instances there is an absolute requirement for one optical isomer rather than another [197]. Thus while alphaxalone is a powerful anaesthetic, its 3β-hydroxy epimer is non-anaesthetic. Though the observed stereoselectivity of anaesthetics is low when compared to enzyme substrate reactions, it nevertheless suggests that there are specific binding sites for the large anaesthetic molecules.

Second, there is evidence that the effectiveness of an anaesthetic in perturbing function can be increased by stimulation. Thus increasing the rate of stimulation of a nerve deepens the nerve block produced by a range of amine local anaesthetics [57, 112]. Similarly, Adams [2] has found that barbiturates bind preferentially to the active form of the nicotinic receptor. These results suggest that certain anaesthetics bind preferentially to particular conformations of functional proteins.

Third, there is evidence that positively charged local anaesthetics which cannot cross the nerve membrane (e.g. quaternary derivatives of lidocaine (lignocaine)) will only block nerve conduction when they are applied directly to the inside of the nerve [85, 266]. As there is no evidence that the inner face of the membrane possesses lipids with special properties, the simplest explanation is that there is a binding site on the proteins of the sodium conductance mechanism that is accessible only from the inner face of the membrane. This is consistent with the finding that the degree of inhibition of the sodium conductance of a nerve during voltage-clamp experiments depends upon the size of the voltage step applied [266].

Fourth, if anaesthetics produced a change in the properties of the membrane lipids that was indirectly sensed by the membrane proteins, we might reasonably expect that a given receptor would show the same functional changes whatever anaesthetic was applied. It is apparent from the previous section (p. 38) that this is not so. For example, the effects of volatile anaesthetics on the Ach muscarinic receptor are qualitatively different to those of alphaxalone [252]. Similarly, short- and long-chain alkanols (C2 and C8) which have similar effects on membrane fluidity have different effects on the neuromuscular nicotinic Ach receptor [92]. These differential effects may be resolved by assuming that the anaesthetics bind directly to the receptors at different sites.

Both Miller and Pang [170] and Lee [154] have faced the problem of differential effects of anaesthetics on specific functions. They have proposed that the local composition of the membrane lipid will determine the effect of an anaesthetic. Miller and Pang have even produced some evidence that, for example, the fluidizing action of pentobarbitone and alphaxalone depends upon the cholesterol content of the membrane. However, such postulates are of little value in the absence of detailed information about the local composition of membrane lipid in nerve membranes. The available evidence suggests that lipid molecules diffuse laterally across the surface of bilayer at a high rate although exchange of lipid between the two surfaces of the bilayer is slow [155, 162]. Furthermore, such an *ad hoc* explanation cannot reconcile all the anomalies of the lipid models (the effects of temperature on anaesthetic potency, the stereospecific binding of certain anaesthetics, the use-dependent inhibition, and differential anaesthetic effects on identical receptors).

Is There a Specific Site of Anaesthetic Action?

Underlying much of the previous discussion has been the idea that there is a specific lesion induced by all anaesthetics, irrespective of their type, that is responsible for anaesthesia. It is surely evident from the physiological experiments that this idea is improbable. However, one could regard the fact that different anaesthetics perturb synaptic transmission by different mechanisms as interesting effects which may be related to anaesthesia but which are not responsible for it. Can this argument be refuted? If not, the concept of a unitary hypothesis may still be valid.

There are four possible models of anaesthetic action:

1. All anaesthetics cause a specific neuronal lesion by the same molecular mechanism.
2. All anaesthetics cause a number of neuronal lesions as the result of a common action on some cellular constituent.
3. All anaesthetics cause a common neuronal lesion by different molecular mechanisms.
4. Anaesthetics cause a number of neuronal lesions by various mechanisms.

Of these four only the first two are in any strict sense unitary hypotheses. Clearly, the first hypothesis is wrong as we have already established that anaesthetics cause a variety of neuronal lesions. The second hypothesis is plausible as it does not specify that one lesion is produced, nor does it necessarily imply that all the lesions that are produced are related to anaesthesia. The third case is clearly a multisite model, i.e. it is not a unitary hypothesis; this is obvious if we consider the mechanisms of local anaesthesia. In this case we define anaesthesia in terms of a specific neuronal lesion, block of nerve impulse conduction, but in so doing we do not assume a common mode of action for all anaesthetics. The final case represents the most extreme example of a multisite model.

Implicit in a unitary hypothesis of anaesthetic action is the assumption that all anaesthetics act in an identical way. Thus all anaesthetics should affect the nervous system by the same series of perturbations which will depend not on the precise chemical constitution of individual anaesthetics but on the concentration they achieve at their actual site of action, i.e. the effect will depend only on the number of anaesthetic molecules in equilibrium with the site of action and not on their type. Such a model predicts that the potency of mixtures of anaesthetics should be directly proportional to the amount of each constituent in the mixture. Thus in a binary mixture the effects of two agents should be strictly additive [254]. Consider the action of two anaesthetics A and B. Let us assume that the concentration of each agent required to reach a given depth of anaesthesia (say loss of righting reflex) is a and b for the two anaesthetics. Then the criteria of additivity require that mixtures of $0{\cdot}5a + 0{\cdot}5b$ or $0{\cdot}25a + 0{\cdot}75b$

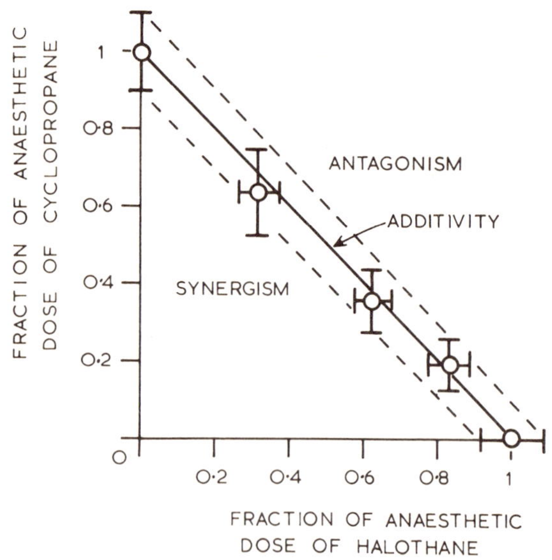

Fig. 1.29. The anaesthetic potency of mixtures of cyclopropane and halothane. The full anaesthetic dose of either anaesthetic was defined as the concentration required to abolish the motor response of rats to a painful stimulus. The same end-point was used to determine the anaesthetic potencies of the mixtures – the concentration of one anaesthetic was held constant at a fraction of its full dose while the other was steadily raised until no motor response could be seen in response to the standard stimulus. The concentration of the second agent was then expressed as a fraction of its full dose. (*From Difazio et al. [69].*)

or $0{\cdot}75a + 0{\cdot}25b$ should produce the same depth of anaesthesia as either agent alone at their full dose. If the effect of the mixtures is greater or less than that of either agent alone at their full dose the unitary hypothesis fails. This is a severe test which should apply for each anaesthetic end-point and for any combination of anaesthetics. Several mixtures of gaseous anaesthetics have been subjected to this test and in general the results support the unitary hypothesis, i.e. the effects are additive [61, 69, 174] (*Fig. 1.29*). However, slight deviations were observed with mixtures of cyclopropane and nitrous oxide and with mixtures of cyclopropane and ethylene. Furthermore, while mixtures of steroid anaesthetics (alphaxalone and alphadalone acetate) had strictly additive effects, mixtures of alphaxalone and methohexitone showed a powerful synergism [17] (*Fig. 1.30*). Thus, the general hypothesis that all anaesthetics work by the

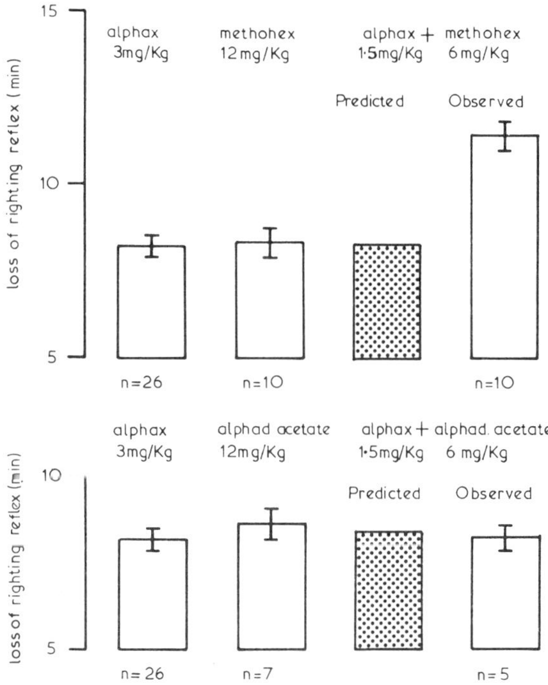

Fig. 1.30. Additive and non-additive effects of mixtures of intravenous anaesthetics. The height of each column represents the duration of the loss of righting reflex of rats (mean ± s.e.m.) that is produced by the intravenous administration of the dose of anaesthetic or combination of anaesthetics shown at the head of each column. The stippled columns indicate the values predicted by the simple membrane occupation theories of anaesthesia. (*From Archer et al. [17].*)

same molecular mechanism cannot be sustained. It is worth noting that additivity of action does not prove identity of action, it is merely consistent with that hypothesis.

A Degenerate Protein Perturbation Hypothesis

The previous discussion has shown that there is no obvious correlation between the potency of anaesthetic agents and their ability to perturb the physical properties of lipid bilayers. We are, therefore, forced to conclude that anaesthetics do not modify the function of membrane proteins indirectly via perturbations of the lipid bilayer but directly by specific interactions between the anaesthetic molecules and the functional membrane proteins themselves. Such a conclusion does not imply that all anaesthetics bind to a single site on one or more of the functional proteins. Indeed, this is very improbable as the previous paragraphs show. It is far more likely that different anaesthetics bind to various sites on the proteins which have the appropriate size and shape. Direct evidence for this postulate comes from work on the binding of xenon and halothane to haemoglobin where it has been shown by X-ray and NMR methods that these molecules bind to hydrophobic clefts of appropriate dimensions within the structure of the protein [32, 242]. The activity-dependent inhibition of the sodium conductance of nerve by amine anaesthetics is further indirect evidence in favour of this idea. Clearly, to affect the function of a protein, the binding must result either in a conformational change that impairs normal activity or in a restriction of the normal conformational changes associated with activity.

Large and complex molecules such as the barbiturates and steroids, which have some specific structural requirements for their anaesthetic activity, will bind to a set of sites having characteristics different from those binding the smaller anaesthetics. There is evidence of synergistic actions between the anaesthetic actions of barbiturates and steroids which suggests cooperative binding to specific sites [17]. This synergism has also been shown for the depressant actions of these anaesthetics on synaptic transmission. Furthermore, there is also evidence of antagonism between the depressant actions of structurally similar anaesthetics on synaptic transmission [219], which also suggests that the steroids bind to specific sites on membrane proteins. Finally, molecules that possess structural features similar to those of the phospholipids (e.g. long-chain alkanols) may compete for the hydrophobic areas of membrane proteins which normally interact with the hydrocarbon chains of the membrane phospholipids. This competition would result in displacement of the annular lipids with a consequent disruption of the normal lipid–protein interactions that are required for the maintenance of function. This appears to be the mechanism whereby dodecanol inhibits the function of the sarcoplasmic reticulum calcium transport protein. In summary, this hypothesis proposes that anaesthetic action is, therefore, highly degenerate at the molecular level and has been called the degenerate perturbation hypothesis of anaesthetic action [217, 220].

While the critical volume hypothesis is not compatible with the hypothesis expounded in the previous paragraphs, there are some common features. The critical volume hypothesis predicts that pressure should reverse the effects of anaesthetics by opposing the volume change caused by anaesthetics and, as we have seen, this is a general feature of anaesthetic action [103, 173]. The degenerate perturbation hypothesis predicts conformational changes in membrane proteins and it is to be expected that these changes would be accompanied by changes in the volume of proteins. If anaesthetics bind directly to the proteins and do not displace some bound component essential to function, the binding of anaesthetics will be accompanied by an increase in volume. The difference between the hypotheses is that unlike the critical volume hypothesis, the degenerate perturbation hypothesis regards these volume changes as secondary and it can accommodate situations in which increased pressure fails to reverse anaesthesia (no volume change) or actually enhances it (e.g. the pressure enhancement of the nerve blocking action of TEMPO [25]). Different anaesthetics require different pressures to reverse their effects, a fact readily accommodated by the degenerate perturbation hypothesis, but not easily reconciled with the critical volume hypothesis, as it implies that different anaesthetics produce different volume changes or act at sites which have different compressibilities or both.

Much has been made of the lack of correlation between anaesthetic potency and lipid solubility as temperature is varied, but how can the degenerate perturbation hypothesis accommodate these results? If the model is correct then temperature will have two effects that will determine the equilibrium between the anaesthetic dissolved in the membrane lipid and that bound to the membrane proteins. First, there is the equilibrium between the aqueous phase and the membrane lipid. Second, there is an equilibrium between the anaesthetic in the membrane lipid and that bound to the membrane protein. The effect of temperature on these equilibria will depend on the sign and magnitude of the energy changes that occur. In general, the binding of anaesthetics to lipid is an endothermic reaction (it requires energy) so that as the temperature is lowered, less anaesthetic is bound. However, the binding between an anaesthetic and a membrane protein will vary according to the nature of the anaesthetic and its binding site. If the reaction is endothermic then the pattern will follow that of the lipid solubility; if it is exothermic then, as temperature decreases, the equilibrium will be shifted in favour of the bound state and potency will tend to increase. Thus the final relationship between anaesthetic potency and temperature will depend on the balance between these two processes and a general prediction is impossible. However, anaesthetics whose potency decreases with temperature can be as readily assimilated into this model as those with the reverse behaviour.

SYNTHESIS

Anaesthetics act by virtue of modifications they cause in the function of membrane proteins. The changes in function occur as a result of direct, reversible, non-covalent binding of anaesthetic molecules to specific sites on membrane proteins and not as a result of their binding to membrane lipid. Anaesthetics of different chemical constitution bind to sites of appropriate size, shape and chemical characteristics. As the membrane proteins are embedded in a lipid matrix, access to the binding sites on the proteins requires a degree of lipid solubility; furthermore most of the binding sites appear to be hydrophobic in nature. Once bound, anaesthetics modify the properties of neural mechanisms such as transmitter release, the binding of released transmitter to the receptor and nerve impulse conduction. For any given anaesthetic some combination of these effects leads to impaired synaptic transmission and so disturbs the normal processing of sensory information and its appreciation by the higher centres of the brain. There is no good evidence that anaesthetics specifically affect one region of the brain rather than another. However, as the cerebral cortex appears to be the site of conscious experience, a direct effect of anaesthetics on cortical activity would appear to be one major factor in producing unconsciousness.

REFERENCES

1. Abrahamian H. A., Allison T., Goff W. R. et al. (1963) Effect of thiopental on human cerebral evoked responses. *Anesthesiology* **24**, 650–657.
2. Adams P. R. (1976) Drug blockade of open end plate channels. *J. Physiol. (Lond.)* **260**, 531–552.
3. Åkerman S. B. A., Camougis G. and Sandberg R. V. (1969) Stereoisomerism and differential activity in excitation block by local anaesthetics. *Eur. J. Pharmacol.* **8**, 337–347.
4. Albaum H. G., Tepperman J. and Bodansky O. (1946) The *in vivo* inactivation by cyanide of brain cytochrome oxidase and its effects on glycolysis and on the high energy phosphate compounds in brain. *J. Biol. Chem.* **164**, 45–51.
5. Alexander S. C., Colton E. T., Smith A. L. et al. (1970) The effects of cyclopropane on cerebral and systemic carbohydrate metabolism. *Anesthesiology* **32**, 236–245.
6. Andersen P., Eccles J. C. and Løyning Y. (1963) Recurrent inhibition in the hippocampus with identification of the inhibitory cell and its synapses. *Nature (Lond.)* **198**, 540–542.
7. Andersen P., Eccles J. C. and Løyning Y. (1964) Pathway of post-synaptic inhibition in the hippocampus. *J. Neurophysiol.* **27**, 608–619.
8. Anderson C. R. and Stevens C. F. (1973) Voltage clamp analysis of acetylcholine produced end plate current fluctuations at frog neuromuscular junction. *J. Physiol. (Lond.)* **235**, 655–691.
9. Andersson S. A., Norrsell K. and Norrsell V. (1972) Spinal pathways projecting to the cerebral first somatosensory area in the monkey. *J. Physiol. (Lond.)* **225**, 589–579.
10. Angel A. (1963) Evidence for cortical inhibition of transmission at the thalamic sensory relay nucleus in the rat. *J. Physiol. (Lond.)* **169**, 108–109P.
11. Angel A. (1977) Processing of sensory information. *Prog. Neurobiol.* 9, 1–122.
12. Angel A. (1977) Modulation of information transmission in the dorsal column–lemniscothalamic pathway by anaesthetic agents. In: Hulsz E. et al. (ed.), *Anesthesiology.* Amsterdam and Oxford, Excerpta-Medica, pp. 82–89.
13. Angel A., Berridge D. A. and Unwin J. (1973) The effect of anaesthetic agents on primary cortical evoked responses. *Br. J. Anaesth.* **45**, 825–836.
14. Angel A. and Clarke K. A. (1975) An analysis of the representation of the forelimb in the ventrobasal thalamic complex of the albino rat. *J. Physiol. (Lond.)* **249**, 399–423.

15. Angel A. and Dawson G. D. (1963) The facilitation of thalamic and cortical responses in the dorsal column pathway by strong peripheral stimulation. *J. Physiol. (Lond.)* **166**, 587–604.
16. Angel A. and Unwin J. (1970) Effect of urethane on transmission along dorsal column sensory pathway in rat. *J. Physiol. (Lond.)* **208**, 32–33P.
17. Archer E. R., Richards C. D. and White A. E. (1977) Non-additive anaesthetic effects of alphaxalone and methohexitone. *Br. J. Pharmacol.* **59**, 508P.
18. Arduini A. and Arduini M. G. (1954) Effect of drugs and metabolic alterations on brain stem arousal mechanism. *J. Pharmacol. Exp. Ther.* **110**, 76–85.
19. Ashcroft R. G., Coster H. G. L. and Smith J. R. (1977) Local anaesthetic benzyl alcohol increases membrane thickness. *Nature (Lond.)* **269**, 819–820.
20. Ashcroft R. G., Coster H. G. L. and Smith J. R. (1977) The molecular organisation of bimolecular lipid membranes: the effect of benzyl alcohol on the structure. *Biochim. Biophys. Acta* **469**, 13–22.
21. Barker J. L. and Ransom B. R. (1978) Pentobarbitone pharmacology of mammalian central neurones grown in tissue culture. *J. Physiol. (Lond.)* **280**, 355–372.
22. Biebuyck J. F., Dedrick D. F. and Scherer Y. (1975) Brain cyclic AMP and putative transmitter amino acids during anesthesia. In: Fink B. R. (ed.), *Molecular Mechanisms of Anesthesia. Progress in Anesthesiology*, vol. 1. New York, Raven Press, pp. 451–470.
23. Biscoe T. J. and Krnjević K. (1963) Chloralose and the activity of Renshaw cells. *Exp. Neurol.* **8**, 395–405.
24. Blaustein M. P. and Ector A. C. (1975) Barbiturate inhibition of calcium uptake by depolarised nerve terminals *in vitro*. *Mol. Pharmacol.* **11**, 369–378.
25. Boggs J. M., Roth S. H., Yoong T. et al. (1976) Site and mechanism of anesthetic action. II. Pressure effect on the nerve conduction-blocking activity of a spin label anesthetic. *Mol. Pharmacol.* **12**, 136–143.
26. Boggs J. M., Yoong T. and Hsia J. C. (1976) Site and mechanism of anesthetic action. I. Effect of anesthetics and pressure on fluidity of spin-labelled lipid vesicles. *Mol. Pharmacol.* **12**, 127–135.
27. Bradford H. F. and Richards C. D. (1976) Specific release of endogenous glutamate from piriform cortex stimulated *in vitro*. *Brain Res.* **105**, 168–172.
28. Bremer F. (1954) The neurophysiological problem of sleep. In: Delafresnaye J. F. (ed.), *Brain Mechanisms and Consciousness*. Oxford, Blackwell, pp. 163–199.
29. Brink F. and Posternak J. M. (1948) Thermodynamic analysis of the relative effectiveness of narcotics. *J. Cell. Comp. Physiol.* **32**, 211–233.
30. Brown A. G., House C. R. and Hume R. B. (1975) Physiology and morphology of identified spinal cord neurones. *J. Physiol. (Lond.)* **244**, 10–12P.
31. Brown A. G. and Short A. D. (1974) Effects from the somatic sensory cortex on transmission through the spino-cervical tract. *Brain Res.* **74**, 338–341.
32. Brown F. F., Halsey M. J. and Richards R. E. (1976) Halothane interactions with haemoglobin. *Proc. R. Soc. Lond. [Biol.]* **193**, 387–411.
33. Brown M. F. and Seelig J. (1978) Influence of cholesterol on the polar region of phosphatidylcholine and phosphatidylethanolamine bilayers. *Biochemistry* **17**, 381–384.
34. Bryan R. N., Coulter J. D. and Willis W. D. (1973) Location and somatotopic organisation of the cells of origin of the spino-cervical tract in the monkey. *Exp. Neurol.* **42**, 574–586.
35. Büch H., Knabe J., Buzello W. et al. (1970) Stereospecificity of anesthetic activity, distribution, inactivation and protein binding of the optical antipodes of two N-methylated barbiturates. *J. Pharmacol. Exp. Ther.* **175**, 709–716.

36. Burns B. D. (1951) Some properties of isolated cerebral cortex in the unanaesthetised cat. *J. Physiol. (Lond.)* **112,** 156–175.
37. Cairns H. (1952) Disturbances of consciousness with lesions of the brain stem and diencephalon. *Brain* **75,** 109–146.
38. Cassano G. B., Chetti B., Gliozzi E. et al. (1967) Autoradiographic distribution study of short acting and long acting barbiturates: ^{35}S thiopentone and ^{14}C phenobarbitone. *Br. J. Anaesth.* **39,** 11–20.
39. Catchlove R. F. H., Krnjević K. and Maretić H. (1972) Similarity between effects of general anaesthetics and dinitrophenol on cortical neurones. *Can. J. Physiol. Pharmacol.* **50,** 1111–1114.
40. Chance B. and Hollunger G. (1963) Inhibition of electron and energy transfer in mitochondria. *J. Biol. Chem.* **238,** 418–431.
41. Chapman D. (1975) Phase transitions and fluidity characteristics of lipids and cell membranes. *Q. Rev. Biophys.* **8,** 185–235.
42. Cherkin A. and Catchpool J. F. (1964) Temperature dependence of anaesthesia in goldfish. *Science* **144,** 1460–1462.
43. Christ D. (1977) Effects of halothane on ganglionic discharges. *J. Pharmacol. Exp. Ther.* **200,** 336–342.
44. Christensen B. N. and Perl E. R. (1970) Spinal neurons specifically excited by noxious or thermal stimuli: marginal zone of the dorsal horn. *J. Neurophysiol.* **33,** 293–307.
45. Clark D., Hughes J. and Gasser H. S. (1935) Afferent function in the group of nerve fibres of slowest conduction velocity. *Am. J. Physiol.* **114,** 69–76.
46. Clark D. L., Butler R. A. and Rosner B. S. (1969) Dissociation of sensation and evoked responses by a general anesthetic in man. *J. Comp. Physiol. Psychol.* **68,** 315–319.
47. Clark D. L., Hosick E. and Rosner B. (1971) Neurophysiological effects of different anaesthetics in unconscious man. *J. Appl. Physiol.* **31,** 884–891.
48. Clark D. L. and Rosner B. S. (1973) Neurophysiologic effects of general anaesthetics. I. The electroencephalogram and sensory evoked responses in man. *Anesthesiology* **38,** 564–582.
49. Clark W. E. Le Gros (1936) The termination of ascending tracts in the thalamus of the Macaque monkey. *J. Anat. (Lond.)* **71,** 7–40.
50. Cobb S. (1948) *Foundations of Neuropsychiatry.* Baltimore, Williams & Wilkins, p. 89.
51. Cohen E. N., Chow K. L. and Mathers L. (1972) Autoradiographic distribution of volatile anesthetics within the brain. *Anesthesiology* **37,** 324–331.
52. Cohen E. N. and Hood N. (1969) Application of low-temperature autoradiography to studies of the uptake and metabolism of volatile anesthetics in the mouse. III. Halothane. *Anesthesiology* **31,** 553–559.
53. Cohen P. J. (1973) Effect of anesthetics on mitochondrial function. *Anesthesiology* **39,** 153–164.
54. Colley C. M. and Metcalfe J. C. (1972) The localisation of small molecules in lipid bilayers. *FEBS Lett.* **24,** 241–246.
55. Connor P., Mangat B. S. and Rao L. S. (1974) The labilization of lecithin liposomes by steroidal anaesthetics: a correlation with anaesthetic activity. *J. Pharm. Pharmacol.* **26,** 120P.
56. Conseiller C., Benoist J. M., Hamann K. F. et al. (1972) Effects of ketamine (CL 581) on cell responses to cutaneous stimulations in laminae IV and V in the cat's dorsal horn. *Eur. J. Pharmacol.* **18,** 346–352.
57. Courtney K. R., Kendig J. J. and Cohen E. N. (1978) Frequency-dependent conduction block: the role of nerve impulse pattern in local anesthetic potency. *Anesthesiology* **48,** 111–117.
58. Crawford J. M. (1970) Anesthetic agents and the chemical sensitivity of cortical neurones. *Neuropharmacology* **9,** 31–46.

59. Crawford J. M. and Curtis D. R. (1966) Pharmacological studies on feline Betz cells. *J. Physiol. (Lond.)* **186**, 121–138.
60. Crossland J. and Merrick A. J. (1954) The effect of anaesthesia on the acetylcholine content of brain. *J. Physiol. (Lond.)* **125**, 56–66.
61. Cullen S. C., Eger E. I., Cullen B. F. et al. (1969) Observations on the anesthetic effect of the combination of xenon and halothane. *Anesthesiology* **31**, 305–309.
62. Cutler R. W. P., Markowitz D. and Dudzinski D. S. (1974) The effect of barbiturates on (^{3}H) GABA transport in rat cerebral cortex slices. *Brain Res.* **81**, 189–197.
63. Davis H. S., Collins W. F., Randt C. T. et al. (1957) Effect of anesthetic agents on evoked central nervous system responses: gaseous agents. *Anesthesiology* **18**, 634–642.
64. Davis H. S., Quitmayer V. E. and Collins W. F. (1961) The effect of halothane (Fluothane) on the thalamus and midbrain reticular formation. *Anaesthesia* **16**, 32–49.
65. Dawson G. D. (1958) The central control of sensory inflow. *Proc. R. Soc. Med.* **51**, 531–535.
66. Dawson G. D., Podachin V. P. and Schatz S. W. (1963) Facilitation of cortical responses by competing stimuli. *J. Physiol. (Lond.)* **166**, 363–381.
67. Dedrick D. F., Scherer Y. D. and Biebuyck J. F. (1975) Use of a rapid brain-sampling technique in a physiologic preparation – effects of morphine, ketamine and halothane on tissue energy intermediates. *Anesthesiology* **42**, 651–657.
68. Dempsey E. W. and Morrison R. S. (1942) The production of rhythmically recurrent cortical potentials after localised thalamic stimulation. *Am. J. Physiol.* **135**, 293–300.
69. Difazio C. A., Brown R. E., Ball C. G. et al. (1972) Additive effects of anesthetics and theories of anesthesia. *Anesthesiology* **36**, 57–63.
70. Domino E. F. (1967) Effects of preanesthetic and anesthetic drugs on visually evoked responses. *Anesthesiology* **28**, 184–191.
71. Domino E. F. and Corssen G. (1964) Visually evoked response of man with and without induced muscle paralysis. *Ann. N.Y. Acad. Sci.* **112**, 226–237.
72. Domino E. F., Corssen G. and Sweet R. B. (1963) Effects of various general anesthetics on the visually evoked response in man. *Anesth. Analg. (Cleve.)* **42**, 735–747.
73. Eccles J. C. (1964) *The Physiology of Synapses.* Berlin, Springer.
74. Eccles J. C., Eccles R. M., Iggo A. et al. (1961) Electrophysiological investigations of Renshaw cells. *J. Physiol. (Lond.)* **159**, 461–478.
75. Eccles J. C., Schmidt R. F. and Willis W. D. (1963) Pharmacological studies on presynaptic inhibition. *J. Physiol. (Lond.)* **168**, 500–530.
76. Evans E. F. and Nelson P. G. (1973) The responses of single neurones in the cochlear nucleus of the cat as a function of their location and their anesthetic state. *Exp. Brain Res.* **17**, 402–427.
77. Feldberg W. (1959) A physiological approach to the problem of general anaesthesia and loss of consciousness. *Br. Med. J.* **2**, 771–782.
78. Feldman S. M. and Waller H. J. (1962) Dissociation of electrocortical activation and behavioural arousal. *Nature (Lond.)* **196**, 1320–1322.
79. Frank G. B. and Ohta M. (1971) Blockade of the reticulospinal inhibitory pathway by anaesthetic agents. *Br. J. Pharmacol.* **42**, 328–342.
80. Frank G. B. and Ohta M. (1972) Blockade of the reticulospinal inhibitory pathway by nitrous oxide and tetrodotoxin. *Br. J. Pharmacol.* **46**, 23–31.
81. Frank G. B. and Sanders H. D. (1963) A proposed common mechanism of action for general and local anaesthetics in the central nervous system. *Br. J. Pharmacol. Chemother.* **21**, 1–9.

82. Frank K. and Fuortes M. G. F. (1957) Presynaptic and postsynaptic inhibition of monosynaptic reflexes. *Fed. Proc.* **16**, 39–40.
83. Franks N. P. and Leib W. R. (1978) Where do general anaesthetics act? *Nature (Lond.)* **274**, 339–342.
84. Frazier D. T., Murayama K., Abbott N. J. et al. (1971) Effects of morphine on internally perfused squid giant axons. *Fed. Proc.* **30**, 205.
85. Frazier D. T., Narahashi T. and Yamada M. (1970) The site of action and active form of local anesthetics. II. Experiments with quaternary compounds. *J. Pharmacol. Exp. Ther.* **171**, 45–51.
86. French J. D., Amerongen F. K. V. and Magoun H. W. (1952) An activating system in brain stem of monkey. *Arch. Neurol. Psychiat. (Chic.)* **68**, 577–590.
87. French J. D., Hernandez-Peón R. and Livingston R. B. (1955) Projections from cortex to cephalic brain stem (reticular formation) in the monkey. *J. Neurophysiol.* **18**, 74–95.
88. French J. D., Verzeano M. and Magoun H. W. (1953) An extralemniscal sensory system in the brain. *Arch. Neurol. Psychiat. (Chic.)* **69**, 505–518.
89. French J. D., Verzeano M. and Magoun H. W. (1953) A neural basis of the anesthetic state. *Arch. Neurol. Psychiat. (Chic.)* **69**, 519–529.
90. Funderburk W. H. and Case T. J. (1951) The effect of atropine on cortical potentials. *Electroencephalogr. Clin. Neurophysiol.* **3**, 213–223.
91. Gage P. W. and Hamill O. P. (1976) Effects of several inhalation anaesthetics on the kinetics of postsynaptic conductance changes in mouse diaphragm. *Br. J. Pharmacol.* **57**, 263–272.
92. Gage P. W., McBurney R. N. and Schneider G. T. (1975) Effects of some aliphatic alcohols on the conductance change caused by a quantum of acetylcholine at the toad end plate. *J. Physiol. (Lond.)* **244**, 409–429.
93. Galindo A. (1969) Effects of procaine, pentobarbital and halothane on synaptic transmission in the central nervous system. *J. Pharmacol. Exp. Ther.* **169**, 185–195.
94. Gasser H. S. and Erlanger J. (1929) The role of fiber size in the establishment of a nerve block by pressure or cocaine. *Am. J. Physiol.* **88**, 581–591.
95. Godfraind J.-M., Kawamura H., Krnjević K. et al. (1971) Actions of dinitrophenol and some other metabolic inhibitors on cortical neurones. *J. Physiol. (Lond.)* **215**, 199–222.
96. Goldberg N. D., Passoneau J. V. and Lowry O. H. (1966) Effects of changes in brain metabolism on the levels of citric acid cycle intermediates. *J. Biol. Chem.* **241**, 3997–4003.
97. Gordon G. and Jukes M. G. M. (1962) Correlation of different excitatory and inhibitory influences on cells in the nucleus gracilis of the cat. *Nature (Lond.)* **196**, 1183–1185.
98. Gordon G. and Paine C. H. (1960) Functional organisation in nucleus gracilis of the cat. *J. Physiol. (Lond.)* **153**, 331–349.
99. Gordon G. S., Guadagni N., Picci J. et al. (1955) Anesthesie steroidienne chez l'homme: effects cliniques et cerebrometaboliques. *Press. Med.* **63**, 1483–1484.
100. Gray J. A. B. (1966) The representation of information about rapid changes in a population of receptor units signalling mechanical events. In: De Rueck A. V. S. and Knight J. (ed.), *Touch, Heat and Pain.* London, Churchill, pp. 209–315.
101. Hall G. M., Kirtland S. J. and Baum H. (1973) The inhibition of mitochondrial respiration by inhalational anaesthetic agents. *Br. J. Anaesth.* **45**, 1005–1009.
102. Hall G. M., Kirtland S. J., Grist E. M. et al. (1973) Calcium-induced loss of respiratory control in rat liver mitochondria in the presence of inhalational anaesthetic agents. *Trans. Biochem. Soc.* **1**, 854–857.

103. Halsey M. J. and Wardley-Smith B. (1975) Pressure reversal of narcosis produced by anaesthetics, narcotics and tranquilizers. *Nature* (*Lond.*) **257**, 811–813.
104. Haycock J. W., Levy W. B. and Cotman C. W. (1977) Pentobarbital depression of stimulus-secretion coupling in brain-selective inhibition of depolarisation-induced calcium dependent release. *Biochem. Pharmacol.* **26**, 159–161.
105. Haydon D. A., Hendry B. M., Levinson S. R. et al. (1977) The molecular mechanisms of anaesthesia. *Nature* (*Lond.*) **268**, 356–358.
106. Haydon D. A., Hendry B. M., Levinson S. R. et al. (1977) Anaesthesia by the *n*-alkanes: a comparative study of nerve impulse blockage and the properties of black lipid bilayer membranes. *Biochim. Biophys. Acta* **470**, 17–34.
107. Heavner J. E. and de Jong R. H. (1974) Modulation of dorsal horn throughput by anesthetics. *Adv. Neurol.* **4**, 179–185.
108. Heinbecker P., Bishop G. H. and O'Leary J. (1933) Pain and touch fibres in peripheral nerves. *Arch. Neurol. Psychiat.* (*Chic.*) **29**, 771–789.
109. Hernandez-Péon R. and Hagbarth K. E. (1955) Interaction between afferent and cortically-induced reticular responses. *J. Neurophysiol.* **18**, 44–55.
110. Hesketh T. R., Smith R. A., Houslay M. D. et al. (1976) Annular lipids determine the ATPase activity of a calcium transport protein complexed with dipalmitoyl lecithin. *Biochemistry* **15**, 4145–4151.
111. Hill M. W. (1974) The effect of anaesthetic-like molecules on the phase transition in smetic mesophases of dipalmitoyl lecithin. I. The normal alcohols up to C = 9 and three inhalational anaesthetics. *Biochim. Biophys. Acta* **356**, 117–124.
112. Hille B., Courtney K. and Dum R. (1975) Rate and site of action of local anesthetics in myelinated nerve fibres. In: Fink B. R. (ed.), *Molecular Mechanisms of Anesthesia. Progress in Anesthesiology*, vol. 1. New York, Raven Press, pp. 13–20.
113. Himwich W. A., Homburger E., Meresca R. et al. (1947) Brain metabolism in man: unanesthetised and in pentobarbital narcosis. *Am. J. Psychiatry* **103**, 689–696.
114. Hosick E. C., Clark D. L., Adam N. et al. (1971) Neurophysiological effects of different anesthetics in conscious man. *J. Appl. Physiol.* **31**, 892–898.
115. Hubbell W. L., Metcalfe J. C., Metcalfe S. M. et al. (1970) The interaction of small molecules with spin-labelled erythrocyte membranes. *Biochim. Biophys. Acta* **219**, 415–427.
116. Hulands G. H., Beard D. J. and Brammall A. (1975) The *in vitro* interaction of inhalational anesthetics with glutamate dehydrogenase and other enzymes. In: Fink B. R. (ed.), *Molecular Mechanisms of Anesthesia. Progress in Anesthesiology*, vol. 1. New York, Raven Press, pp. 501–507.
117. Humphrey N. K. (1970) What the frog's eye tells the monkey's brain. *Brain Behav. Evol.* **3**, 324–337.
118. Iwama K. and Yamamoto C. (1961) Impulse transmission of thalamic somatosensory relay nuclei as modified by electrical stimulation of the cerebral cortex. *Jpn. J. Physiol.* **11**, 169–182.
119. Jain N. K. and Wu N. Y.-M. (1977) Effect of small molecules on the dipalmitoyl lecithin liposomal bilayer. III Phase transition in lipid bilayer. *J. Membr. Biol.* **34**, 157–201.
120. Jain N. K., Wu N. Y.-M and Wray L. V. (1975) Drug-induced phase change in bilayer as possible mode of action of membrane expanding drugs. *Nature* (*Lond.*) **255**, 494–495.
121. Jessel T. M. and Richards C. D. (1977) Barbiturate potentiation of hippocampal ipsps is not mediated by blockade of GABA uptake. *J. Physiol.* (*Lond.*) **269**, 42–44P.
122. Johnson F. H., Brown D. E. S. and Marsland D. A. (1942) Pressure reversal of the action of certain narcotics. *J. Cell. Comp. Physiol.* **20**, 269–276.

123. Johnson F. H. and Flager E. A. (1950) Hydrostatic pressure reversal of narcosis in tadpoles. *Science* **112,** 91–92.

124. Jones E. G. and Powell T. P. S. (1970) Connections of the somatic sensory cortex of the rhesus monkey. III Thalamic connections. *Brain* **93,** 37–56.

125. de Jong R. H., Freund F. G., Robles R. et al. (1968) Anesthetic potency determined by depression of synaptic transmission. *Anesthesiology* **29,** 1139–1144.

126. de Jong R. H. and Nace R. A. (1967) Nerve impulse conduction and cutaneous receptor responses during general anesthesia. *Anesthesiology* **28,** 851–855.

127. de Jong R. H., Robles R., Corbin R. W. et al. (1968) Effect of inhalation anesthetics on monosynaptic and polysynaptic transmission in the spinal cord. *J. Pharmacol. Exp. Ther.* **162,** 326–330.

128. de Jong R. H. and Wagman I. H. (1968) Block of afferent impulses in the dorsal horn of monkey. A possible mechanism of anesthesia. *Exp. Neurol.* **20,** 352–358.

129. Katz B. (1969) *The Release of Neural Transmitter Substances.* Liverpool, Liverpool University Press.

130. Katz B. and Miledi R. (1966) Input–output relation of a single synapse. *Nature* (*Lond.*) **212,** 1242–1245.

131. Katz B. and Miledi R. (1970) Membrane noise produced by acetylcholine. *Nature* (*Lond.*) **226,** 962–963.

132. Kendig J. J., Trudell J. R. and Cohen E. N. (1973) Halothane stereoisomers, lack of stereospecificity in two model systems. *Anesthesiology* **39,** 518–524.

133. King E. E. (1956) Differential action of anesthetics and interneuron depressants upon E.E.G. arousal and recruitment responses. *J. Pharmacol. Exp. Ther.* **116,** 404–417.

134. King E. E., Naquet R. and Magoun H. W. (1957) Alterations in somatic afferent transmission through thalamus by central mechanisms and barbiturates. *J. Pharmacol. Exp. Ther.* **119,** 48–63.

135. Kitahata L. M. (1968) Effects of halothane on neuronal tissue – neurophysiological aspects. *Clin. Anesth.* **6,** 62–78.

136. Kitahata L. M., Ghazi-Saidi K., Yamashita M. et al. (1975) The depressant effect of halothane and sodium thiopental on spontaneous and evoked activity of dorsal horn cells: lamina specificity, time course and dose dependence. *J. Pharmacol. Exp. Ther.* **195,** 515–521.

137. Kitahata L. M., Taub A. and Kosaka Y. (1973) Lamina-specific suppression of dorsal horn unit activity by ketamine hydrochloride. *Anesthesiology* **38,** 4–11.

138. Krnjević K. (1974) Chemical nature of synaptic transmission in vertebrates. *Physiol. Rev.* **54,** 418–540.

139. Krnjević K. (1974) Central actions of general anaesthetics. In: Halsey M. J., Millar R. A. and Sutton J. A. (ed.), *Molecular Mechanisms in General Anaesthesia,* ch. 5. London, Churchill Livingstone, pp. 65–89.

140. Krnjević K. and Morris M. E. (1976) Input–output relation of transmission through cuneate nucleus. *J. Physiol.* (*Lond.*) **257,** 791–815.

141. Krnjević K., Pumain R. and Renaud L. (1971) The mechanism of excitation by acetylcholine in the cerebral cortex. *J. Physiol.* (*Lond.*) **215,** 247–268.

142. Kuffler S. W. and Nicholls J. G. (1976) *From Neuron to Brain.* Sunderland, Mass., USA, Sinauer Associates.

143. Laasberg L. H. and Hedley-White J. (1971) Optical rotary dispersion of hemoglobin and polypeptides: effect of halothane. *J. Biol. Chem.* **246,** 4886–4893.

144. Ladbrooke B. D., Williams R. M. and Chapman D. (1968) Studies on lecithin–cholesterol–water interaction by DSC and X-ray diffraction. *Biochim. Biophys. Acta* **150,** 333–340.

145. Landau W. M., Freygang W. H., Rowland L. P. et al. (1955) The local circulation of the living brain, values in the unanesthetised and anesthetised cat. *Trans. Am Neurol. Assoc.* **80,** 125–129.
146. Landgren S., Nordwall A. and Wengstrom C. (1965) The location of the thalamic relay in the spino-cervical lemniscal path. *Acta Physiol. Scand.* **65,** 164–175.
147. Larrabee M. G., Garcia-Ramos J. and Bülbring E. (1952) Effects of anesthetics on oxygen consumption and on synaptic transmission in sympathetic ganglia. *J. Cell. Comp. Physiol.* **40,** 461–495.
148. Larrabee M. G. and Posternak J. M. (1952) Selective action of anesthetics on synapses and axons in mammalian sympathetic ganglia. *J. Neurophysiol.* **15,** 91–114.
149. Larson M. D. and Major M. A. (1970) The effect of hexobarbital on the duration of the recurrent IPSP in cat motoneurones. *Brain Res.* **21,** 309–311.
150. Lawrence D. K. and Gill E. W. (1975) Structurally specific effects of some steroid anesthetics on spin-labelled liposomes. *Mol. Pharmacol.* **11,** 280–286.
151. Lawrence D. K. and Gill E. W. (1975) The effects of Δ' tetrahydrocannabinol and other cannabinoids on spin-labelled liposomes and their relationship to mechanisms of general anesthesia. *Mol. Pharmacol.* **11,** 595–602.
152. Lee A. G. (1976) Model for action of local anaesthetics. *Nature* (*Lond.*) **262,** 545–548.
153. Lee A. G. (1976) Interactions between phospholipids and barbiturates. *Biochim. Biophys. Acta* **455,** 102–108.
154. Lee A. G. (1977) Local anesthesia: the interaction between phospholipids and chlorpromazine, propanol and practalol. *Mol. Pharmacol.* **13,** 474–487.
155. Lee A. G., Birdsall N. J. M. and Metcalfe J. C. (1973) Measurement of fast lateral diffusion of lipids in vesicles and in biological membranes by ^1H nuclear magnetic resonance. *Biochemistry* **12,** 1650–1659.
156. Lever M. J., Miller K. W., Paton W. D. M. et al. (1971) Pressure reversal of anaesthesia. *Nature* (*Lond.*) **231,** 368–371.
157. Lidbrink P. (1974) The effect of lesions of ascending noradrenergic pathways on sleep and waking in the rat. *Brain Res.* **74,** 19–40.
158. Lodge D. and Curtis D. R. (1978) Time course of GABA and glycine actions on cat spinal neurones: effect of pentobarbitone. *Neurosci. Lett.* **8,** 125–129.
159. McDowall D. G. (1967) The effects of clinical concentrations of halothane on the blood flow and oxygen uptake of the cerebral cortex. *Br. J. Anaesth.* **39,** 186–196.
160. Magni F., Morruzzi G., Rossi G. F. et al. (1959) EEG arousal following inactivation of the lower brain stem by selective injection of barbiturate into lower brain stem circulation. *Arch. Ital. Biol.* **97,** 33–46.
161. Mapleson W. W. (1972) Absorption, distribution and excretion. Kinetics. In: Chenoweth M. B. (ed.), *Modern Inhalational Anesthetics.* Berlin, Springer, pp. 326–344.
162. Marsh D. (1975) Spectroscopic studies of membrane structure. *Essays Biochem.* **11,** 139–180.
163. Matthews E. K. and Quilliam J. P. (1964) Effects of central depressant drugs upon acetylcholine release. *Br. J. Pharmacol.* **22,** 415–440.
164. Matthews P. B. C. and Rushworth G. (1957) The relative sensitivity of muscle nerve fibres to procaine. *J. Physiol.* (*Lond.*) **135,** 263–269.
165. Meech R. W. (1972) Intracellular calcium injection causes increased potassium conductance in *Aplysia* nerve cells. *Comp. Biochem. Physiol. A* **42,** 493–499.
166. Metcalfe J. C. and Richards C. D. (1978) The effects of temperature on the local anaesthetic action of primary alcohols. *J. Physiol.* (*Lond.*) **281,** 35–36P.
167. Metcalfe J. C., Seeman P. and Burgen A. S. V. (1968) The proton relaxation of benzyl alcohol in erythrocyte membranes. *Mol. Pharmacol.* **4,** 87–95.

168. Meyer K. H. (1937) Contributions to the theory of narcosis. *Trans. Faraday Soc.* **33,** 1062–1068.
169. Meyer-Lohman J., Hagenah R., Hellweg C. et al. (1972) The action of ethyl alcohol on the activity of individual Renshaw cells. *Arch. Pharmacol.* **272,** 131–142.
170. Miller K. W. and Pang K.-Y. Y. (1976) General anaesthetics can selectively perturb lipid bilayer membranes. *Nature* (*Lond.*) **263,** 253–255.
171. Miller K. W., Paton W. D. M., Smith E. B. et al. (1972) Physico-chemical approaches to the mode of action of general anesthetics. *Anesthesiology* **36,** 339–351.
172. Miller K. W., Paton W. D. M., Smith R. A. et al. (1973) The pressure reversal of general anesthesia and the critical volume hypothesis. *Mol. Pharmacol.* **9,** 131–143.
173. Miller K. W. and Wilson M. W. (1978) The pressure reversal of a variety of anesthetic agents in mice. *Anesthesiology* **48,** 104–110.
174. Miller R. D., Wahrenbrock E. A., Schroeder C. F. et al. (1969) Ethylene–halothane anesthesia: addition or synergism? *Anesthesiology* **31,** 301–304.
175. Miller R. N. and Hunter F. E. (1970) The effect of halothane on electron transport, oxidative phosphorylation and swelling in rat liver mitochondria. *Mol. Pharmacol.* **6,** 67–77.
176. Miller S. L. (1961) A theory of gaseous anesthetics. *Proc. Natl Acad. Sci. USA* **47,** 1515–1524.
177. Mizuno N., Nakano K., Imaizumi M. et al. (1967) The lateral cervical nucleus of the Japanese monkey (*Macaca fuscata*). *J. Comp. Neurol.* **129,** 375–381.
178. Modak A. T., Weintraub S. T., McCoy T. H. et al. (1976) Use of 300 msec. microwave irradiation for enzyme inactivation: a study of effects of sodium pentobarbital on acetylcholine concentration in mouse brain regions. *J. Pharmacol. Exp. Ther.* **197,** 245–252.
179. Mori K., Winters W. D. and Spooner C. E. (1968) Comparison of reticular and cochlear multiple unit activity with auditory evoked responses during various stages induced by anesthetic agents. II. *Electroencephalogr. Clin. Neurophysiol.* **24,** 242–248.
180. Morin F., Schwartz H. G. and O'Leary J. L. (1951) Experimental study of the spinothalamic and related tracts. *Acta Psychiatr. Neurol.* **26,** 371–396.
181. Moruzzi G. and Magoun H. W. (1949) Brain stem reticular formation and activation of the EEG. *Electroencephalogr. Clin. Neurophysiol.* **1,** 455–473.
182. Mueller P. and Rudin D. O. (1967) Action potential phenomena in experimental bimolecular lipid membranes. *Nature* (*Lond.*) **213,** 603–604.
183. Mullins L. J. (1954) Some physical mechanisms in narcosis. *Chem. Rev.* **54,** 289–323.
184. Nafstad P. H. J. (1967) An electron microscopic study on the termination of the perforant path fibres in the hippocampus and the fascia dentata. *Z. Mikrosk. Anat. Forsch.* **76,** 532–542.
185. Narahashi T., Frazier D. T. and Yamada M. (1970) The site of action and active form of local anesthetics. I. Theory and pH experiments with tertiary compounds. *J. Pharmacol. Exp. Ther.* **171,** 32–44.
186. Nathan P. W. and Sears T. A. (1961) Some factors concerned in differential nerve block by local anaesthetics. *J. Physiol.* (*Lond.*) **157,** 565–580.
187. Ngai S. H., Cheney D. L. and Fink A. D. (1978) Acetylcholine concentrations and turnover in rat brain structures during anesthesia with halothane, enflurane and ketamine. *Anesthesiology* **48,** 4–10.
188. Nicoll R. A. (1972) The effect of anaesthetics on synaptic excitation and inhibition in the olfactory bulb. *J. Physiol.* (*Lond.*) **223,** 803–814.
189. Nicoll R. A. (1975) Pentobarbital: action on frog motoneurones. *Brain Res.* **96,** 119–123.

190. Nicoll R. A., Eccles J. C., Oshima T. et al. (1975) Prolongation of hippocampal inhibitory post synaptic potentials by barbiturates. *Nature (Lond.)* **258**, 625–627.
191. Nilsson L. and Seisjö B. K. (1974) Influence of anaesthetics on the balance between production and utilisation of energy in the brain. *J. Neurochem.* **23**, 29–36.
192. Olsen N. S. and Klein J. R. (1947) Effect of cyanide on the concentration of lactate and phosphates in brain. *J. Biol. Chem.* **167**, 739–746.
193. Overath P. and Thilo L. (1978) Structural and functional aspects of biological membranes revealed by lipid phase transitions. *Int. Rev. Biochem.* **19**, 1–44.
194. Paolo T. D., Kier L. B. and Hall L. H. (1977) Molecular connectivity and structure–activity relationship of general anesthetics. *Mol. Pharmacol.* **13**, 31–37.
195. Pauling L. (1961) A molecular theory of general anesthesia. *Science* **134**, 15–21.
196. Perl E. R., Whitlock D. G. and Gentry J. R. (1962) Cutaneous projection to second order neurones of the dorsal column system. *J. Neurophysiol.* **25**, 337–358.
197. Phillipps G. H. (1974) Structure–activity relationships in steroidal anaesthetics. In: Halsey M. J., Millar R. A. and Sutton J. A. (ed.), *Molecular Mechanisms in General Anaesthesia,* ch. 3. London, Churchill Livingstone.
198. Pierce E. C., Lambersen C. J., Deutsch S. et al. (1962) Cerebral circulation and metabolism during thiopental anesthesia and hyperventilation in man. *J. Clin. Invest.* **41**, 1664–1671.
199. Pomeranz B. (1973) Specific nociceptive fibres projecting from spinal cord neurones to the brain: a possible pathway for pain. *Brain Res.* **50**, 447–451.
200. Ponten U., Ratcheson R. A., Salford L. G. et al. (1973) Optimal freezing conditions for cerebral metabolites in rats. *J. Neurochem.* **21**, 1127–1138.
201. Pöppel E., Held R. and Frost D. (1973) Residual visual function after brain wounds involving the central visual pathway in man. *Nature (Lond.)* **243**, 295–296.
202. Price J. L. and Sprich W. W. (1975) Observations on the lateral olfactory tract of the rat. *J. Comp. Neurol.* **162**, 321–336.
203. Pritz W. and Stockinger L. (1971) Uber den Zahnschmertz. *Oster. Z. Ztomat.* **5**, 170–178.
204. Procter W. R. and Weakly J. N. (1976) A comparison of the presynaptic and postsynaptic actions of pentobarbitone and phenobarbitone in the neuromuscular junction of the frog. *J. Physiol. (Lond.)* **258**, 257–268.
205. Quastel D. J. M. and Linder T. M. (1975) Pre and post synaptic actions of central depressants at the mammalian neuromuscular junction. In: Fink B. R. (ed.), *Molecular Mechanisms of Anesthesia. Progress in Anesthesiology,* vol. 1. Raven Press, New York, pp. 157–165.
206. Quastel J. H. (1965) Effects of drugs on metabolism of the brain *in vitro. Br. Med. Bull.* **21**, 49–56.
207. Ransom B. R. and Barker J. L. (1975) Pentobarbital modulates transmitter effects on mouse spinal neurones grown in tissue culture. *Nature (Lond.)* **254**, 703–705.
208. Ransom B. R. and Barker J. L. (1976) Pentobarbital selectively enhances GABA-mediated post synaptic inhibition in tissue cultured mouse spinal neurons. *Brain Res.* **114**, 530–535.
209. Rassmusen A. T. and Peyton W. T. (1948) The course and termination of the medial lemniscus in man. *J. Comp. Neurol.* **88**, 411–424.
210. Reivich M. (1974) Blood flow metabolism couple in brain. In: Plum F. (ed.), *Brain Dysfunctions in Metabolic Disorders.* (*Res. Publ. Assoc. Res. Nerv. Ment. Dis.* **53**.) New York, Raven Press, pp. 125–140.

211. Reivich M., Jehle J., Sokoloff L. et al. (1969) Measurement of regional cerebral blood flow with antipyrine ^{14}C in awake cats. *J. Appl. Physiol.* **27**, 296–300.
212. Rexed B. and Ström G. (1952) Afferent nervous connections of the lateral cervical nucleus. *Acta Physiol. Scand.* **25**, 219–229.
213. Richards C. D. (1972) On the mechanism of barbiturate anaesthesia. *J. Physiol. (Lond.)* **227**, 749–767.
214. Richards C. D. (1973) On the mechanism of halothane anaesthesia. *J. Physiol. (Lond.)* **233**, 439–456.
215. Richards C. D. (1974) The action of general anaesthetics on synaptic transmission within the central nervous system. In: Halsey M. J., Millar R. A. and Sutton J. A. (ed.), *Molecular Mechanisms of General Anaesthesia,* ch. 6. London, Churchill Livingstone.
216. Richards C. D. (1978) Evidence of localisation of glutamate receptors in layer 1a of the dendritic field of neurones in the prepiriform cortex. In: Ryall R. W. and Kelly J. S. (ed.), *Iontophoresis and Transmitter Mechanisms in the Mammalian Central Nervous System.* Amsterdam, Elsevier and North Holland, pp. 185–187.
217. Richards C. D. (1978) Anesthetics and membranes. *Int. Rev. Biochem.* **19**, 157–220.
218. Richards C. D. (1979) The actions of pentobarbitone, procaine, propanidid and tetrodotoxin on impulse conduction and synaptic transmission in the olfactory cortex: further evidence of a specific synaptic blockade by barbiturates. In preparation.
219. Richards C. D. and Hesketh T. R. (1975) Implications for theories of anaesthesia of antagonism between anaesthetic and non-anaesthetic steroids. *Nature (Lond.)* **256**, 179–182.
220. Richards C. D., Martin K., Gregory S. et al. (1978) Degenerate perturbations of protein structure as the mechanism of anaesthetic action. *Nature (Lond.)* **276**, 775–779.
221. Richards C. D., Russell W. J. and Smaje J. C. (1975) The action of ether and methoxyflurane on synaptic transmission in isolated preparations of the mammalian cortex. *J. Physiol. (Lond.)* **248**, 121–142.
222. Richards C. D. and Sercombe R. (1968) Electrical activity observed in guinea-pig olfactory cortex maintained *in vitro. J. Physiol. (Lond.)* **197**, 667–683.
223. Richards C. D. and Sercombe R. (1970) Calcium, magnesium and the electrical activity of guinea-pig olfactory cortex *in vitro. J. Physiol. (Lond.)* **211**, 571–584.
224. Richards C. D. and Smaje J. C. (1974) The actions of halothane and pentobarbitone on the sensitivity of neurones in the guinea-pig prepiriform cortex to iontophoretically applied L-glutamate. *J. Physiol. (Lond.)* **239**, 103–105P.
225. Richards C. D. and Smaje J. C. (1976) Anaesthetics depress the sensitivity of cortical neurones to L-glutamate. *Br. J. Pharmacol.* **58**, 347–357.
226. Richards C. D. and White A. E. (1975) The actions of volatile anaesthetics on synaptic transmission in the dentate gyrus. *J. Physiol. (Lond.)* **252**, 241–257.
227. Richards W. (1973) Visual processing in scotoma. *Exp. Brain Res.* **17**, 333–347.
228. Richens A. (1969) The action of general anaesthetic agents on root responses of the frog isolated spinal cord. *Br. J. Pharmacol.* **36**, 294–311.
229. Richter J. A. and Waller M. B. (1977) Effects of pentobarbitone on the regulation of acetylcholine content and release in different regions of the rat brain. *Biochem. Pharmacol.* **26**, 609–615.
230. Rinvik E. (1968) The corticothalamic projection from the pericruciate and coronal gyri in the cat. An experimental study with silver impregnation methods. *Brain Res.* **10**, 79–119.

231. Roizen M. F., Kopin I. J., Palkovitz M. et al. (1975) The effect of two diverse inhalation anesthetic agents on serotonin in discrete regions of the rat brain. *Exp. Brain Res.* **24,** 203–207.
232. Roizen M. F., Kopin I. J., Thoa N. B. et al. (1976) The effect of two anesthetic agents on norepinephrinc and dopamine in discrete brain nuclei, fibre tracts and terminal regions of the rat. *Brain Res.* **110,** 515–522.
233. Rosenberg P. H., Eibl H. and Steir A. (1975) Biphasic effects of halothane on phospholipid and synaptic plasma membranes: a spin label study. *Mol. Pharmacol.* **11,** 879–882.
234. Rosenberg P. H., Jansson S. E. and Gripenberg J. (1977) Effects of halothane, thiopental and lidocaine on fluidity of synaptic plasma membranes and artificial phospholipid membranes. *Anesthesiology* **46,** 322–326.
235. Rosner B. S. and Clark D. L. (1973) Neurophysiological effects of general anesthetics. II. Sequential regional actions in the brain. *Anesthesiology* **39,** 59–81.
236. Rosner B. S., Clark D. L. and Beck C. (1971) Inhalational anesthetics and conduction velocity of human peripheral nerve. *Electroencephalogr. Clin. Neurophysiol.* **31,** 109–114.
237. Roth S. and Seeman P. (1971) All lipid soluble anaesthetics protect red cells. *Nature* [*New Biol.*] **231,** 284–285.
238. Roth S. and Seeman P. (1972) Anesthetics expand erythrocyte membranes without causing loss of K^+. *Biochim. Biophys. Acta* **255,** 190–198.
239. Ruff R. L. (1977) A quantal analysis of local anaesthetic alteration of miniature end plate currents and end plate current fluctuations. *J. Physiol.* (*Lond.*) **264,** 89–124.
240. Sanders M. D., Warrington E. K., Marshall J. et al. (1974) 'Blindsight': vision in a field defect. *Lancet* **1,** 707–708.
241. Schmidt R. F. (1963) Pharmacological studies on the primary afferent depolarisation of the toad spinal cord. *Pfluegers Arch.* **277,** 325–346.
242. Schoenborn B. P. (1968) Binding of anesthetics to protein: an X-ray crystallographic investigation. *Fed. Proc.* **27,** 888–894.
243. Schwartzkroin P. A., Duijn H. Van and Prince D. A. (1974) Effects of projected cortical epileptiform discharges on unit activity in the cat cuneate nucleus. *Exp. Neurol.* **43,** 106–123.
244. Seeman P. (1972) The membrane actions of anesthetics and tranquilisers. *Pharmacol. Rev.* **24,** 583–655.
245. Seeman P. (1974) The membrane expansion theory of anesthesia: direct evidence using ethanol and a high precision density meter. *Experientia* **30,** 759–760.
246. Seeman P. and Roth S. (1972) General anesthetics expand cell membranes at surgical concentrations. *Biochim. Biophys. Acta* **255,** 171–177.
247. Seyama I. and Narahashi T. (1975) Mechanism of blockade of neuromuscular transmission by pentobarbital. *J. Pharmacol. Exp. Ther.* **192,** 95–104.
248. Shapiro H. M., Greenberg J. H., Reivich M. et al. (1978) Local cerebral glucose uptake in awake and halothane-anesthetised primates. *Anesthesiology* **48,** 97–103.
249. Sherrington C. S. (1906) *The Integrative Action of the Nervous System.* New Haven, Yale University Press.
250. Shimshick E. J. and McConnell H. M. (1973) Lateral phase separation in phospholipid membranes. *Biochemistry* **12,** 2351–2360.
251. Singer S. J. and Nicholson G. L. (1972) The fluid-mosaic model of the structure of cell membranes. *Science* **175,** 720–731.
252. Smaje J. C. (1976) General anaesthetics and the acetylcholine sensitivity of cortical neurones. *Br. J. Pharmacol.* **58,** 359–366.
253. Smith A. L. and Wollman H. (1972) Cerebral blood flow and metabolism: effects of anesthetic drugs and techniques. *Anesthesiology* **36,** 378–400.

254. Smith E. B. (1974) Physical chemical investigations of the mechanisms of general anaesthesia. In: Halsey M. J., Millar R. A. and Sutton J. A. (ed.), *Molecular Mechanisms of General Anaesthesia,* ch. 7. London, Churchill Livingstone.
255. Sokoloff L. (1959) The action of drugs on the cerebral circulation. *Pharmacol. Rev.* **11,** 1–85.
256. Sokoloff L. (1977) Relation between physiological function and energy metabolism in the central nervous system. *J. Neurochem.* **29,** 13–26.
257. Sokoloff L., Reivich M., Kennedy C. et al. (1977) The (^{14}C) deoxyglucose method for the measurement of local cerebral glucose utilisation: theory, procedure and normal values in the conscious and anaesthetised albino rat. *J. Neurochem.* **28,** 897–916.
258. Somjen G. G. (1963) Effects of ether and thiopental on spinal presynaptic terminals. *J. Pharmacol. Exp. Ther.* **140,** 396–402.
259. Somjen G. G. (1967) Effects of anesthetics on spinal cord of mammals. *Anesthesiology* **28,** 135–143.
260. Somjen G. G. and Gill M. (1963) The mechanism of the blockade of synaptic transmission in the mammalian spinal cord by diethyl ether and by thiopental. *J. Pharmacol. Exp. Ther.* **140,** 19–30.
261. Sperry R. W. (1967) Mental unity following surgical disconnection of the cerebral hemispheres. *Harvey Lect.* **62,** 293–323.
262. Sperry R. W. (1968) Hemisphere deconnection and unity in conscious awareness. *Am. Psychol.* **23,** 723–733.
263. Staiman A. and Seeman P. (1974) The impulse-blocking concentrations of anesthetics, alcohols, anticonvulsants, barbiturates and narcotics on phrenic and sciatic nerves. *Can. J. Physiol. Pharmacol.* **52,** 535–550.
264. Stewart W. B. and Scott J. W. (1976) Anesthetic-dependent field potential interactions in the olfactory bulb. *Brain Res.* **103,** 487–499.
265. Stokinger L. and Pritz W. (1970) Morphologische Aspekte des schmerzemp Findung in Zahn. *Dtsch Zahnärztl.* **25,** 557–565.
266. Strichartz G. R. (1973) The inhibition of sodium currents in myelinated nerve by quaternary derivatives of lidocaine. *J. Gen. Physiol.* **62,** 37–57.
267. Takeshita H., Okuda Y. and Sari A. (1972) The effects of ketamine on cerebral circulation and metabolism in man. *Anesthesiology* **36,** 69–75.
268. Takeuchi A. and Takeuchi N. (1962) Electrical changes in pre and post synaptic axons of the giant synapse of *Loligo. J. Gen. Physiol.* **45,** 1181–1193.
269. Theye R. A. and Michenfelder J. D. (1973) Effects of methoxyflurane on canine cerebral metabolism. *Anesthesiology* **38,** 123–127.
270. Thilo L. and Overath P. (1976) Randomisation of membrane lipids in relation to transport system assembly in *Escherichia coli. Biochemistry* **15,** 328–334.
271. Thompson T. D. and Turkanis S. A. (1973) Barbiturate-induced transmitter release at a frog neuromuscular junction. *Br. J. Pharmacol.* **48,** 48–58.
272. Thornton J. A., Whelpton D. and Brown B. H. (1968) The effect of general anaesthetic agents on nerve conduction velocities. *Br. J. Anaesth.* **40,** 583–586.
273. Torda T. A. and Gage P. W. (1977) Post synaptic effect of i.v. anaesthetic agents at the neuromuscular junction. *Br. J. Anaesth.* **49,** 771–776.
274. Towe A. L. and Jabbur S. J. (1961) Cortical inhibition of neurones in dorsal column nuclei of cat. *J. Neurophysiol.* **24,** 488–498.
275. Treveno D. L., Coulter J. D. and Willis W. D. (1973) Location of cells of origin of spinothalamic tract in lumbar enlargement of the monkey. *J. Neurophysiol.* **36,** 750–761.
276. Trudell J. R. (1977) The membrane volume occupied by anesthetic molecules: a reinterpretation of the erythrocyte expansion data. *Biochim. Biophys. Acta* **470,** 509–510.

277. Trudell J. R. (1977) A unitary theory of anesthesia based on lateral phase separations in nerve membranes. *Anesthesiology* **46,** 5–10.
278. Trudell J. R., Hubbell W. L. and Cohen E. N. (1973) The effect of two inhalation anesthetics on the order of spin-labelled phospholipid vesicles. *Biochim. Biophys. Acta* **291,** 321–327.
279. Trudell J. R., Hubbell W. L. and Cohen E. N. (1973) Pressure reversal of inhalation anesthetic induced disorder in spin labelled phospholipid vesicles. *Biochim. Biophys. Acta* **291,** 328–334.
280. Ueda I., Shieh D. D. and Eyring H. (1974) Anesthetic interaction with a model cell membrane: expansion, phase transition and melting of the lecithin monolayer. *Anesthesiology* **41,** 217–225.
281. Ueda I., Shieh D. D. and Eyring H. (1975) Disordering effects of anesthetics in firefly luciferase and in lecithin surface monolayer. In: Fink B. R. (ed.), *Molecular Mechanisms of Anesthesia.* New York, Raven Press, pp. 291–305.
282. Ueda I., Tashiro C. and Arakawa K. (1977) Depression of phase transition temperatures in a model cell membrane by local anesthetics. *Anesthesiology* **46,** 327–332.
283. Verveen A. A. and Derksen H. E. (1968) Fluctuation phenomena in nerve membrane. *Proc. IEEE* **56,** 906–916.
284. Verworn M. (1912) Narcosis. *Harvey Lect.* (1911–1912) pp. 52–75.
285. Wahlströom G., Busch H. and Buzello T. W. (1970) Unequal anesthetic potency despite equal brain concentrations of hexobarbital antipodes. *Acta Pharmacol. Toxicol.* **28,** 493–498.
286. Wall P. D. (1960) Cord cells responding to touch, damage and temperature of skin. *J. Neurophysiol.* **23,** 197–210.
287. Wall P. D. (1967) The laminar organisation of the dorsal horn and effects of descending inputs. *J. Physiol. (Lond.)* **188,** 403–424
288. Walshe F. M. R. (1948) *Critical Studies in Neurology.* Edinburgh, Livingstone.
289. Warren G. B., Houslay M. D., Metcalfe J. C. et al. (1975) Cholesterol is excluded from the phospholipid annulus surrounding an active calcium transport protein. *Nature (Lond.)* **255,** 684–687.
290. Warren G. B., Toon P. A., Birdsall N. J. M. et al. (1974) Reversible lipid titrations of the activity of pure adenosine-triphosphatase–lipid complexes. *Biochemistry* **13,** 5501–5507.
291. Waxman S. G. and Bennett M. V. L. (1972) Relative conduction velocities of small myelinated and non-myelinated fibres in the central nervous system. *Nature [New Biol.]* **238,** 217–219.
292. Weakly J. N. (1969) Effect of barbiturates on quantal synaptic transmission in spinal motoneurones. *J. Physiol. (Lond.)* **204,** 63–77.
293. Weakly J. N., Esplin D. W. and Zablocká B. (1968) Criteria for assessing effects of drugs on postsynaptic inhibition. *Arch. Int. Pharmacodyn. Ther.* **171,** 385–393.
294. Weight F. F. (1974) Synaptic potentials resulting from conductance decreases. In: *Synaptic Transmission and Neuronal Interaction.* New York, Raven Press, pp. 141–152.
295. Weiskrantz L. (1972) Behavioural analysis of the monkey's visual nervous system. *Proc. R. Soc. Lond. [Biol.]* **182,** 427–455.
296. Westmoreland B. F., Ward D. and Johns T. R. (1971) The effect of methohexital at the neuromuscular junction. *Brain Res.* **26,** 465–468.
297. Wickler A. (1952) Pharmacologic dissociation of behaviour and EEG 'sleep patterns' in dogs: morphine, *n*-allyl morphine and atropine. *Proc. Soc. Exp. Biol. Med.* **79,** 261–265.
298. Willis W. D., Trevino D. L., Coulter J. D. et al. (1974) Responses of primate spinothalamic tract neurones to natural stimulation of the hind limb. *J. Neurophysiol.* **37,** 358–372.

299. Winter P. M., Smith R. A., Smith M. et al. (1976) Pressure antagonism of barbiturate anesthesia. *Anesthesiology* **44**, 416–419.
300. Winters W. D. (1976) Effects of drugs on the electrical activity of the brain: anesthetics. *Ann. Rev. Pharmacol.* **16**, 413–426.
301. Wishnia A. (1962) The solubility of hydrocarbon gases in protein solutions. *Proc. Natl Acad. Sci. USA* **48**, 2200–2204.
302. Wolfson L. I., Sakurada O. and Sokoloff L. (1977) Effects of γ-butyrolactone on local cerebral glucose utilisation in the rat. *J. Neurochem.* **29**, 777–783.
303. Wright E. B. (1954) Effect of mephenesin and other depressants on spinal cord transmission in frog and cat. *Am. J. Physiol.* **179**, 390–401.
304. Wulf R. J. and Featherstone R. M. (1957) A correlation of Van der Waals' constants with anesthetic potency. *Anesthesiology* **18**, 97–105.
305. Zamyatnin A. A. (1972) Protein volume in solution. *Prog. Biophys. Mol. Biol.* **24**, 107–123.
306. Zorychta E., Esplin D. W. and Capek R. (1975) Action of halothane on transmitter release in the spinal monosynaptic pathway. *Fed. Proc.* **34**, 749.
307. Zotterman Y. (1933) Studies in the peripheral nervous mechanism of pain. *Acta Med. Scand.* **80**, 185–242.

Benjamin G. Covino

2 The Mechanisms of Local Anaesthesia

INTRODUCTION

Local anaesthetic agents have been utilized clinically for approximately 100 years. Although cocaine was isolated from the leaves of the *Erythroxylon coca* bush by Niemann in 1860, its clinical utility was not appreciated until Koller reported the production of corneal anaesthesia following topical application of cocaine in 1884. The following year Halstead utilized cocaine by injection for infiltration anaesthesia and in 1898 subarachnoid block in man was performed by Bier with this remarkable new substance. Since these initial studies, a large number of chemical entities have been synthesized, specifically for use as local anaesthetic agents. However, the ability to produce a localized state of insensibility is present in a variety of chemical entities employed for a number of different clinical purposes, such as antihistaminics, antiarrhythmic agents, beta-adrenergic receptor blocking agents, and some of the tranquillizers.

During the past 100 years various research efforts have been exerted in the field of local and regional anaesthesia. Safer, more efficacious, and more varied types of local anaesthetic agents have been developed. Numerous animal and clinical studies have been carried out to elucidate the physiological changes following regional anaesthesia and to develop improved methods of regional anaesthesia. Concomitant with these studies of a more practical clinical nature, a number of investigators have concerned themselves with the basic nature of local anaesthesia. These investigations have mainly been directed at answering the following questions: (*a*) How do local anaesthetic agents inhibit the generation and propagation of a nerve impulse? (*b*) Where is the site of action of local anaesthetics in the nerve? (*c*) How do local anaesthetics reach their site of action? The purpose of this present review is to assimilate the available scientific data and attempt to formulate a unified theory of the process by which local anaesthetic drugs inhibit nerve conduction. Of necessity, such a review must be interdisciplinary in nature, since it must consider the interrelationship of the morphology, chemistry, and physiology of peripheral nerves with the pharmacology of the local anaesthetic drugs.

HOW DO LOCAL ANAESTHETICS BLOCK NERVE CONDUCTION?

The Excitation–Conduction Process

The basic pharmacological action of local anaesthetic drugs is to inhibit the excitation–conduction process of peripheral nerve fibres and nerve endings. The use of intracellular electrodes has made possible a number of studies of a biophysical nature concerning the generation and propagation of nerve impulses. This technique of microelectrodes was perfected by Ling and Gerard who described the use of glass electrodes of <1 μm in diameter, which could be inserted intracellularly without detectable damage to the nerve membrane [48]. The use of this KCl-filled microelectrode and the proper electronic equipment made possible the recording of the electrical potential between the inside and outside of a nerve cell. At rest, a negative electrical potential of approximately -60 to -90 mV

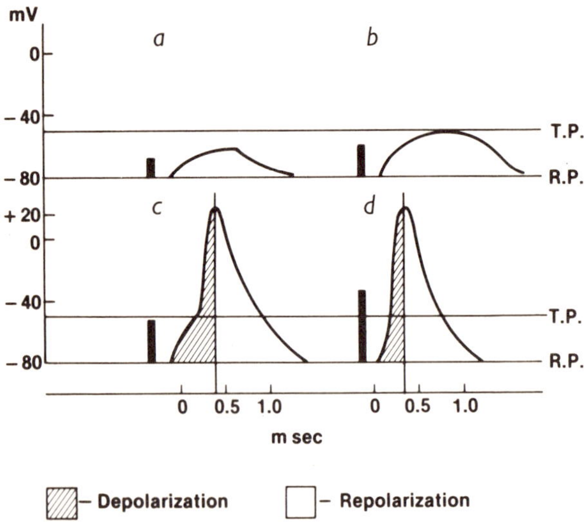

Fig. 2.1. Relationship of stimulus strength to generation of nerve impulse. Height of bar in *a, b, c, d* indicates increasing strength of electrical stimulus (mA). Depolarization in *a* and *b* is insufficient to reduce membrane potential from resting level (RP) to threshold potential (TP). In *c* and *d* stimulus strength is sufficient to achieve TP resulting in complete depolarization.

was found to exist across the nerve cell membrane. This represents the 'resting potential' when the cell is considered to be in a state of polarization. If a stimulus is applied to the nerve at this time, the interior of the cell becomes progressively less negative with respect to the exterior, resulting in a state of depolarization (*Fig. 2.1*). The decrease in potential difference between the interior and the exterior surface of the cell membrane is dependent on the strength of stimulus applied to the nerve. The cell membrane possesses a critical threshold potential or firing level which must be achieved before complete depolarization can occur. Normally, the threshold potential level is approximately 20 mV less than the resting potential. A cell with a resting potential level of −70 mV will have a threshold potential or firing level of approximately −50 mV. If the stimulus applied to the nerve is not sufficient to decrease the potential difference across the cell membrane from the resting to the threshold potential level, then a localized incomplete state of depolarization occurs which is not adequate to produce a propagated action potential. If the stimulus is sufficient in strength to raise the intracellular potential to the firing level, then a complete state of depolarization will occur. Once the threshold potential level is achieved, an extremely rapid phase of depolarization commences, which is spontaneous in nature and not dependent on the strength of the applied stimulus. The nerve membrane essentially follows the 'all-or-none' rule, i.e. an applied stimulus of sufficient strength is required to achieve the threshold potential level which, in turn, will result in complete depolarization (*Fig. 2.1*). Any additional increase in stimulus intensity has no effect on the degree of depolarization or the amplitude of the action potential. Complete depolarization of the cell membrane results in a reversal of the electrical potential, such that at the end of the depolarization phase, the interior of the cell actually has a positive electrical potential of +40 mV as compared to the exterior of the cell. Under normal conditions the height of the action potential is approximately 110 mV, i.e. the potential difference across the membrane has changed from a resting potential level of −70 mV to a peak level of +40 mV at the end of depolarization.

At the conclusion of the depolarization phase, repolarization of the cell membrane begins. During this time period, the electrical potential within the cell again becomes progressively more negative until such time as the original resting potential of −60 to −90 mV is re-established. The rate of repolarization occurs more slowly than the rate of depolarization. For example, in a series of studies on the giant squid axon, the maximum rate of depolarization varied from 423 to 532 V/sec, while the maximum rate of repolarization averaged 335–440 V/sec [71]. The period of repolarization is important electrophysiologically since during this phase the membrane is in a state of refractoriness. During the early portion of the repolarization phase, the refractoriness is absolute in nature such that the cell will not respond to a stimulus regardless of strength. During the latter phase of repolarization, the cell is in a state of relative refractoriness. During this time period, the cell will only respond to a stimulus whose intensity is greater than that normally required to produce depolarization. The refractory period is important, since it limits the number of impulses that can be conducted along a nerve fibre per unit time. The entire process of depolarization and repolarization occurs within 1 msec. The depolarization phase occupies approximately 30 per cent of the entire action potential, whereas repolarization accounts for the remaining 70 per cent. Frequently, a brief period of hyperpolarization may be observed following the end of the repolarization phase. During this time, the potential difference across the cell membrane is actually more negative than during the resting potential.

Propagation of the action potential from the area of initial excitation along the entire length of a nerve fibre does not require sequential stimulation of individual segments of the nerve. Once initial excitation occurs in a localized area of the nerve, a spontaneous and self-perpetuating system propagates the impulse along the entire length of the nerve fibre. This process is dependent on the change of electrical potential across the cell membrane at the area of excitation and the ability of the nerve to function as an electrical cable. Following depolarization of one segment of the nerve fibre, current will flow from the polarized inactive region in the extracellular fluid into the adjacent depolarized segment and then return by way of the axoplasm (*Fig. 2.2*). This current flow will thereby reduce

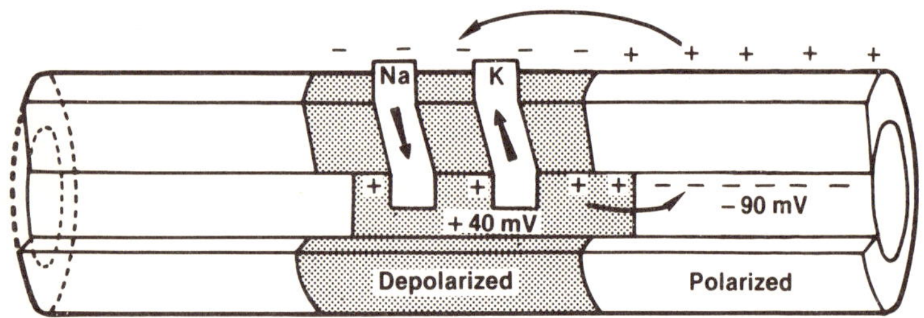

Fig. 2.2. Schematic representation of a nerve showing current flows (arrows) between adjacent areas of polarized and depolarized membrane.

the charge and voltage in the inactive region which is sufficient to decrease the intracellular potential to the threshold level required for depolarization. Therefore, the local circuit flow of current between immediate adjacent areas of polarized and depolarized membrane results in spontaneous propagation of the impulse along the fibre at a constant velocity.

Electrophysiological Effect of Local Anaesthetics

A consideration of the factors involved in impulse generation and propagation suggests that local anaesthetic agents may alter the excitation–conduction process in one or more of the following ways: (*a*) alteration of the resting membrane potential; (*b*) alteration of the threshold potential; (*c*) decrease in the rate of depolarization; (*d*) prolongation of the rate of repolarization; (*e*) inhibition of local current flow from inactive to active regions.

A number of studies have clearly shown that the resting membrane potential of isolated nerves is not altered following exposure to various concentrations of local anaesthetic agents, such as procaine or lidocaine (lignocaine) [1, 71, 86]. In addition, these same studies have failed to reveal any change in the threshold potential or firing level following application of local anaesthetic agents to an isolated nerve.

The primary electrophysiological effect of local anaesthetic agents involves the depolarization phase of the action potential. A decrease in the rate and degree of depolarization is observed as the concentration of local anaesthetic agent applied to an isolated nerve is increased. Although a subminimal concentration of local anaesthetic agents will not prevent the development of a propagated action potential, rates of depolarization and repolarization are decreased, refractory period is prolonged and conduction velocity is decreased. As a result, the number of impulses transmitted per unit time in an isolated nerve exposed to a subminimal concentration of local anaesthetic agent will be decreased. When the minimum concentration of a local anaesthetic agent required to cause complete conduction blockade is achieved, then the rate and degree of depolarization is sufficiently depressed that the threshold potential level is not achieved. Studies by Aceves and Machne have shown a decrease in the maximum rate of rise of the action potential of the isolated lumbar spinal ganglion of the frog from a control value of 134 to 55 V/sec after exposure to 0·005–0·04 per cent procaine [1]. Similarly Shanes and co-workers reported that the maximum rate of depolarization of the squid axon decreased from a mean of 532 to 308 V/sec, following exposure to 0·1 per cent cocaine or procaine [71]. In both studies, a concomitant decrease in the rate of repolarization was also observed following local anaesthetic application. In the lumbar spinal ganglion preparation, the rate of repolarization decreased from 86 to 54 V/sec, while in the squid axon, the rate of repolarization decreased from 440 to 197 V/sec following local anaesthetic application. The prolonged repolarization phase may reflect a direct local anaesthetic action or may be indicative of a direct relationship between the rate of repolarization and the rate of depolarization. In general, one can conclude that, electrophysiologically, local anaesthetics cause conduction blockade by preventing impulse generation subsequent to inhibition of membrane depolarization with no change in either the threshold or resting potential (*Fig. 2.3*). Prolongation of the repolarization phase and the refractory period may also play a role in the anaesthetic action of these agents in man.

Membrane Electrochemistry

The classical studies of Hodgkin and Huxley revealed that the electrophysiological properties of the nerve membrane are dependent on (*a*) the concentration of electrolytes in nerve cytoplasm and extracellular fluid and (*b*) the permeability of the cell membrane to various ions – particularly sodium and potassium [40, 41]. The ionic composition of the cytoplasm and the extracellular fluid differs markedly. The intracellular concentration of potassium is approximately 110–170 mmol/l, whereas the intracellular concentration of sodium and chloride ions is approximately 5–10 mmol/l.

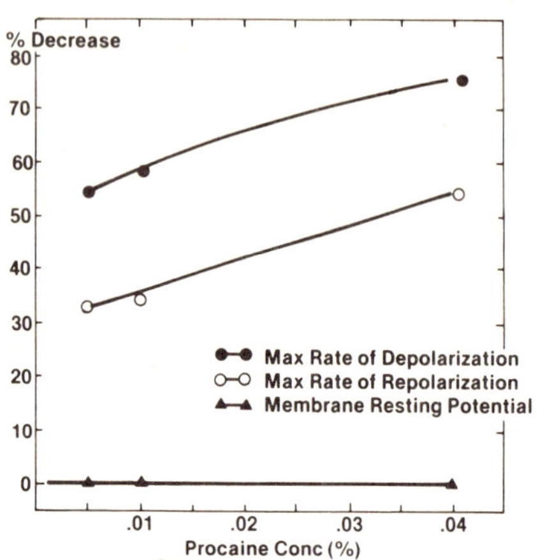

Fig. 2.3. Effect of procaine on resting potential, maximum rate of depolarization and maximum rate of repolarization of isolated nerve. (*Data derived from Aceves and Machne [1].*)

In extracellular fluid the situation is reversed. The concentration of sodium is approximately 140 mmol/l and the concentration of chloride is 110 mmol/l. On the other hand, the extracellular concentration of potassium is only 3–5 mmol/l. The ionic asymmetry on either side of the cell membrane is due in part to the selective permeability characteristics of the membrane. At rest, potassium ions may diffuse easily across the cell membrane indicating that the membrane is fully permeable to this particular ion. On the other hand, only limited diffusion of sodium ions across the membrane occurs at rest, indicating that the membrane is relatively impermeable to sodium, which accounts for the high extracellular concentration and low intracellular concentration of sodium. Although the membrane is permeable to potassium ions, a high intracellular concentration of this ion is maintained by the attractive forces of the negative charges mainly on proteins which exist within the cell. These large, negatively charged proteins are unable to diffuse across the cell membrane. The attraction of the negative charges on the proteins tends to counterbalance the tendency of the positively charged potassium ions to diffuse out of the cell by passive movement along a concentration gradient and through a freely permeable membrane. The electrical potential which should exist across the membranes separating two concentrations of the same ion (A) was predicted by the Nernst equation:

$$E = -\frac{RT}{nF} \ln \frac{[A]_i}{[A]_o}.$$

E = membrane potential between inside and outside of cell.
R = gas constant in joules (8·315).

T = absolute temperature.
n = valence of the ion.
F = Faraday's constant (96 500 coulombs).
ln = natural logarithm.

At room temperature (18 °C) and assuming a K_i/K_o ratio across the nerve membrane of 30, the Nernst equation would predict the following:

$$E = -58 \log \frac{[30\text{K}]_i}{[\text{K}]_o}$$

$$E = -85{\cdot}7 \text{ mV}.$$

This predicted resting membrane potential of −85·7 mV agrees closely with the measured resting potential values of −60 to −90 mV obtained from nerve preparations with intracellular electrodes. At rest, it would appear that the nerve cell behaves as a potassium electrode, which should react to changes in intra- or extracellular potassium concentration. Indeed, it has been clearly shown that changes in the intracellular or extracellular concentration of potassium will markedly alter the resting membrane potential. For example, as the extracellular concentration of potassium is increased, the resting membrane potential will tend to decrease. Studies have indicated that a decrease of 58 mV in resting potential occurs for a tenfold change in external potassium concentration. On the other hand, changes in sodium concentration appear to have little, if any, effect on the resting membrane potential.

Excitation of a nerve results in marked changes in the permeability of the cell membrane and ionic fluxes across the membrane. Various methods have been used to study the changes in ionic permeability during activity, such as (*a*) altering the extracellular concentration of sodium or potassium and determining the effect on the action potential, (*b*) utilizing radioisotopes to determine ionic fluxes during excitation and (*c*) use of voltage-clamp techniques which allow measurement of membrane current as a function of time while the transmembrane potential is fixed. The most detailed studies of ionic conductance during nerve activity have been based on voltage-clamp techniques. Application of a stimulus to a nerve results in a decrease in the electrical potential difference across the membrane, an increase in membrane permeability to sodium and an increase in sodium conductance. A direct correlation exists between the strength of stimulus, the decrease in potential difference across the membrane and the increase in sodium conductance until such time as the threshold potential is achieved. At the threshold potential or firing level, the net influx of sodium ions just balances the net outflow of potassium and chloride ions. However, when threshold potential is exceeded, a maximum increase in the permeability of the cell membrane to sodium ions occurs and an explosively rapid influx of sodium ions into the axoplasm follows. This marked increase of sodium conductance is responsible for the rapid depolarization of the cell. As the potential difference changes from the threshold level of approximately −50 to +40 mV at the peak of the action potential, inactivation of sodium conductance occurs. It is this sodium inactivation that ultimately terminates the depolarization phase. At the end of depolarization or at the peak of the action potential, the nerve membrane is essentially transformed from a potassium electrode to a sodium electrode, and the positive membrane potential of +40 mV can be calculated again from the Nernst equation by substituting the ratio of sodium ions between the inside and the outside of the nerve membrane (Na_i/Na_o) for the potassium ion ratio (K_i/K_o).

At the conclusion of the depolarization phase, the membrane starts to repolarize. The initial phase of repolarization and the absolute refractory period are related mainly to inactivation of sodium conductance. However, the remaining portion of the repolarization phase is a function of an increase in potassium conductance and efflux of this ion from the interior to the exterior of the cell. Potassium conductance is still somewhat greater than normal when repolarization is complete, which accounts for the phase of membrane hyperpolarization. When the membrane potential returns to its normal resting level, potassium and sodium conductances have also returned to their normal resting states.

Although the fluxes of sodium and potassium are high during the depolarization and repolarization phases, the actual concentration changes across the cell membrane are very small, since time during which these flows occur is very short. Therefore, following return of the membrane to the resting potential level, only a slight excess of sodium ions is present within the cell and a slight excess of potassium ions exists outside the nerve cell. At the conclusion of the excitation period, a metabolically active period begins, although electrically the nerve cell is quiescent. Restoration of the normal ionic gradient across the nerve membrane requires the expenditure of energy for the active transport of sodium from the inside to the outside of the nerve cell against a concentration gradient. This active transport of sodium ions is made possible by the so-called 'sodium pump'. The energy required to drive the sodium pump is derived from the oxidative metabolism of adenosine triphosphate. It has been shown that dinitrophenol, which interferes with oxidative phosphorylation, can prevent the active transport of sodium, suggesting that the sodium pump is dependent on phosphorylation mechanisms. Addition of excess adenosine triphosphate to a dinitrophenol-treated axon can reverse the inhibition of sodium efflux and restore the rate of sodium extrusion to normal. This metabolic pump, which actively extrudes intracellular sodium ions, also is believed responsible, in part, for the transport of potassium ions from the extracellular space to the interior of the nerve cell.

The return of potassium to the interior of the nerve cell occurs against a concentration gradient, but down an electrogenic gradient. Thus, re-establishment of the potassium gradient across the cell membrane may be partly an active process and partly a passive phenomenon. Potassium will continue to return to the interior of the cell until the electrostatic attraction of the negative charges on the intracellular proteins balances the chemical concentration gradient. *Fig. 2.4* summarizes the relationship between electrical activity in nerve and the alterations in ionic fluxes across the membrane.

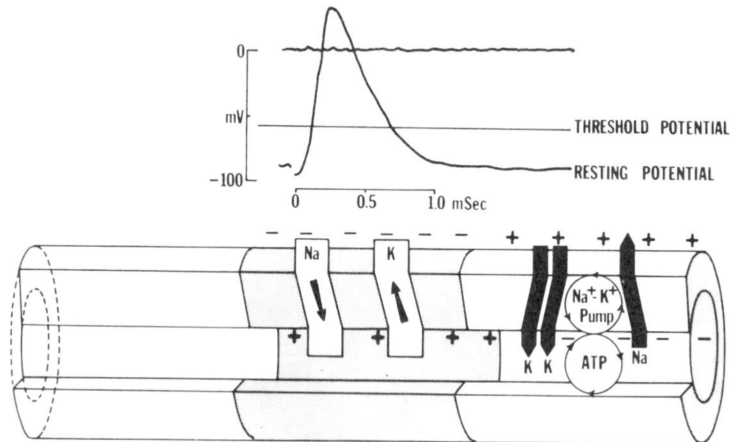

Fig. 2.4. Relationship between nerve action potential and ionic fluxes across the nerve membrane. (*Reproduced by permission from Covino and Vassallo [20].*)

Effect of Local Anaesthetics on Membrane Permeability

Since depolarization and repolarization of the nerve action potential are related to changes in cell permeability and conductance of sodium and potassium ions, it was reasonable to assume that decreases in rate of depolarization and repolarization observed in isolated nerves exposed to local anaesthetic agents reflected a primary action on ionic fluxes across the nerve membrane. A variety of studies have been carried out to evaluate the relationship between local anaesthetics and sodium and potassium conductance. Condouris constructed a series of dose–response curves relating concentration of cocaine and the height of the spike potential recorded from the surface of the isolated frog sciatic–peroneal nerve trunk to the sodium concentration of the Ringer's solution [16]. A direct correlation was observed between the concentration of sodium in the bathing solution and the concentration of cocaine required to reduce the height of the spike potential. For example, at a normal sodium concentration of 116 mmol, approximately 3·2 mmol of cocaine were required to produce a 50 per cent decrease in the height of the spike potential. When the sodium concentration was lowered to 12 mmol, only 0·15 mmol of cocaine were necessary to cause a similar reduction of 50 per cent in the amplitude of the spike potential.

The most direct evidence concerning the effect of local anaesthetic agents on both sodium and potassium conductance has been obtained by means of voltage-clamp techniques. Studies on the squid giant axon by Taylor [86] and Shanes and co-workers [71] demonstrated that procaine and cocaine are capable of decreasing the inward flow of sodium currents and the outward flow of potassium currents during voltage clamping of the membrane. However, both studies demonstrated a greater inhibitory effect on sodium conductance (g_{Na}) than on potassium conductance (g_K) (*Fig. 2.5*). For example, 0·05–0·1 per cent cocaine produced a 31–64 per cent

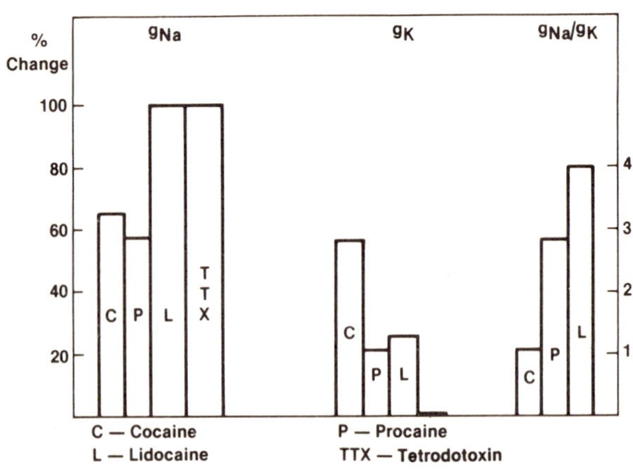

Fig. 2.5. Effect of various local anaesthetics on sodium (g_{Na}) and potassium (g_K) conductance. Ratio of g_{Na}/g_K indicates predominant action on g_{Na}. Tetrodotoxin (TTX) exerts no effect on g_K. (*Data derived from references 34, 71, 86.*)

decrease in g_{Na} compared to a 22–57 per cent decrease in g_K [71]. Procaine (0·1 per cent) resulted in a 58 per cent decrease in g_{Na}, while at the same time reducing g_K by 21 per cent [86]. Furthermore, studies on the isolated frog sciatic nerve by Hille [34] in which the membrane potential was held at the normal resting potential of −75 mV demonstrated complete loss of sodium currents in the presence of 10^{-3} M lidocaine with no discernible effect on outward potassium current. A concentration of $3{\cdot}5 \times 10^{-3}$ M of lidocaine was required to produce a 25 per cent decrease in g_K (*Fig. 2.5*). In a subsequent study, Strichartz also demonstrated almost complete inhibition of g_{Na} with minimal change in g_K following application of lidocaine to a single myelinated frog sciatic nerve preparation [82]. These studies clearly suggest that the primary action of local anaesthetics is to decrease the permeability of the cell membrane to sodium ions and thereby decrease sodium conductance and prevent cellular depolarization. The partial decrease in potassium permeability and conductance by local anaesthetics, particularly procaine and cocaine, is probably not involved in the inhibition of impulse generation by this class of drugs. Definitive proof that decrease in g_K is unrelated to the development of conduction blockade was forthcoming from investigations with the biotoxins, tetrodotoxin (TTX) and saxitoxin (STX). TTX is derived mainly from the ovaries of the Japanese puffer fish, while STX is produced by certain marine dinoflagellates. These two substances are the most potent nerve conduction blockers found to date. TTX will prevent excitation of the isolated squid axon at a concentration of 10^{-7} M [52].

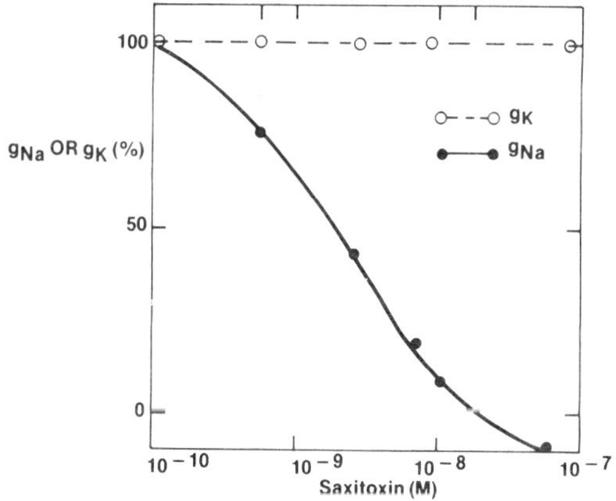

Fig. 2.6. Per cent reduction in g_{Na} and g_K by various concentrations of saxitoxin. (*Data derived from Hille [36].*)

In vivo studies have shown that TTX can produce spinal anaesthesia in sheep for 17–23 hr at a dose of 4 μg [20]. In terms of ionic membrane permeability, these two biotoxins have been demonstrated in various biological preparations to specifically inhibit sodium conductance without any effect on potassium conductance. For example, Hille reported that 3×10^{-7} M TTX completely inhibited g_{Na} in the isolated frog sciatic nerve without any discernible effect on g_K [34]. Similarly, STX caused a dose-related decrease in g_{Na} with complete blockade occurring at approximately 10^{-7} M, while no change in g_K was observed at any concentration of STX (*Fig. 2.6*) [36]. Conversely, tetraethylammonium (TEA) specifically inhibits g_K without altering g_{Na} [35]. Although TEA is an effective ganglionic blocking agent, it exerts no significant conduction blocking activity on isolated nerve and no local anaesthetic action *in vivo*.

The other potential effect of local anaesthetic agents on ionic fluxes involves the sodium–potassium pump. A decrease in the active extrusion of sodium at the end of the action potential would cause an accumulation of intracellular sodium and a reduction in the concentration gradient of sodium across the membrane. This would ultimately lead to a decrease in sodium conductance. Metabolic inhibitors are capable of producing conduction blockade, although the nature of the block is considerably different from that produced by local anaesthetic agents [91]. Adenosine triphosphate (ATP) which is intimately involved in re-establishment of the normal sodium–potassium gradient across the nerve membrane has been reported to prevent and reverse conduction block by procaine in the isolated frog sciatic nerve [46]. This would suggest that local anaesthetics may exert a metabolic inhibitory effect on the sodium pump. However, this antagonism between ATP and procaine was not found to be competitive in nature, since an increase in procaine concentration was not able to overcome the ATP antagonism. Moreover, conduction blockade due to an impairment of the sodium pump by an inhibitory effect on ATP should have been accompanied by a change in the membrane resting potential. As indicated previously, local anaesthetic activity is not associated with a change in the resting membrane potential. Although the explanation for the ATP–procaine interaction is not clear, ATP inhibition is not believed to be responsible for the conduction-blocking properties of local anaesthetic drugs. Moreover, direct studies involving cellular metabolism of nerves have not revealed any significant metabolic depression by local anaesthetic compounds at concentrations which produce conduction blockade. Finally, little or no effect was observed on the electrogenic component of the sodium pump in non-myelinated fibres of the desheathed rabbit vagus nerve exposed to concentrations of lidocaine varying from 0·2 to 3 mmol, while the action potential amplitude was reduced by 89–100 per cent. Only when the concentration of lidocaine was elevated to 10 mmol did a significant reduction in the electrogenic component of the sodium pump occur [23].

In summary, the evidence is overwhelming that the primary action of local anaesthetic agents involves direct depression of membrane permeability to sodium ions. This decrease in sodium conductance prevents the normal depolarization response to an applied stimulus, so that generation of a propagated impulse fails to occur which ultimately results in conduction blockade. Changes in potassium permeability observed, particularly, with agents such as procaine and cocaine, and metabolic inhibition of the sodium pump are not involved in the basic mechanism of action of local anaesthetic agents.

Interaction between Calcium and Local Anaesthetics

A major controversy existed several years ago concerning the role of calcium ions in the mechanism of conduction blockade produced by local anaesthetic agents. Calcium is believed by some investigators to play a critical role in the generation of the nerve impulse. At rest, calcium ions are bound to phospholipids in the cell membrane and in this state act as a barrier to the movement of sodium ions across the nerve membrane.

Application of a stimulus to the membrane may displace calcium from this phospholipid-binding site which would then represent the initial step in the increased permeability of the membrane to sodium ions. Support for the role of calcium as a membrane stabilizer obtains from studies which demonstrated that increases in calcium concentration raise the electrical threshold of the nerve membrane, reduce the frequency of spontaneous discharges and abolish propagated impulses without changing the resting potential level [71]. The similarity in the membrane-stabilizing effect of calcium and local anaesthetic agents was suggestive of a similar site of action in the nerve membrane [61]. The hypothesis was advanced that local anaesthetic agents acted by inhibition or displacement of calcium from a phospholipid-binding site in the membrane and that a competitive type of antagonism existed between local anaesthetics and calcium [6, 25]. The following evidence tended to support this hypothesis. The decrease in the rate of depolarization and amplitude of the action potential of isolated nerves by various local anaesthetics could be reversed by a tenfold increase in calcium concentration bathing the nerve preparation [1]. Moreover, direct measurements of sodium conductance in the lobster giant axon by voltage-clamp techniques have shown that the local anaesthetic inhibition of sodium conductance can be reversed by increasing the calcium ion concentration, and conversely, reduction in calcium concentration accentuates the inhibitory effect of local anaesthetic drugs on sodium conductance [6]. The concept of a displacement of calcium from a membrane-binding site by local anaesthetic agents was forthcoming from experiments in isolated nerves, skeletal muscle, and *in vitro* phospholipid models. For example, procaine and tetracaine (amethocaine) were found to increase the rate of calcium efflux from isolated frog sciatic nerves and isolated sartorius muscle preparations which were equilibrated with labelled calcium for 8 hr [45]. Moreover, tetracaine was 10 times more potent than procaine in terms of increasing the rate of calcium efflux from sartorius muscle, which correlates well with the relative anaesthetic potency of these two drugs. Finally, Blaustein and Goldman showed that calcium binds to an *in vitro* phospholipid model, namely, phosphatidyl-*l*-serine [6a]. Addition of various local anaesthetic agents to a test-tube containing phosphatidyl-*l*-serine inhibited the binding of calcium to this particular phospholipid. A rough correlation existed between the degree of inhibition of calcium binding and the local anaesthetic potency of the various agents as determined on an isolated frog sciatic nerve. Thus, lidocaine was found to be 3·5 times as potent as procaine in terms of inhibiting calcium binding to phosphatidyl-*l*-serine and 3·8 times as potent as procaine in terms of blocking conduction in the isolated frog sciatic nerve. Tetracaine was approximately 10 times more potent than procaine as a blocker of nerve conduction and 30 times as potent in the prevention of calcium binding to phospholipids. On the basis of these results, it was proposed that the interaction of calcium and local anaesthetics represents the initial step in the mechanism of action of local anaesthetic drugs. Feinstein suggested that local anaesthetics may inhibit the release of calcium from binding sites in the membrane, which, in turn, would prevent the increased permeability of the cell membrane to sodium following application of a stimulus [61]. Blaustein and Goldman, on the other hand, theorized that, in fact, local anaesthetics may release calcium from the cell membrane and the local anaesthetics themselves may then attach to phospholipid-binding sites resulting in a greater degree of membrane stabilization and an inhibition of sodium permeability and sodium conductance. Although the above studies clearly indicate an interaction between calcium and local anaesthetics, they do not necessarily demonstrate that calcium inhibition or release from a binding site in the nerve membrane represents the initial step in the mechanism of action of local anaesthetic drugs. More recent studies would suggest that calcium is not essential to the action of local anaesthetic drugs and that the antagonistic effect of calcium and local anaesthetics is due to actions at different sites in the nerve membrane. The rationale for rejecting the hypothesis that an interaction between calcium and local anaesthetics represents the initial step in conduction blockade was critically reviewed by Strichartz [83]. As pointed out by the latter author, local anaesthetics depress sodium permeability with minimal effects on the voltage-dependence of sodium permeability, whereas calcium markedly shifts the voltage-dependence of sodium permeability. In addition, local anaesthetic blockade can be enhanced by increasing the frequency of nerve stimulation, whereas an increased frequency of stimulation tends to overcome calcium blockade. Finally, discrepancies exist concerning the antagonistic effect of calcium and local anaesthetics on impulse generation and sodium conductance. The reversal of the inhibitory action of procaine on sodium conductance by calcium in the lobster giant axon reported by Blaustein and Goldman [6] could not be confirmed by Narahashi et al. in the squid axon [56]. The latter investigators observed no difference in the dose–response curve relating concentration of procaine to percent suppression of sodium conductance when the squid axon was exposed to sea water containing either 10 mM or 100 mM of calcium. Strichartz has attempted to explain this discrepancy on the basis of a morphological difference between the various nerve preparations [83]. Lobster axons are tightly bound by a giant sheath through which local anaesthetics must diffuse in order to reach their site of action. Calcium may interfere with the passage of local anaesthetics through this giant sheath and, thereby, block their action. A similar diffusion barrier does not appear to exist in the squid axon.

Although most investigators at the present time do not believe that local anaesthetic agents act by means of a direct calcium inhibition or displacement mechanism, an indirect action between calcium and local anaesthetics obviously does exist. The ability of calcium to antagonize the action potential blockade of local anaesthetics in frog spinal ganglion cells was ascribed by Aceves and Machne to an action at different sites in the membrane [1]. The effect of calcium may be similar to that of membrane hyperpolarization on the slow inactivation of sodium [83]. As indicated previously, the degree of membrane depolarization is self-limiting due to spontaneous sodium inactivation, i.e. decrease in sodium permeability. Local anaesthetics enhance the degree of sodium inactivation, whereas hyperpolarization of the membrane by 30–40 mV and an increase in calcium concentration will tend to inhibit the process of sodium inactivation. Thus, hyperpolarization and calcium excess may counteract the action of local anaesthetics, but in a non-specific manner.

WHERE IS THE SITE OF ACTION OF LOCAL ANAESTHETIC AGENTS?

Although it is generally accepted that local anaesthetics act by decreasing sodium conductance across the nerve membrane, most studies in recent years have attempted to determine the specific site in the nerve membrane at which local anaesthetics exert their inhibitory action. Three specific sites have been suggested as possible locations for the action of local anaesthetics: (*a*) the surface of the nerve membrane; (*b*) within the nerve membrane; (*c*) specific receptors within the sodium channel. A brief review of the structure of the membrane may be appropriate to allow a clearer interpretation of these various theories concerning the possible site of action of local anaesthetics.

Morphology of the Nerve Membrane

Various molecular structures have been proposed for biological membranes including the axonal membrane. Danielli and Davson originally suggested that the cell membrane consisted of a lipid core arranged in such a fashion that the polar lipid heads were oriented in an outward direction and were covered by a non-lipid monolayer which was probably protein in nature [22] (*Fig. 2.7a*). Several modifications of this basic model have been proposed. For example, in 1959, Robertson advocated the term ‘the unit membrane’ as the fundamental unit of all biological membranes [65]. The unit membrane was visualized as consisting of a bimolecular leaflet of unspecified lipids at the centre, with the polar lipid heads pointing outward and covered on both exposed surfaces by a monolayer of non-lipids (*Fig. 2.7b*). This model differed from that of Danielli and Davson in that the non-lipid layers covering the internal and external surface of the polar lipid heads were believed to differ in chemical composition.

The basic features of these original membrane models were: (*a*) the concept that lipids represented the essential organizational elements of the membrane and (*b*) the bimolecular lipid layer and, therefore, the membrane itself was rigid in nature. Support for the importance of lipids in cell membranes derives from studies of the chemical composition of various types of membranes. For example, Camejo and co-workers [11] attempted an analysis of the axolemma of the first stellar nerve of the giant squid by extruding the axoplasm and subjecting the remaining material, presumably axolemma, to centrifugation. These investigators concluded that the protein to lipid ratio for the squid axolemma was 0·13, indicating that approximately 90 per cent of the axolemma consisted of lipids. Most of the lipids existed in the form of phospholipids such as phosphatidylcholine, phosphatidylethanolamine, phosphatidylserine and sphingomyelin.

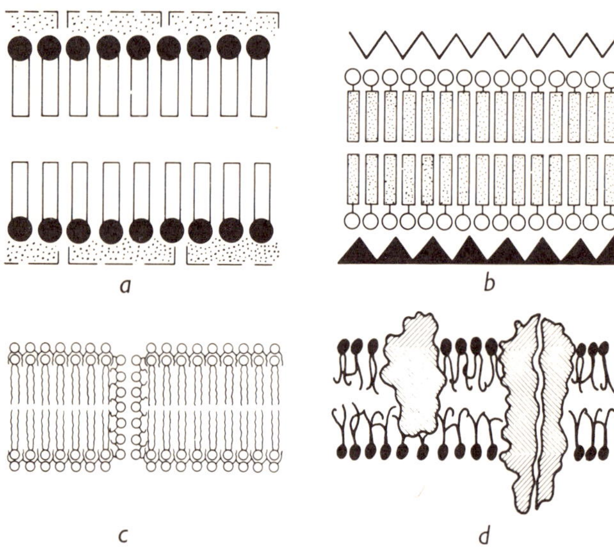

Fig. 2.7. Representative membrane models. *a* depicts the original bilipid leaflet model. Model *b* suggests that the internal and external surfaces of polar lipid heads differ in chemical composition. Model *c* incorporates the concept of membrane pore. Model *d* depicts the heterogeneous non-rigid membrane model with pore extending through protein globule.

The concept of a rigid membrane was consistent with the original belief that the function of membranes was to act as barriers. In an effort to explain the rapid movement of ions and other molecular substances across cell membranes, the intact lipid-bilayer model was modified to include pores through which ionic fluxes could occur. These pores were visualized as channels lined with proteins and extending from the extracellular to the intracellular surface of the membrane (*Fig. 2.7c*).

The second generation of membrane models resulted when proteins rather than lipids were suggested as the basic molecular components of membranes [51]. Singer stated that 50–75 per cent by weight of nearly all membranes with the exception of myelin consisted of proteins [75]. In addition, these recent concepts of membrane structure differed from the original models since they were visualized as more heterogeneous in nature [75] (*Fig. 2.7d*). The proteins were conceived as globular molecules of varying size. Some of the protein globules transversed the entire width of the membrane, while others extended only partway through the membrane. These protein globular structures were believed to be partly hydrophobic. The hydrophobic portion was that embedded in the lipid bilayer, while the hydrophilic end (or ends) would project out into the extracellular or intracellular aqueous medium. Furthermore, Singer and Nicholson conceived of the membrane as a fluid mosaic which could change its configuration, rather than a rigid structure [76]. Ionic transport across the membrane is visualized as occurring through water-filled channels formed by the clustering of protein subunits [75]. At rest, the diameter of these channels would be of such a size as to restrict the movement of sodium ions. Upon activation of the membrane, a conformational change would occur which would result in dilation of the channels to permit the passage of sodium ions and so lead to membrane depolarization. The movement of ions such as sodium could either occur by diffusion following channel dilation, or following activation, the membrane could change its conformation so as to trap the sodium ion on the extracellular surface, 'squeeze' it through the membrane, and expel it into the intracellular space. Irrespective of the precise structure and composition of the nerve membrane, it is apparent that lipids and proteins play an essential role in the molecular organization of the membrane and that local anaesthetic agents must interact in some way with them to impede neural conduction.

Membrane Surface Location

This location has been implicated in the so-called 'surface charge theory' of local anaesthetic activity. The resting potential of a nerve membrane determined by placement of electrodes in the axoplasm and in solution bathing an isolated nerve reflects the relative bulk concentration of intra- and extracellular ions. However, the surface of the cell membrane contains an excess of fixed negative charges due to the proteins and phospholipids in the cell membrane. The relative negativity of the exterior and interior surfaces of the cell membrane is responsible for the actual potential difference across the membrane, which determines the rate of sodium and potassium current during the action potential (*Fig. 2.8*). The potential difference across the membrane itself is less than the potential difference between the intra- and extracellular space. Changes in the degree of negativity at the surface of the membrane can alter the transmembrane potential and influence sodium conductance without altering the resting potential inside the nerve cell.

The surface charge theory postulates that local anaesthetic agents penetrate and are bound to the membrane in such a way that the lipophilic aromatic end of the molecule is embedded in the membrane, while the positively charged polar end extends into the extracellular aqueous medium

(*Fig. 2.8*). As a result of this alignment, the fixed negative charges on the membrane surface are partially neutralized, resulting in an increase in the transmembrane potential, while the resting intracellular potential is unaltered. If the increase in transmembrane potential is of sufficient magnitude, electrotonic currents from neighbouring unanaesthetized portions of the nerve membrane would be incapable of reducing the membrane potential to its threshold or firing level such that depolarization would be inhibited and conduction blockade would ensue. Support for the

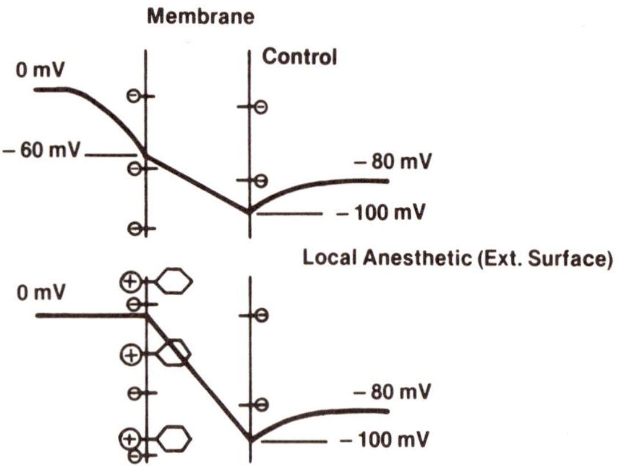

Fig. 2.8. Alteration in transmembrane potential difference by penetration of local anaesthetics into the membrane with their charged polar ends extending onto aqueous surface of the membrane.

surface charge theory has emanated mainly from studies involving *in vitro* monolayer and phospholipid-bilayer membranes. Skou originally showed a correlation between the anaesthetic potency of various tertiary amine compounds and their ability to penetrate a monolayer of lipids from peripheral nerves [79]. More recently, Hendrickson demonstrated that the relative penetration into monolayers of didecanoylphosphatidylcholine of various local anaesthetics was correlated with their conduction-blocking potency and their lipid solubility [33]. Subsequently, dibucaine (cinchocaine), tetracaine, cocaine, lidocaine and procaine were found to inhibit the efflux of sodium ions across phosphatidylserine vesicles [60]. Finally, Singer [73, 74] and McLaughlin [49] demonstrated that local anaesthetics such as lidocaine and dibucaine were capable of decreasing the negative surface charge and inhibiting the cationic permeability of phospholipid-bilayer membranes. The correlation between the anaesthetic activity of various agents and their ability to penetrate, inhibit sodium permeability, and decrease the surface charge of phospholipid membranes is presented in Table 2.1.

Table 2.1. C_m of Various Local Anaesthetics for Conduction Blockade and Depression of Cation Conductance in Phospholipid Bilayer Membranes

Agent	Conduction blockade (frog sciatic nerve)	Inhibition of cation conductance		
		Phosphatidyl-ethanolamine	*Phosphatidyl-glycerol*	*Phosphatidyl-serine*
Procaine	1×10^{-3}	6×10^{-2}	3×10^{-3}	2×10^{-3}
Lidocaine	3×10^{-4}	1×10^{-2}	1×10^{-3}	6×10^{-4}
Tetracaine	3×10^{-5}	4×10^{-4}	2×10^{-5}	3×10^{-5}
Dibucaine	2×10^{-5}	2×10^{-4}	1×10^{-5}	2×10^{-5}

Data derived from McLaughlin [49].

The surface charge theory requires that the cationic form of local anaesthetics represents the active conduction-blocking moiety. As will be described later, this has been demonstrated by Ritchie and Greengard [61]. In addition, the membrane surface location is also consistent with the direct relationship between anaesthetic potency and lipid solubility, and would also explain the apparent antagonism between calcium and local anaesthetic agents without requiring a direct interaction between them as an essential component of conduction blockade. This hypothesis, however, is incapable of explaining the anaesthetic activity of agents such as benzocaine which exist only in an uncharged form.

Location within the Nerve Membrane

The highly lipid nature of the nerve membrane and the relationship between local anaesthetic potency and lipid solubility has led some investigators to conclude that the site of action of local anaesthetic agents resides within the lipid component of the nerve membrane. Seeman studied a number of different agents capable of producing conduction blockade and reported that an inverse correlation existed between the membrane/buffer partition coefficient of the agents and the concentration required in the membrane to cause conduction block [69].

An intramembranal site of action of local anaesthetic agents is visualized as involving some type of conformational change in the organization of the membrane. The alteration most commonly postulated is membrane expansion or change in critical volume. The membrane expansion theory of local anaesthesia is basically an extension of the Meyer–Overton law for general anaesthesia, which stated that the physicochemical combination of an anaesthetic substance with cell lipids causes a change in the relationship between cell constituents which, in turn, leads to an inhibition of cell function. Originally the membrane expansion theory of local anaesthesia suggested a constriction of the sodium channels due to increased lateral pressure within the membrane [70]. *In vitro* studies by Skou, in which the surface pressure of monomolecular layers of lipids increased following placement of local anaesthetics into the solution below the lipid layer, served as the basis for this concept of lateral expansion within the membrane [78]. Seeman has attempted to quantitate the actual change in volume of membranes during conditions of local anaesthesia [69]. In general, membrane concentrations of 0·04 mol/kg of membrane are required for the production of conduction blockade. This concentration occupies a volume of 0·3 per cent of the membrane which results in a 2–3 per cent expansion of the membrane. The membrane expansion theory holds a certain attraction for several reasons. It would readily explain the site and mechanism of action of local anaesthetic agents that exist only in an uncharged form, such as benzocaine and benzyl alcohol. Moreover, it would also provide a single theory for the site and mechanism of action of both general and local anaesthetic drugs. With regard to general anaesthetic agents, one of the critical experiments that has been quoted to support the concept of membrane expansion or increase in volume involves reversal of anaesthesia by exposure to elevated atmospheric pressures. This can be dramatically demonstrated in the following fashion: addition of general anaesthetics to a bath containing tadpoles abolishes the spontaneous swimming of the tadpoles. When the bath containing the anaesthetized tadpoles is exposed to hydrostatic pressures of 150–350 atm, swimming motion is again re-established indicating a removal of the state of anaesthesia. In addition, emulsions of general anaesthetics can produce conduction block in a variety of peripheral nerves, which can then be antagonized by an increase in atmospheric pressure. Similar studies with local anaesthetic agents are limited and contradictory in nature. Roth et al. reported that high pressure could reverse the depression of action potential amplitude in frog sciatic nerves produced by chloroform, diethyl ether (anaesthetic ether) and halothane. However, no pressure-induced antagonism of action potential depression due to procaine or dibucaine was observed [66]. Similar studies were conducted by Kendig and Cohen utilizing the preganglionic sympathetic nerve of the superior cervical ganglion of the rat [44]. Depression of action potential amplitude was induced following exposure to the general anaesthetics, halothane and methoxyflurane, the local anaesthetics, lidocaine, procaine and benzocaine, the biotoxin, TTX, a quaternary amine analogue of lidocaine, QX-572, and the spin-label molecule, TEMPO. Subsequent exposure of the blocked nerves to high pressure helium resulted in partial, but significant antagonism of the halothane, methoxyflurane, benzocaine, lidocaine and TEMPO induced action potential depression.

However, no pressure reversal of procaine, QX-572 or TTX induced depression was observed. These findings are consistent with the hypothesis that conduction blockade may be related, in part, to membrane expansion following penetration of the uncharged form of local anaesthetic into the interior of the cell membrane. Since QX-572 and TTX exist only in a charged form, these agents presumably are incapable of membrane expansion. The absence of pressure antagonism to procaine is probably related to the high pK_a of this agent [5], which means that at a pH of 7·4, less than 5 per cent of procaine exists in an uncharged form. These findings by Kendig and Cohen differ from the results of Boggs and co-workers [7]. The latter investigators utilized the rat phrenic nerve and desheathed frog sciatic nerve to study the interaction of high pressure and local anaesthetic blockade. The spin-label molecule, TEMPO, produced a 68 per cent decrease in action potential amplitude at normal atmospheric pressure. Upon application of 100 atm of helium pressure, a further reduction of 14 per cent in action potential height occurred. High pressure had no observable effect on the action potential depression produced by lidocaine and benzyl alcohol. Thus, it appears that high pressure may enhance, antagonize, or exert no effect on conduction blockade produced in peripheral nerves by various local anaesthetic substances.

A number of modifications of the membrane expansion theory have been proposed, all of which are based on an intramembrane site of anaesthetic action. A variety of experimental techniques such as nuclear magnetic resonance have been employed to study changes in the fluidity of model membranes following exposure to local anaesthetic agents. Phospholipid membranes may undergo a transition from a gel–crystalline to a liquid–crystalline state. Various clinically useful local anaesthetics such as procaine, lidocaine, tetracaine and bupivacaine have been shown to increase the fluidity of these phospholipid membranes [90]. This increase in the freedom of movement of lipid molecules within the membrane may occur with or without a concomitant increase in the volume of the membrane. For example, the increase in fluidity or disorder of the lipid molecules may result in conformational changes in the membrane proteins which are closely associated with the lipids. The concept of increased fluidity of lipid molecules resulting either in an expansion of the membrane or a conformational change in membrane proteins is consistent with the fluid mosaic membrane model proposed by Singer.

Irrespective of the precise membrane perturbation produced by local anaesthetics, the common feature of these various theories involves a decrease in the diameter of the sodium channel or a prevention of sodium channel dilation upon membrane activation. Therefore, the local anaesthetics are perceived as penetrating the interior of the cell membrane, producing a conformational change in the membrane which results in a decreased sodium permeability and ultimately conduction blockade. Although the site of local anaesthetic action within the nerve membrane is attractive from a theoretical point of view, it is difficult to prove experimentally that membrane conformational changes can produce conduction blockade. In addition, although the suggestive evidence is strong that uncharged forms of local anaesthetics may act from within the cell membrane, the data are not equally strong regarding charged local anaesthetics. Finally, some data exist which indicate that local anaesthetics stabilize and inhibit conformational changes in certain membranes (rat liver mitochondria) rather than inducing alterations in membrane configuration [42].

Specific Receptor Sites within the Sodium Channel

The third and most common site proposed for the action of local anaesthetic agents involves specific receptors within the sodium channel. The concept of a drug–receptor interaction has been considered essential to the mechanism of most pharmacological agents. Thus, it is not surprising that attempts have been made to demonstrate that local anaesthetics also act by combining with a specific receptor site in the nerve membrane. Neither of the previous two theories concerning the site and mechanism of action of local anaesthetics implied a drug–receptor interaction. Both the surface charge and membrane expansion or perturbation hypotheses simply require penetration of the anaesthetic substance into the lipoprotein matrix of the membrane. The concept of a specific receptor site for local anaesthetic activity is based on the following information: (*a*) *in vitro* biochemical evidence that local anaesthetic agents can bind to phospholipids and/or proteins; (*b*) demonstration that the cationic form of local anaesthetics is essential for conduction blockade; (*c*) specificity of optical isomers of local anaesthetic drugs; (*d*) selectivity of binding of the biotoxins, TTX and STX; (*e*) modulation of local anaesthesia by the frequency of nerve stimulation.

In Vitro *Binding Studies*

It has been demonstrated that local anaesthetic agents are capable of binding both to phospholipids and proteins. Feinstein has suggested that one local anaesthetic molecule may serve as an electrostatic bond between the negatively charged phosphate groups of two phospholipid molecules [25]. In addition, evidence exists for the formation of hydrogen bonds between local anaesthetics and phospholipids [67]. Protein binding of local anaesthetics has also been well documented. Studies on nerve homogenates revealed that approximately 75 per cent of tetracaine is bound to proteins as compared to 6 per cent for procaine [88]. Subsequent studies with plasma proteins have shown that all amide-type local anaesthetics are capable of binding to protein, but to varying degrees [89]. A direct correlation exists between the degree of protein binding and the duration of conduction blockade. For example, action potentials recorded from the surface of an isolated frog sciatic nerve are depressed by 50 per cent following exposure to 20 mM of lidocaine, but return to their control height within 30 min following removal of lidocaine from the bathing solution. Similar experiments with bupivacaine or etidocaine show that approximately 2 hr is required for complete reversal of conduction blockade. In terms of protein binding, lidocaine is 55 per cent bound to plasma proteins, whereas bupivacaine and etidocaine are 95 per cent protein bound. It is acknowledged that these studies do not prove that local anaesthetics combine with a specific receptor in the membrane. Nevertheless, the fact that these agents can bind to lipoproteins, the lipoprotein composition of the nerve membrane and the relationship between protein binding and anaesthetic activity are certainly suggestive of a local anaesthetic–lipoprotein receptor interaction.

Cationic Anaesthetic Moiety Causes Conduction Blockade at the Internal Surface of the Nerve Membrane

In solution, the clinically useful local anaesthetic agents exist both in the form of uncharged molecules (B) and as positively charged cations (BH^+). The relative proportion between the uncharged base (B) and the charged cation (BH^+) is dependent on the pH of the solution and the pK_a of the specific chemical compound and can be determined by the Henderson–Hasselbalch equation:

$$pH = pK_a + \log [B]/[BH^+].$$

Since the pK_a is constant for any specific compound, the relative proportion of free base and charged cation in a local anaesthetic solution is basically dependent on the pH of the solution ($BH^+ \rightleftharpoons B + H^+$). As the pH of the solution is decreased and hydrogen ion concentration is increased, the equilibrium will shift toward the charged cationic form. Conversely, an increase in pH and decrease in hydrogen ions will result in the formation of relatively greater amounts of the free base form. Ritchie et al. used this knowledge to design a series of experiments which evaluated the relationship between the pH of solutions of lidocaine and dibucaine and local anaesthetic activity in isolated desheathed mammalian and amphibian nerves [62, 63]. At a pH of 7·2, dibucaine (10 μM) produced a 90 per cent reduction in spike potential amplitude, whereas only a 10 per cent depression in spike potential occurred when the pH was elevated to 9·2. Similarly, 300 μM of lidocaine produced almost complete abolition of the spike potential at a pH of 7·2. In an alkaline solution (pH = 9·2–10·7), the same concentration of lidocaine resulted in only a 50 per cent decrease in action potential amplitude (*Fig. 2.9*).

Under these experimental conditions, the less alkaline local anaesthetic solution, which would contain a relatively greater amount of the charged cation (BH^+), clearly was more active in terms of conduction blockade. When nerves were exposed to *n*-butanol or benzyl alcohol, which exist only in the uncharged form regardless of pH, depression of action potential amplitude was unaffected by pH changes between 7·0 and 9·0. However, an increase in pH to 10·5 did enhance the anaesthetic effect of these agents. The results of these studies strongly support the charged cationic form of conventional local anaesthetics as the active moiety responsible for conduction blockade. Demonstration of the charged cationic form as the active anaesthetic entity is important to the theory of a specific local

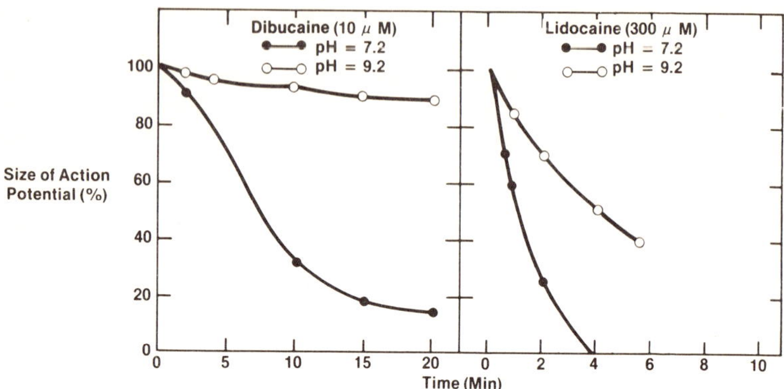

Fig. 2.9. Effect of pH on the reduction in action potential amplitude of desheathed rabbit vagus nerve produced by dibucaine and lidocaine. (*Data derived from references 62 and 63.*)

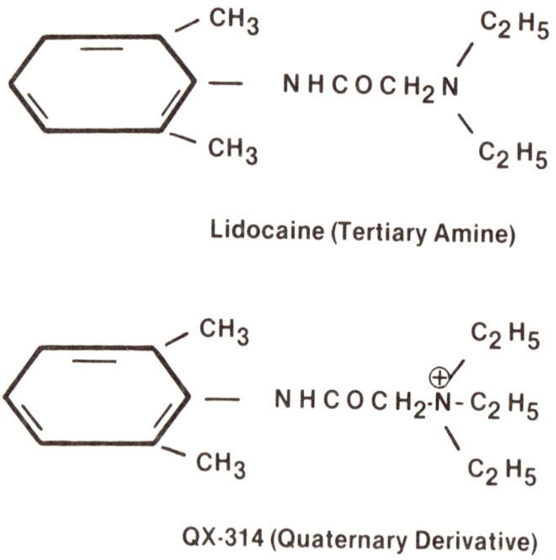

CH_3 C_2H_5

— $NHCOCH_2N$

CH_3 C_2H_5

Lidocaine (Tertiary Amine)

CH_3 C_2H_5

— $NHCOCH_2\text{-}\overset{\oplus}{N}\text{-}C_2H_5$

CH_3 C_2H_5

QX-314 (Quaternary Derivative)

Fig. 2.10. Comparative chemical structures of a tertiary amine local anaesthetic, lidocaine, and its quaternary derivative, QX–314.

anaesthetic receptor, since electrostatic binding is probably involved in the interaction between anaesthetic agent and a lipoprotein receptor. However, these studies do not indicate where the receptor site is located.

Narahashi and co-workers conducted a series of experiments in which the squid giant axon was perfused either externally or internally with various local anaesthetic solutions [27, 57, 58]. Initially, two tertiary and two quaternary derivatives of lidocaine were studied. The tertiary amine derivatives can exist partially in a charged and uncharged form, whereas the quaternary compounds possess only a charged configuration (*Fig. 2.10*). Experiments were performed in which the axon was perfused either internally or externally with the local anaesthetic agents and the pH of the perfusing solution was varied from 7·0 to 9·0. When the tertiary amine compound, 6211, was applied externally at a concentration of 1 mM, a 13 per cent decrease in the maximum rate of rise of the action potential (dV/dt) was observed. Increasing the pH from 7·0 to 9·0 did not affect the degree of reduction in dV/dt. Internal perfusion with 1 mM of 6211 at a pH of 7·0 caused a 57 per cent decrease in dV/dt. The same concentration of 6211 produced only a 20 per cent reduction in dV/dt when the pH of the internal perfusion medium was elevated to 8·0. Since the increase in pH would tend to lower the relative concentration of the cationic form of 6211, these results again demonstrate that the charged moiety is responsible for conduction blockade (Table 2.2). In addition, these data suggest that

Table 2.2. Effects of Internal Perfusion of 1 mM of Tertiary (6211) and Quaternary (QX–314) Derivatives of Lidocaine on the Maximum Rate of Rise of the Action Potential (dV/dt) of the Squid Giant Axon

Parameters	*6211 (1 mM)*		*QX–314 (10 mM)*	
Chemical structure	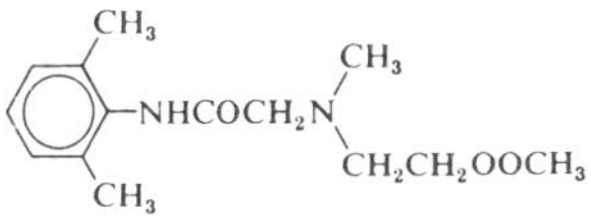 2,6-dimethylphenyl–$NHCOCH_2N(CH_3)CH_2CH_2OOCH_3$		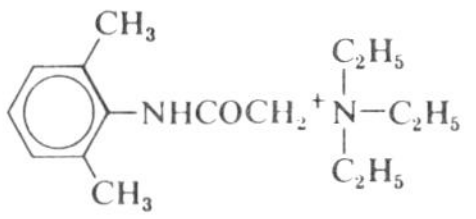 2,6-dimethylphenyl–$NHCOCH_2{}^{+}N(C_2H_5)_3$	
Internal pH	7·0	8·0	7·0	8·0
Percentage in dV/dt	57	20	33	37

Data derived from Narahashi et al. [57] and Frazier et al. [27].

the local anaesthetic receptor was located on the inner surface of the nerve membrane, since internal perfusion with 6211 was more efficacious in reducing dV/dt than external perfusion. However, tertiary amines are capable of diffusing across membranes so that they are effective conduction blockers following either external or internal application. In order to overcome the problem of diffusion, quaternary derivatives of lidocaine were utilized. Since these compounds exist only as cations, they do not diffuse readily across membranes. External application of 10 mM of the quaternary compound, QX-314 (*Fig. 2.10*), produced less than a 10 per cent decrease in dV/dt in the squid axon. Internal perfusion of 1 mM of QX-314 caused a mean reduction of 67 per cent in dV/dt (Table 2.2). Strichartz extended the studies of Narahashi and co-workers by determining the effects of the quaternary derivatives of lidocaine on sodium permeability of the frog sciatic nerve [81]. External application of 5 mM of QX-314 decreased the amplitude of the inward sodium currents by 7 per cent. By contrast, internal application of only 0·5 mM of QX-314 diminished the sodium currents by almost 90 per cent. These results indicate that the receptor site for local anaesthetic activity is not only located at the inner surface of the membrane, but probably in close association with the opening of the sodium channel on the inside of the membrane. Since all the above studies were carried out with lidocaine and its derivatives, Narahashi and Frazier investigated the effects of internal and external perfusion of procaine at different pH levels on the sodium permeability of the squid axon. The results demonstrated that procaine also acts primarily in the cationic form at the internal opening of the sodium channel [55].

Specificity of Optical Isomers of Local Anaesthetics

The differential action of optical isomers of a drug is usually accepted as proof of the existence of a stereospecific receptor. Akerman studied the optical isomers of a series of different local anaesthetics including certain agents which are employed clinically, e.g. prilocaine, mepivacaine and bupivacaine [4]. For example, the levo form of prilocaine was twice as potent as the dextro form in terms of producing corneal anaesthesia in rabbits and cutaneous anaesthesia in guinea-pigs. Studies on the isolated sheathed and desheathed frog sciatic nerve showed as much as a fivefold difference in conduction-blocking activity between the isomers of different local anaesthetics, e.g. levo-bupivacaine was approximately four times more potent than dextro-bupivacaine. The most detailed study concerning site and mechanism of action of optical isomers was carried out with an experimental compound, RAC 109 (Table 2.3). This local anaesthetic

Table 2.3. Relative Activity of the Isomers of RAC 109 on Action Potential Amplitude (AP) and Sodium Conductance (g_{Na}) of Frog Sciatic Nerve and Maximum Rate of Rise of Action Potential (dV/dt) of Squid Giant Axon

Parameters	*RAC 109 I*	*RAC 109 II*	*Ratio I/II*
C_m for AP sheathed nerve	$1{\cdot}7 \times 10^{-4}$	$8{\cdot}0 \times 10^{-4}$	4·7
C_m for AP desheathed nerve	$8{\cdot}0 \times 10^{-5}$	$2{\cdot}4 \times 10^{-4}$	3·0
Percentage decrease in g_{Na} (0·28 mM)	76	47	1·6
Percentage decrease in dV/dt (1·0 mM)	86	70	1·2

Data derived from Akerman [4].

substance is a succinimide derivative (*Fig. 2.11*), in contrast to an agent such as lidocaine which is an anilide derivative. The enantiomers of RAC 109 were designated simply RAC 109 I and RAC 109 II. Although the absolute configuration of these two isomers is not known, they do possess opposite steric configurations. Measurements of the maximum rate of rise of the action potential of the squid axon revealed that 1·0 mM of RAC 109 I caused an 88 per cent reduction in dV/dt following internal perfusion, while the same concentration of RAC 109 II produced only a 53 per cent decrease in dV/dt. Subsequent voltage-clamp studies on the frog sciatic nerve demonstrated a 76 per cent reduction in sodium conductance following application of 0·28 mM of RAC 109 I, but only 42–57 per cent decrease in sodium permeability when RAC 109 II was used. Although these results were strongly indicative of the presence of a stereospecific local anaesthetic receptor, the possibility remained that the difference in activity between isomers might be related to differential uptake and

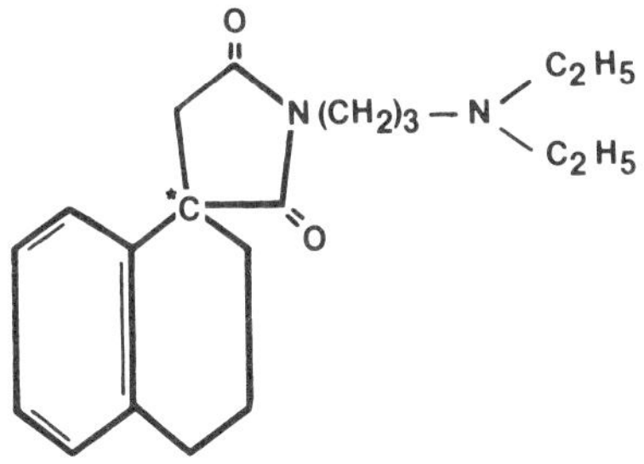

O
N(CH2)3 — N
C2H5
C2H5
*C
O

RAC 109 I and II

* = Asymmetrical Carbon

Fig. 2.11. Chemical structure of RAC 109 which can exist as optical isomer I and II.

penetration of the membrane. This possibility was evaluated by Akerman in several ways. The uptake of radioactive RAC 109 I and II by both sheathed and desheathed frog sciatic nerves was measured and no difference was observed in the uptake of the two isomers by the isolated sciatic nerve. Additional studies also failed to reveal any difference between the uptake and binding of radioactive RAC 109 I and II to erythrocyte and synaptosome membranes or to the phospholipid, phosphatidylserine, which is known to be a component of nerve membrane. Since the isomers of RAC 109 penetrate membranes to the same extent, possess similar physical–chemical properties and similar proportions of charged and uncharged forms, their differential anaesthetic potencies would be difficult to explain in terms of the surface charge theory or change in membrane volume or configuration hypothesis. The action of the optical isomers of RAC 109 are consistent with the concept of differential binding to stereospecific receptors located at the opening of the sodium channel on the inner surface of the nerve membrane.

Selectivity of Binding of Biotoxins, Tetrodotoxin and Saxitoxin

Other agents exist which are capable of causing conduction blockade and which may act at specific receptor sites other than that described for the conventional type of local anaesthetic drug. Specifically, several naturally occurring biotoxins, namely saxitoxin (STX) and tetrodotoxin (TTX) (*Fig. 2.12*), exist which are capable of producing profound conduction blockade in isolated nerves, but appear to act at the external surface of the nerve membrane rather than the internal surface. TTX is a product mainly of the ovaries of the puffer fish located along the coast of Japan [43], while STX is produced by certain marine dinoflagellates and is believed to

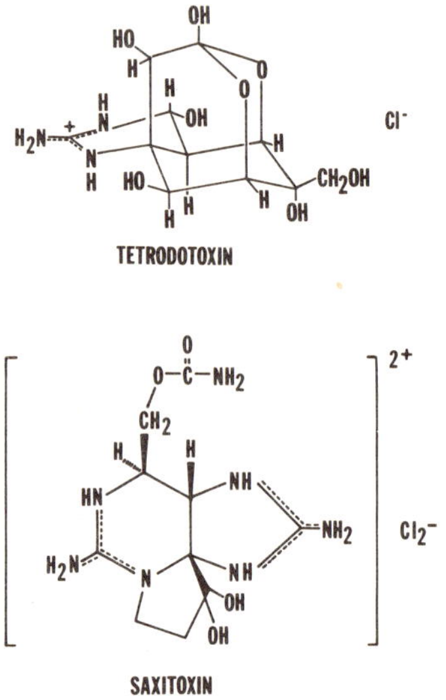

TETRODOTOXIN

SAXITOXIN

Fig. 2.12. Chemical structures of tetrodotoxin and saxitoxin.

be the agent contaminating certain shellfish which may lead to paralytic shellfish poisoning in man [72]. These substances are unique biologically, since they act specifically on the sodium channel to inhibit sodium conductance. Their site of action appears to be located on the external surface of the sodium channel [53], since internal and external perfusion of the giant squid axon with solutions of TTX revealed that external perfusion with 1×10^{-7} M resulted in inhibition of a propagated action potential within 3–6 min. On the other hand, axoplasmic perfusion with 1×10^{-6} M and 1×10^{-5} M TTX for as long as 17–37 min had no effect on the maximum rate of rise of the action potential. Further evidence that these substances act at the external surface of the sodium channel obtained from studies in which conventional local anaesthetics such as lidocaine, which act at the internal surface of the nerve membrane, failed to alter the binding of the biotoxins to the membrane [14, 32].

On the other hand, a competitive antagonism does exist between TTX and STX. Henderson et al. demonstrated that the specific binding of 4 nM of STX to frog myelinated fibres was reduced by 95 per cent when 500 nM of TTX was added to the perfusion medium [32]. Divalent ions such as calcium which are believed to act at the external surface of the nerve membrane also are capable of displacing TTX and STX from membrane binding sites. For example, in the absence of calcium, 100 per cent of TTX and STX are bound to solubilized garfish membrane preparations. In the presence of 50 nM of calcium, only 28 per cent of TTX and 34 per cent of STX were bound to the garfish membrane preparation.

The receptors of TTX and STX are believed to be located at the opening of the sodium channels at the external surface of the membrane. As mentioned previously, Hille has provided quantitative data on the degree of sodium conductance inhibition produced by TTX and STX in the frog sciatic nerve [36]. The binding of the biotoxins to the external opening of the sodium channel is so specific that these agents have been utilized to determine the size and number of sodium channels in various nerve preparations. Hille has calculated that the external opening of the sodium channel is a space 3 Å wide by 5 Å long lined by six oxygen atoms [37]. One molecule of TTX or STX will occupy one sodium channel opening. On the basis of the studies with TTX and STX, it was concluded that approximately 30 sodium channels/cm^2 exist in the rabbit vagus nerve, whereas in the non-myelinated fibres of the garfish olfactory nerve, there are only 6 sodium channels/cm^2 [14, 32]. However, studies utilizing an improved method for labelling STX indicated a significantly greater density of sodium channels [64]. Data presented by Ritchie et al. based on STX-binding sites calculated 110 sodium channels/cm^2 in garfish nerves [64]. In summary, the investigations with the biotoxins provide additional evidence that the basic mechanism of local anaesthesia involves combination with a specific membrane receptor which is located at the sodium channel. The only difference between the biotoxins and the conventional local anaesthetics such as lidocaine is the receptor site location. The biotoxin receptor apparently is located at the external opening of the sodium channel, while the receptor for the conventional local anaesthetics is present at the internal opening of the sodium channel.

Modulation of Local Anaesthesia by Frequency of Nerve Stimulation

The studies described so far have provided evidence that the local anaesthetic receptor is actually located within the sodium channel. As indicated previously, Strichartz demonstrated that the quaternary derivative of lidocaine, QX-314, could inhibit sodium currents by more than 90 per cent following axoplasmic perfusion of the frog sciatic nerve [81]. Application of depolarizing pulses of 5 msec duration at 1 sec intervals enhanced the rate and degree of sodium permeability inhibition produced by QX-314. This phenomenon has been referred to as 'use-dependent inhibition' [83]. An increase in frequency of stimulation without a local anaesthetic does not affect the sodium currents. In the absence of depolarizing pulses, QX-314 requires 20–30 min to produce a maximum inhibition of sodium permeability. A combination of internal perfusion of the membrane with QX-314 and application of 20 depolarizing pulses to a level of +75 mV will cause maximal inhibition of sodium permeability within 5 min. In addition, a direct correlation exists between the frequency of nerve stimulation and the degree of sodium conductance blockade (*Fig. 2.13*).

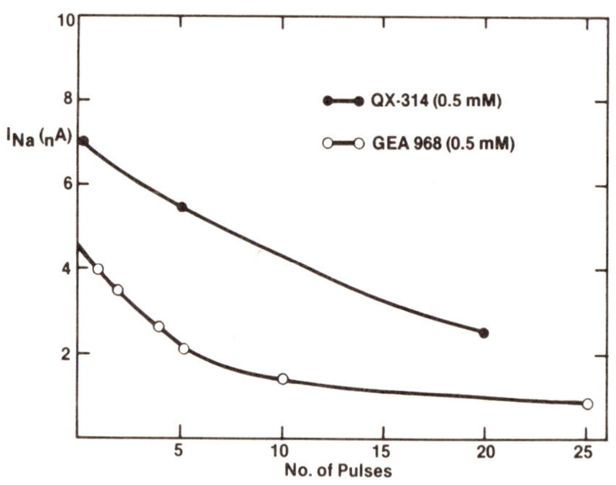

Fig. 2.13. Relationship between frequency of nerve stimulation and inhibition of inward sodium current (I_{Na}) by QX-314 and GEA 968. (*Data derived from Strichartz [81] and Courtney [18].*)

Similar studies were conducted by Courtney with the tertiary amine type of local anaesthetic agents [18]. Most of the experiments were performed with an experimental tertiary amine compound, GEA 968, which is structurally related to lidocaine (*Fig. 2.14*). Again, a direct correlation was found between the frequency of stimulation and the degree of inhibition of inward sodium currents in myelinated frog nerves. In the presence of 0·5 mM of GEA 968, repetitive depolarization at the rate of 2 pulses/sec resulted in a progressive decrease in sodium conductance, such that inward sodium current was decreased by 76 per cent after 25 pulses (*Fig. 2.13*). Similar frequency-dependent inhibition of sodium permeability was observed with procaine and lidocaine, although frequencies of, at least, 2 pulses/sec were required to clearly demonstrate this relationship with lidocaine.

Following maximal depression of sodium permeability and a period of rest, the inhibitory effect of both tertiary amine and quaternary type local anaesthetics can be reversed by an increase in the frequency of nerve stimulation. Under conditions in which a large hyperpolarizing prepulse is applied to the nerve followed by a series of depolarizing pulses, the rate of reversal of local anaesthetic activity is directly related to the frequency of stimulation. This phenomenon of use- or frequency-dependent inhibition has been interpreted in the following manner. The sodium channel contains two gates, the h and m^3 gates as designated by Hodgkin and Huxley. At rest, these gates are closed which prevents sodium flux across the membrane. During nerve stimulation, the gates are open to allow the influx of sodium ions which is essential for membrane depolarization. An increase in the frequency of stimulation will permit the h and m^3 gates to remain in an open state for a longer period of time. In addition, the degree of the

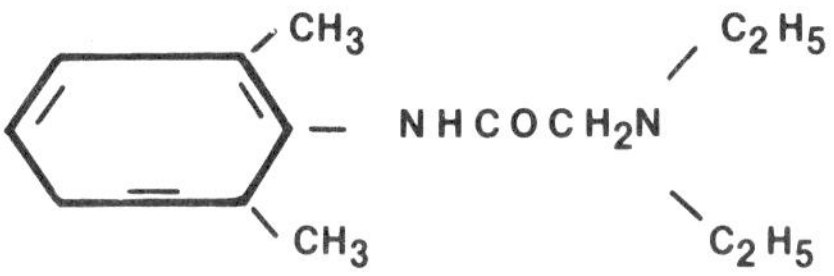

CH_3 C_2H_5
— $NHCOCH_2N$
CH_3 C_2H_5

Lidocaine

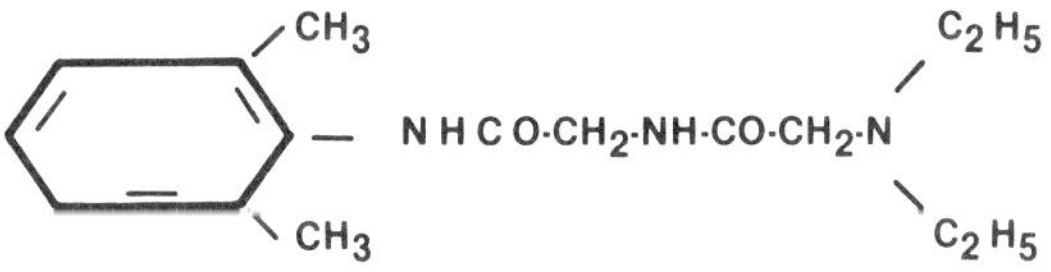

CH_3 C_2H_5
— $NHCO\text{-}CH_2\text{-}NH\text{-}CO\text{-}CH_2\text{-}N$
CH_3 C_2H_5

GEA-968

Fig. 2.14. Comparison of chemical structures of lidocaine and GEA 968.

depolarization pulses will determine the number of channels that are open. The size and number of depolarizing pulses basically effect the phase of sodium activation. Application of a hyperpolarizing prepulse to the membrane is believed to prevent the phase of sodium inactivation. Thus, the combination of a hyperpolarizing prepulse and a series of depolarizing pulses of optimal size will maximize the number and duration of sodium channels opened. Both tertiary and quaternary local anaesthetic activity is enhanced, has a shorter latency, and also is dissipated more rapidly when the gates of the sodium channels are open. This strongly supports the concept that a specific local anaesthetic receptor is located within the sodium channel which is readily accessible when sodium gates are in the open position.

Multiple vs Single Site of Anaesthetic Action

On the basis of studies with various substances that can produce conduction blockade in peripheral nerve, two theories have currently evolved concerning the site of action of local anaesthetic agents. Takman has summarized the various sites of action proposed by different authors for various substances that can cause conduction blockade and attempted to provide a biological classification of local anaesthetic agents based on these different sites of action [84]. According to Takman's classification, local anaesthetic type substances can be categorized in the following manner:

CLASS A Agents acting at a receptor site on the external surface of the sodium channel. This would include the biotoxin substances, TTX and STX.

CLASS B Agents acting at a receptor site at the axoplasmic side of the sodium channel. These would include the quaternary derivatives of lidocaine such as QX-314, QX-572 and QX-222.

CLASS C Agents acting within the nerve membrane causing an increase in the volume and expansion of the membrane or a change in membrane configuration. Such agents would include benzocaine, *n*-butanol and benzyl alcohol, i.e. the neutral type of local anaesthetic drugs.

CLASS D Agents which may act both at the axoplasmic side of the sodium channel and also within the membrane through a physicochemical mechanism. This would include most of the clinically useful local anaesthetic agents, since they exist both in charged and uncharged form, e.g. procaine, tetracaine, lidocaine, mepivacaine, prilocaine, bupivacaine and etidocaine. The cationic form of these drugs would interact with a specific receptor in the axoplasmic portion of the sodium channel while the base uncharged form would act by a physicochemical mechanism within the membrane. Narahashi and Frazier have suggested that approximately 90 per cent of the blocking action of an agent such as lidocaine is referable to its cationic form and 10 per cent is due to the base form [54].

More recently, Hille has attempted to provide a unified theory for the site of action of both charged and uncharged forms of local anaesthetic drugs [38, 39]. Since it is generally accepted that local anaesthetics act by decreasing sodium permeability, Hille employed a voltage-clamp technique to study the action of tertiary amine, quaternary and neutral type local anaesthetics on sodium conductance in myelinated fibres of the isolated frog sciatic nerve. Hille's theory was based on re-evaluation of the relationship between lipid solubility, pH, voltage and frequency-dependent modulation and the rate, degree and reversal of local anaesthetic depression of sodium permeability. The time required to block half of the sodium currents varied as a function of the pK_a and the lipid solubility of the compounds and the pH of the bathing solution (Table 2.4). In general, low pK_a and high lipid solubility and pH enhance the onset of blockade. The results again demonstrated that the onset of action of neutral and charged agents is pH independent and the quaternary compounds which exist only in the charged form are relatively inactive when applied to the external surface of the nerve. In addition, tertiary amine and quaternary molecules demonstrate voltage- and frequency-dependent inhibition, but the neutral agent, benzocaine, did not show a similar effect.

Table 2.4. Relationship of pK_a, Lipid Solubility of Various Local Anaesthetics and pH to Onset of Depression of Sodium Conductance in Myelinated Mammalian Nerve Fibres

Agent	pK_a	*Partition coefficient**	*Onset of depression of inward sodium current (I_{Na}) (sec)†*	
			pH = 6·0	*pH = 8·3*
Benzocaine	2·9	41	1·0	1·0
GEA 968	7·7	1·3	>200	1·1–2·0
Lidocaine	7·9	225	1·1–1·5	0–0·7
Tetracaine	8·5	273	>15	1·3
Procaine	8·9	45	3·3–>4·5	0·5
RAC 109	9·4	260	2·0	0·9–1·1

*Oil or alcohol/buffer partition coefficient.
†Time required to reduce INa by 50 per cent.
Data derived from Hille [38].

The model proposed by Hille involves a single receptor in the sodium channel for neutral, tertiary and quaternary types of local anaesthetics. However, differences do exist in the pathways which these various substances use to reach the receptor site. The sodium channel exists either in a resting, open, or inactivated state (*Fig. 2.15*). The h and m^3 gates are closed at rest and opened during the active state. The h gate is closed also during the state of sodium inactivation. At rest, approximately 60 per cent of the sodium channels are believed to be closed and 40 per cent in the inactivated state. Following nerve stimulation, the closed channels open to allow the passage of sodium ions and then proceed to the inactivated state which terminates the depolarization phase. During and following repolarization, the majority of the inactivated sodium channels return to the closed resting state. The hydrophilic quaternary molecules such as QX-314, are unable to penetrate the lipid-rich membrane. Thus, these agents can only reach the receptor site from the internal aqueous medium when the sodium gates are open. The neutral lipophilic agents, such as benzocaine, penetrate into the core of the lipid membrane and use the hydrophobic pathway to reach the receptor site even when sodium gates are in the closed or inactive state. Since tertiary amines such as procaine and lidocaine exist both in a charged hydrophilic and uncharged lipophilic form, they may reach the receptor site by both the hydrophilic and hydrophobic pathways. The uncharged base utilizes the hydrophobic path

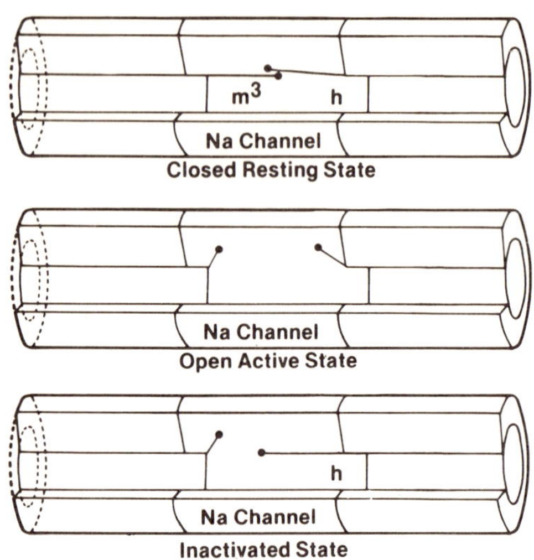

Fig. 2.15. Schematic representation of the status of the h and m³ gates in the sodium channel before (rest), during (open) and following (inactivated) nerve stimulation.

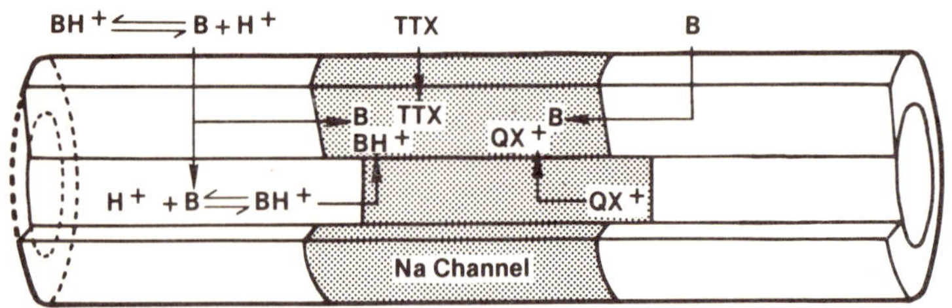

Fig. 2.16. Schematic representation of unified receptor site within sodium channel for all local anaesthetic agents. Uncharged form of conventional agents like lidocaine or neutral agents like benzocaine (B) reach receptor site via hydrophobic pathway. Charged form of conventional agents or quaternary compounds like QX–314 (BH^+ or QX^+) reach receptor site via hydrophilic path when axoplasmic sodium gates are open. Tetrodotoxin (TTX) and saxitoxin (STX) may reach receptor via external opening of sodium channel.

and so can reach the receptor site while the sodium channel is in the closed or inactivated state. The cationic form must use the hydrophilic pathway and so can only reach the receptor when the sodium gates are open (*Fig. 2.16*). Hille's hypothesis does not account for the action of the biotoxins at the external surface of the sodium channel. However, the chemical configuration of the biotoxins is sufficiently different from other types of local anaesthetic agents that they may be unable to enter the inner aperture of the sodium channel even when the gates are open, but may be able to reach the local anaesthetic receptor from the external surface of the sodium channel.

HOW DO LOCAL ANAESTHETICS DIFFUSE TO THE SITE OF ACTION?

Thus far the basic mechanism by which local anaesthetics cause conduction blockade and site of action of local anaesthetics has been reviewed. However, under clinical conditions, local anaesthetic agents are not administered within the axoplasm and rarely within a nerve sheath. Usually, the local anaesthetic solution is deposited outside a nerve trunk and the agent must then diffuse to the site of action.

Peripheral nerves possess a distinctive organizational pattern (*Fig. 2.17*). Each individual axon is surrounded by a connective tissue sheath known as

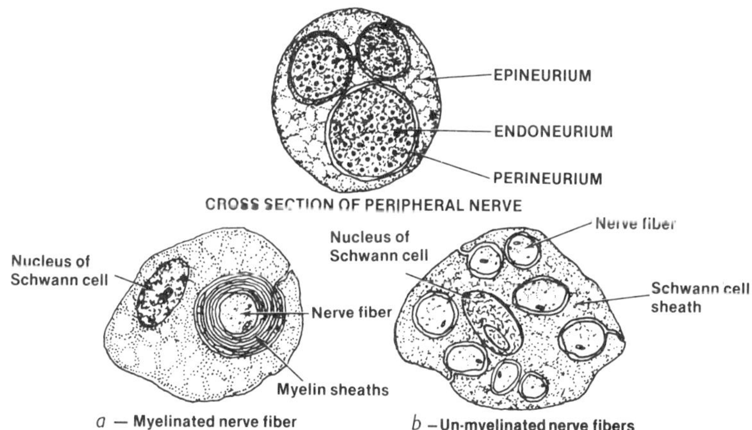

Fig. 2.17. Cross-section of peripheral nerve, myelinated nerve fibre, and unmyelinated nerve fibres.

the endoneurium. Groups of axons are then enclosed in an additional connective sheath called the perineurium. Finally, a number of axonal groups are encased in an external connective tissue sheath, the epineurium. A local anaesthetic must diffuse through these connective tissue layers to the individual axonal fibre and ultimately to the site of action within the sodium channel or the lipoprotein membrane. The axon itself possesses certain anatomical barriers to the movement of local anaesthetics. All nerve fibres are either myelinated or unmyelinated in nature (*Fig. 2.17*). Unmyelinated fibres are surrounded by a single wrapping, the Schwann cell sheath. Groups of unmyelinated fibres share the same Schwann cell. Myelinated fibres are enclosed in spirally wrapped layers of lipoprotein myelin sheaths which are actually a specialized form of a Schwann cell. Each myelinated fibre is enclosed in its own myelin sheath. The outermost layer of myelin essentially consists of the Schwann cell cytoplasm and its nucleus. The myelin sheath surrounding a myelinated nerve fibre is interrupted at intervals by the nodes of Ranvier. The size of the individual Schwann cell determines the distance between adjacent nodes. These myelin sheaths are essentially lipid in nature (75 per cent), but also contain some protein (20 per cent) and carbohydrate (5 per cent) material [30].

Individual nerve fibres have been traditionally classified into A, B and C fibres depending on degree of myelination, diameter size, rate of impulse propagation, and physiological function (Table 2.5) [24]. A fibres are

Table 2.5. Traditional Classification of Nerve Fibres According to Anatomical and Physiological Properties

Class	*Diameter (μm)*	*Myelinated*	*Function*	*Conduction velocity (m/sec)*	C_m	*Order of block*	*Order of recovery*
A Fibres	22	+		10–120	Highest	3	1
	α		Motor				
	β		Motor				
	γ		Sensory				
	δ		Sensory				
B Fibres	1–3	+	Pre-ganglionic autonomic	10–20	Inter-mediate	2	2
C Fibres	0·5–1	–	Sensory post-ganglionic autonomic	0·5–2·0	Lowest	1	3

largest in diameter, heavily myelinated, and conduct both sensory and motor impulses at the highest velocity. The A fibres are further subdivided into alpha, beta, gamma and delta fibres in order of decreasing size and decreasing conduction velocity. The A alpha, beta and gamma fibres are motor in nature, while the A delta fibres are responsible for fast pain sensation. B fibres are lightly myelinated and found in preganglionic autonomic nerves. C fibres consist of unmyelinated sensory and post-ganglionic autonomic fibres. Whitwam has reviewed the classification of peripheral nerve fibres and suggested a more uniform method of description [92].

Following diffusion through the epineurium, perineurium and endoneurium, local anaesthetic agents may reach their site of action by penetration of unmyelinated nerve fibres anywhere along the axonal membrane. However, in myelinated fibres, the local anaesthetics presumably enter the membrane at the exposed nodes of Ranvier. Classically, the size of the nerve fibre was considered to be directly related to anaesthetic potency, i.e. a greater concentration of local anaesthetic agent is required to block nerves of large diameter [28, 50]. This relationship between fibre size and anaesthetic sensitivity in myelinated nerves may be a function of the length of nerve fibre and number of nodes exposed to the local anaesthetic solution [26]. Exposure of 4 mm of myelinated nerves to 0·2 per cent procaine results in complete blockade of all fibres. However, reduction in the length of fibre exposure to 2 mm causes blockade of the A delta fibres, but not the A alpha fibres. Since the number of nodes of Ranvier is inversely proportional to the diameter size of the fibre, more nodes would be exposed to local anaesthetic solution per mm of fibre length in the A delta fibres as compared to the A alpha fibres. If a critical number of nodes must be blocked to ensure complete inhibition of a propagated action potential, the conduction in the smaller A delta fibres will be blocked at a lower minimal anaesthetic concentration (C_m) than the larger myelinated fibres. Although a relationship between fibre size and anaesthetic sensitivity may exist within fibres of the same classification, i.e. A, B or C fibres, data has been presented which indicate that a similar relationship may not exist between fibres of different types. For example, C fibres may continue to transmit impulses when conduction blockade by a local anaesthetic is complete in A gamma and delta fibres [26, 59]. In addition, the C_m of myelinated B fibres was found to be significantly lower than the C_m for unmyelinated C fibres [31, 68]. In fact, the C_m for 50 per cent suppression of action potential amplitude of B fibres was only 25–30 per cent of that required for C fibres, e.g. C_m for tetracaine and prilocaine for B fibres was 5 and 100 μM respectively compared to concentrations of 20 and 300 μM for C fibres. Condouris et al. used a computer simulation of local anaesthetic blockade to study the characteristics of blockade produced by TTX and lidocaine. The computer model indicated that myelinated nerves were more susceptible to local anaesthetic blockade than unmyelinated nerve fibres [17]. Recent investigations have been carried out in our laboratories to re-evaluate the C_m of various local anaesthetics in mammalian A, B and C fibres [29]. The C_m of lidocaine, tetracaine, etidocaine and bupivacaine required to produce a 50 per cent decrease in the amplitude of the action potential of A and B fibres from the desheathed rabbit vagus nerve was significantly less than the C_m required for unmyelinated C fibres (Table 2.6). The results suggest that local anaesthetics may be able to reach their site of action more easily via the nodes of myelinated fibres than through unmyelinated fibres. The other possibility to explain these findings may involve the relative location of the various fibres within the nerve bundle. If the myelinated C fibres are located mainly within the core area of the nerve trunk, a greater concentration of local anaesthetic may be required to ensure adequate diffusion to the centre of the nerve trunk in order to block conduction in these C fibres.

Table 2.6. Minimum Anaesthetic Concentration (C_m) of Various Local Anaesthetics Required to Produce a 50 per cent Decrease in Action Potential Amplitude of A, B and C Fibres of Desheathed Rabbit Vagus Nerve

	C_m (mM)	
Agent	*A & B fibres*	*C fibres*
Lidocaine	0·29	0·55
Tetracaine	0·01	0·025
Bupivacaine	0·11	0·21
Etidocaine	0·09	0·20

Data derived from Gissen et al. [29].

The most definitive studies regarding diffusion and penetration of local anaesthetics to the site of action were carried out by Ritchie and co-workers [62, 63]. Early investigations on isolated intact peripheral nerves indicated that local anaesthetic agents tended to be more efficacious when prepared as alkaline solutions [77, 87]. Since, as indicated previously, the uncharged base form of the drug is present in relatively greater proportion in alkaline solutions, these results did suggest that the base form diffused more readily to the site of action. However, these early results were interpreted as indicating that the base form was the active anaesthetic moiety. Ritchie and co-workers evaluated the interrelationship between pH of solutions of local anaesthetics, such as lidocaine and dubucaine, presence or absence of the nerve sheath, and anaesthetic activity. When isolated nerves possessing an intact sheath were studied, it was found that as the pH of the bathing solution containing either lidocaine or dibucaine was raised from 7·2 to 9·2, the rate of conduction blockade was markedly increased, indicating again that the uncharged base form of the drug was capable of penetrating to the site of anaesthetic action more readily than the charged form. However, when the experiment was repeated utilizing desheathed frog sciatic and rabbit vagus nerve preparations, the results differed. The rate of conduction blockade occurred more rapidly in desheathed nerves when the pH of the local anaesthetic solution was decreased, which indicated that the charged form of the local anaesthetic reached the site of action more readily.

On the basis of these observations, Ritchie and co-workers postulated that the uncharged base form of local anaesthetics is responsible for optimal diffusion through the nerve sheath. After penetration of the nerve sheath and the nerve membrane, re-equilibrium occurs between the base and cationic form in the axoplasm and the charged cationic form of the drug then diffuses to the receptor site within the sodium channel. Additional evidence that the uncharged base form diffuses more readily through nerve sheaths was obtained from studies with quaternary derivatives of lidocaine and the biotoxins, TTX and STX, which exist only in charged forms. *In vitro* experiments on isolated sheathed nerves and *in vivo* studies in animals involving peripheral nerve blocks and epidural anaesthesia indicate that these charged compounds are almost devoid of anaesthetic activity. However, absence of the nerve sheath reveals the high anaesthetic potency of these agents. For example, 80 nM of TTX will produce a 50 per cent reduction in the action potential amplitude of the desheathed rabbit vagus nerve, which indicates that TTX has an intrinsic anaesthetic potency which is approximately 250 000 times greater than that of procaine [14, 15]. Administration of 4 μg of TTX into the subarachnoid space of sheep where no neural sheath covers the spinal cord results in complete sensory analgesia and motor blockade. This dose of TTX is approximately 10 000 times less than that required to produce spinal anaesthesia with a drug such as lidocaine [20]. Interestingly, Adams et al. have shown that the combination of TTX or STX with conventional

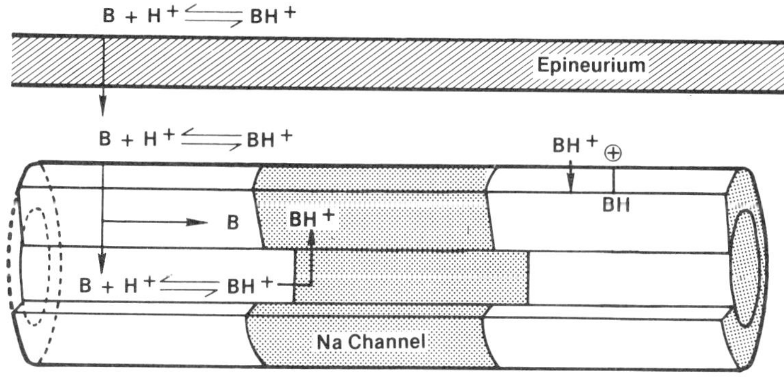

Fig. 2.18. Schematic representation of diffusibility and possible sites of action of conventional local anaesthetic agents. Base form (B) diffuses most easily through epineurium and axonal membrane. B may contribute to anaesthetic action by an action within the membrane. Charged form (BH^+) may diffuse into membrane and cause a change in surface charge or may diffuse through axoplasmic sodium gates to attach to receptor site in sodium channel.

local anaesthetics such as procaine, lidocaine, mepivacaine, cocaine or dibucaine for peripheral nerve blockade in rats, will produce a long duration of anaesthesia which is characteristic of the biotoxins [2, 3]. These results demonstrate that charged forms of local anaesthetics diffuse with great difficulty through neural sheaths and the axonal membrane. The mechanism by which the addition of a partially uncharged agent, e.g. lidocaine or procaine, can increase the diffusibility of a charged compound (TTX or STX) is unknown. Finally, Catchlove has studied the permeability of isolated nerve sheaths to local anaesthetic agents and has reported that the permeability of these agents is a linear function of the fraction of non-ionized drug present in solution [12].

The mechanism of local anaesthesia *in vivo* must include a consideration of diffusion through nerve sheaths and penetrability of the axonal membrane before inhibition of sodium conductance by a surface charge change, membrane alteration, or receptor binding can occur. *Fig. 2.18* attempts to summarize the diffusibility and possible sites of action of a conventional local anaesthetic agent, such as procaine or lidocaine in a sheathed peripheral nerve.

CLINICAL RELEVANCE OF THE MECHANISM OF LOCAL ANAESTHESIA

Knowledge of the factors involved in the mechanism of local anaesthesia has assisted in the elucidation of the differential pharmacological effects of various local anaesthetics and the clinical factors which influence local anaesthetic activity.

Structure–Activity Relationship of Local Anaesthetics

Compounds that demonstrate clinical utility as local anaesthetic agents, in general, possess the following chemical arrangement:

Aromatic portion – Intermediate – chain Amine portion

$$(CH_3)_2C_6H_3{-}NHCOCH_2{-}N(C_2H_5)_2 \quad \text{(lidocaine).}$$

The aromatic portion of the molecule is believed responsible for the lipophilic properties, whereas the amine end is associated with hydrophilicity. Alterations in the aromatic portion, amine portion, or intermediate chain of a specific chemical compound will modify its anaesthetic activity. For example, an increase in molecular weight within an homologous series of compounds, achieved by lengthening the intermediate chain or by the addition of carbon atoms to either the aromatic or amine portion of the molecule, will tend to increase intrinsic anaesthetic potency up to a maximum, beyond which a further increase in molecular weight results in a decrease in anaesthetic activity [85]. Changes in the aromatic or amine portion of a local anaesthetic substance will alter its lipid/water distribution coefficient and its protein-binding characteristics which, in turn, will markedly alter the anaesthetic profile within a series of homologous compounds. A comparison between procaine and tetracaine, which are both ester derivatives of para-amino-benzoic acid, reveals that the addition of a butyl group to the aromatic end of the procaine molecule produces a greater than 100-fold increase in lipid solubility and a tenfold increase in protein binding [88]. Such changes in physicochemical properties are reflected in marked alterations in biological activity. For example, the intrinsic anaesthetic potency of tetracaine as determined on an isolated nerve is approximately 16 times greater than that of procaine, whereas the duration of its anaesthetic activity as determined *in vivo* in the rat sciatic nerve preparation is approximately 4 times longer than that of procaine.

Similar relationships exist in the amide series of compounds. The addition of a butyl group to the amine end of mepivacaine, forming bupivacaine, results in a 35-fold increase in partition coefficient [89] and a significantly greater degree of protein binding as compared to mepivacaine. The chemical alterations of mepivacaine to bupivacaine and the subsequent modification of physicochemical properties result in a fourfold increase in intrinsic anaesthetic activity and a significant prolongation of anaesthetic duration.

Another example of the relationship between modification of chemical structure and biological activity is found in the comparison of lidocaine and etidocaine. Substitution in the lidocaine molecule of a propyl for an ethyl group at the amine end and the addition of an ethyl group at the alpha carbon in the intermediate chain yields etidocaine. These chemical changes in structure produce an increase in partition coefficient of approximately 50-fold and a significant increase in protein binding [20]. As in the previous examples, these alterations in chemical structure and physicochemical properties are reflected in significant changes in biological activity, such that etidocaine possesses an intrinsic anaesthetic potency 4 times greater than that of lidocaine and a duration of anaesthetic action approximately twice that of lidocaine.

One of the important clinical parameters in regional anaesthesia is the rapidity with which conduction blockade occurs. This pharmacological property of local anaesthetic agents can be evaluated quite accurately in an isolated nerve preparation. Onset time is probably related to the physicochemical properties of these various local anaesthetic agents, e.g. pK_a and lipid solubility. For example, a comparison of agents with similar pK_a values such as lidocaine, prilocaine and etidocaine reveals that the most lipid-soluble drug, etidocaine, demonstrates the most rapid onset of action whereas the least lipid-soluble agent, prilocaine, has the longest latency. Lidocaine occupies an intermediate position both in terms of lipid solubility and onset time. A comparison of highly lipid-soluble compounds with varying pK_a values, e.g. etidocaine, bupivacaine and tetracaine, indicates that etidocaine, which possesses the lowest pK_a, has the most rapid onset of action, whereas tetracaine possesses the highest pK_a value and the slowest onset time. The pK_a and latency values for bupivacaine lie between the two extremes [19, 88]. These observations concerning onset time are consistent with the known relationships between pH, pK_a, relative proportion of analgesic agents in the base and cationic form, lipid solubility and lipid composition of the cell membrane. The relationship between lipid solubility, protein binding and intrinsic anaesthetic potency and duration are also consistent with the morphology and physiology of the nerve membrane.

Acid–Base Status

The interrelationship between pH, the diffusion of the base form of local anaesthetics across nerve sheaths and the ultimate potency of local anaesthetic drugs suggests that the acid–base status of the patient would be important in determining the clinical action of local anaesthetic agents. A clinical state of acidosis would clearly favour formation of the charged form of the local anaesthetic drug. Since this form diffuses poorly across nerve sheaths, the onset of anaesthesia may be delayed and the depth of anaesthesia may be less than expected due to the decreased number of local anaesthetic molecules at the ultimate site of action. Conversely, a state of alkalosis may result in a more rapid onset of anaesthesia and a more profound state of anaesthesia. Bromage and Gertel have observed that the duration of brachial plexus anaesthesia was reduced by an average of 38 per cent in patients with chronic renal failure which may reflect a decreased tissue pH and decreased concentration of local anaesthetic base required for diffusion to the site of action [9]. In addition, injection of local anaesthetic agents into infected areas whose tissue pH is reduced, generally results in an inadequate degree of anaesthesia based again presumably on a change in the relative proportion of the base and cationic form of the drug.

A specific clinical problem which may be related to a localized change in hydrogen ion concentration is tachyphylaxis. The continuous infusion or intermittent injection of local anaesthetic agents into the epidural or subdural space has been employed for prolonged surgical procedures or to provide an extended period of postoperative pain relief. However, tachyphylaxis, or rapid tolerance, has been observed to occur following the continuous or repeated administration of local anaesthetic agents into the subarachnoid or epidural space [10, 80]. Tachyphylaxis is defined as a rapidly developing decreased analgesic response to a constant repeated dose of a specific local anaesthetic drug. Bromage and associates have carefully described the development of tachyphylaxis in a group of patients undergoing epidural anaesthesia [10]. A progressive decrease in duration and spread of anaesthesia was observed as the interval between the return of sensation and the subsequent injection was increased from 10 to 60 min, reaching a constant degree of tachyphylaxis when the interanalgesic interval exceeded 60 min. A constant 30 per cent reduction in response to each successive injection occurred at maximum tolerance.

The aetiology of local anaesthetic tachyphylaxis has not been completely resolved. Cohen and associates have proposed that the development of tolerance following repetitive subarachnoid administration is related to changes in the pH of cerebrospinal fluid (CSF) [13]. A significant increase in the H^+ content of CSF was observed when multiple subarachnoid injections of acidic solutions of lidocaine and procaine were made. This greater H^+ content (lower pH) of CSF would tend to increase the amount of ionized form of a local anaesthetic agent and conversely produce a relative decrease in the base form, which is responsible for diffusion through the nerve membrane. Such an alteration would be manifested clinically as a reduced analgesic response. Consistent with this hypothesis was the observation that a correlation existed between the rate of development of tachyphylaxis and the pK_a of the local anaesthetic agent. For example, tolerance occurred more rapidly when an agent with a lower pK_a, e.g. mepivacaine was used. The relative proportion of base and cationic form of such a drug would be affected to a greater degree by alterations in the pH of CSF than would an agent with a higher pK_a. These studies suggest that the development of tachyphylaxis may be retarded by the use of agents with intrinsically longer durations of action, use of agents with higher pK_a values, and use of a buffer to prevent the decrease in pH of CSF.

Electrolyte Disturbances

Membrane excitability is clearly dependent on extracellular and axoplasmic ionic concentration, particularly sodium and potassium. It is conceivable that clinical states involving electrolyte disturbances might alter the action of local anaesthetics. For example, Condouris clearly showed that, in an isolated nerve, a decrease in the sodium concentration in the bathing solution increased the blocking potency of cocaine, whereas an increase in the sodium concentration tended to decrease the potency of cocaine [16]. Unfortunately, little clinical data exists concerning the effect of hypo- or hypernatraemia on the action of local anaesthetic agents. Similarly, changes in extra- or intracellular potassium may also alter the action of local anaesthetics. Again, it is not known whether clinical states of hypo- or hyperpotassaemia alter local anaesthetic activity. However, studies have been reported in which potassium chloride has been added to solutions of local anaesthetic agents in an attempt to combine the conduction blocking effects of a reduced resting potential and an anaesthetic drug. For example, the duration of action and quality of anaesthesia produced by procaine can be increased by the concomitant use of potassium chloride in a concentration of 135–150 mM [47]. Moreover, the addition of potassium chloride to solutions of lidocaine can decrease the onset time and improve the quality of epidural anaesthesia and prolong the duration of digital and ulnar nerve blocks in man [5, 8].

As mentioned previously, studies on isolated nerve have shown that an inverse correlation exists between concentration of calcium in the bathing solution and the conduction-blocking properties of local anaesthetics. Thus, an increase in extracellular calcium tends to inhibit or reverse the blocking action of local anaesthetics, whereas a decrease in extracellular calcium tends to enhance the potency of local anaesthetics. Although the evidence now favours that calcium and local anaesthetics act at different sites in the membrane, it still is possible that under clinical conditions alterations in calcium concentration in extracellular fluid might alter local anaesthetic activity.

Influence of Frequency of Nerve Stimulation

The studies by Strichartz and others suggest that the frequency of nerve stimulation may enhance the activity of local anaesthetics [18, 83]. This could have important clinical ramifications, particularly in the treatment of chronic pain patients. It might be feasible to utilize conventional local anaesthetic drugs and nerve stimulators such as transcutaneous or dorsal cord stimulators to augment the degree of local anaesthesia. The concomitant use of a nerve stimulator and local anaesthetic injections conceivably would make more sodium channels available to the local anaesthetic drug resulting in an increased onset and depth of anaesthesia. On the other hand, the results of Strichartz would suggest that following the establishment of a conduction block, it might be possible to reduce the duration of anaesthesia by stimulating the area of conduction blockade. This observation of use-dependent inhibition and reversal of blockade may explain the clinical observation, particularly in extradural anaesthesia in obstetrics, in which patients who have initially a satisfactory degree of anaesthesia suddenly appear to experience pain as the degree and frequency of uterine contractility increases, resulting presumably in an increased number of impulses delivered over pain pathways. This phenomenon of 'unblocked segments' described by Crawford may be explainable on a physiological basis [21].

SUMMARY

Detailed studies concerning the mechanism of action of local anaesthetic agents have been carried out by a variety of investigators during the past 25 years. The concepts regarding the action of local anaesthetic agents have undergone considerable changes based in part on a greater knowledge of the morphology and physiology of the nerve membrane and the development of more refined experimental techniques to study membrane excitability. Peripheral nerves are enclosed in connective tissue sheaths, the endoneurium, perineurium and epineurium, which essentially act as barriers through which local anaesthetic agents must diffuse. In addition, certain nerve fibres contain a highly lipid myelin sheath and the cell membrane itself is composed primarily of lipids and proteins. Pores are also believed to exist in the lipoprotein axonal membrane through which cations such as sodium may pass. The cell membrane is also believed to undergo conformational changes between the resting and active state. No longer is the cell membrane considered to be a static structure. At rest, an electrical potential difference of approximately −60 to −80 mV exists across the cell membrane due primarily to the excess concentration of potassium ions within the axoplasm. Application of a threshold stimulus to the nerve membrane results in conformational changes which allow channels in the membrane to change from a closed resting state to an open active state. Sodium ions can then pass through the membrane along its concentration gradient to cause depolarization. In turn, the membrane is repolarized by the passive flow of potassium ions out of the cell to the extracellular space.

Local anaesthetic agents inhibit neural excitation by decreasing the permeability of the cell membrane to sodium ions which prevents depolarization of the cell membrane. The sodium channel is believed to be the site at which the local anaesthetics exert their inhibitory effect on sodium permeability. At the present time, most authorities favour the existence of a specific receptor for local anaesthetic agents within the sodium channel for the clinically useful anaesthetic agents, such as lidocaine. This receptor is believed to be present at the internal opening of the sodium channel. The sequence by which local anaesthetic agents administered under clinical conditions produce inhibition of neural conduction is as follows:

1. The clinically useful local anaesthetic agents exist in solution in both a charged and uncharged base form. The relative proportion of the charged and uncharged form is dependent upon the pH of the anaesthetic solution, the pH at the site of injection and the specific pK_a of the chemical substance employed.
2. The uncharged base form diffuses more readily through neural sheaths and across the axonal membrane to reach the axoplasmic surface of the sodium channel. In the axoplasm, the base combines with hydrogen ions to form the charged cation of the local anaesthetic agent which passes through open gates of the sodium channel and attaches to a receptor site inside the internal opening of the sodium channel. The local anaesthetic drug–receptor interaction results in a decrease in the permeability of the cell membrane to sodium ions thereby decreasing sodium conductance and preventing depolarization of the cell membrane, which ultimately is responsible for prevention of a propagated action potential.
3. Although the clinically useful injectable local anaesthetics are believed to act primarily by attachment to a receptor at the internal opening of the sodium channel, other sites of action may exist. The uncharged agents such as benzocaine and the base form of drugs such as procaine and lidocaine may act by penetrating the cell membrane and causing an expansion of the membrane or a conformational change in the membrane which would tend to decrease the diameter of the sodium channel. An alternative explanation for the action of uncharged agents involves diffusion via hydrophobic pathways to the same receptor within the sodium channel with which the charged form of local

anaesthetics interact. This would favour a single site of action for all forms of local anaesthetic agents.

4. The biotoxins, tetrodotoxin and saxitoxin, also interact with a receptor site in the sodium channel. However, these substances which diffuse poorly through nerve sheaths and membrane reach the receptor site via the external opening rather than the internal opening of the sodium channel.
5. A third possible site and mechanism of local anaesthesia is still favoured by some investigators. Penetration of local anaesthetics into the axonal membrane and reduction of surface charges on the membrane would obviate the necessity of a specific local anaesthetic receptor.

Further studies concerning the mechanism of local anaesthesia will probably be directed at attempting to reconcile the concept of multiple versus a single site of anaesthetic action in the nerve membrane. In addition, investigations are also required to elucidate factors which can alter the basic action of local anaesthetics and thereby provide useful information regarding techniques of modifying local anaesthetic activity in specific clinical situations.

REFERENCES

1. Aceves J. and Machne X. (1963) The action of calcium and local anesthetics on nerve cells and their interaction during excitation. *J. Pharmacol. Exp. Ther.* **140**, 138–148.
2. Adams H. J., Blair M. R. and Takman B. H. (1976) The local anesthetic activity of tetrodotoxin alone and in combination with vasoconstrictors and local anesthetics. *Anesth. Analg.* **55**, 568–573.
3. Adams H. J., Blair M. R. and Takman B. H. (1976) The local anesthetic activity of saxitoxin alone and with vasoconstrictor and local anesthetic agents. *Arch. Int. Pharmacodyn. Ther.* **224**, 275–282.
4. Akerman B. (1973) Studies on the relative pharmacological effects of enantiomers of local anesthetics with special regard to block of nervous excitation. Doctoral dissertation, Uppsala, Sweden.
5. Aldrete J. A., Barnes D. R., Sidon M. A. et al. (1969) Studies on effects of addition of potassium chloride to lidocaine. *Anesth. Analg.* **48**, 269–276.
6. Blaustein M. P. and Goldman D. E. (1966) Competitive action of calcium and procaine on lobster axon. *J. Gen. Physiol.* **49**, 1043–1063.

6*a*. Blaustein M. P. and Goldman D. E. (1966) Action of anionic and cationic nerve blocking agents: experiment and interpretation. *Science* **153**, 429–432.

7. Boggs J. M., Roth S. H., Yoong T. et al. (1976) Site and mechanism of anesthetic action. II. Pressure effect on the nerve conduction-blocking activity of a spin-label anesthetic. *Mol. Pharmacol.* **12**, 136–143.
8. Bromage P. R. and Burfoot M. F. (1966) Quality of epidural blockade. II. Influence of physico-chemical factors; hyaluronidase and potassium. *Br. J. Anaesth.* **38**, 857–865.
9. Bromage P. R. and Gertel M. (1972) Brachial plexus anesthesia in chronic renal failure. *Anesthesiology* **36**, 488–493.
10. Bromage P. R., Pettigrew R. T. and Crowell D. E. (1969) Tachyphylaxis in epidural analgesia. I. Augmentation and decay of local anesthesia. *J. Clin. Pharmacol.* **9**, 30–38.

11. Camejo G., Villegas G. M., Barnola F. V. et al. (1969) Characterization of two different membrane fractions isolated from the first stellar nerves of squid *Dosidieus gigas*. *Biochim. Biophys. Acta* **193**, 247–259.
12. Catchlove R. F. H. (1972) The influence of CO_2 and pH on local anesthetic action. *J. Pharmacol. Exp. Ther.* **181**, 298–309.
13. Cohen E. N., Levine D. A., Colliss J. E. et al. (1968) The role of pH in the development of tachyphylaxis to local anesthetic agents. *Anesthesiology* **29**, 994–1001.
14. Colquhoun D. and Ritchie J. M. (1972) The interaction at equilibration between tetrodotoxin and mammalian non-myelinated nerve fibers. *J. Physiol.* **221**, 533–553.
15. Colquhoun D. and Ritchie J. M. (1972) The kinetics of the interaction between tetrodotoxin and mammalian non-myelinated fibers. *Mol. Pharmacol.* 8, 285–292.
16. Condouris G. A. (1961) A study of the mechanism of action of cocaine on amphibian peripheral nerve. *J. Pharmacol. Exp. Ther.* **131**, 243–249.
17. Condouris G. A., Goebel R. H. and Brady T. (1976) Computer simulation of local anesthetic effects using a mathematical model of myelinated nerve. *J. Pharmacol. Exp. Ther.* **196**, 737–745.
18. Courtney K. R. (1975) Mechanism of frequency-dependent inhibition of sodium currents in frog myelinated nerve by the lidocaine derivative GEA 968. *J. Pharmacol. Exp. Ther.* **195**, 225–236.
19. Covino B. G. (1974) New local anesthetics for pain therapy. *Adv. Neurol.* **4**, 463–470.
20. Covino B. G. and Vassallo H. G. (1976) *Local Anesthetics: Mechanism of Action and Clinical Use.* New York, Grune and Stratton, p. 51.
21. Crawford J. S. (1972) The second thousand epidural blocks in an obstetric hospital practice. *Br. J. Anaesth.* **44**, 1277–1287.
22. Danielli J. F. and Davson H. A. (1936) A contribution to the theory of permeability of thin films. *J. Cell. Physiol.* **9**, 89–98.
23. den Hertog A. and Ritchie J. M. (1969) The effect of some quaternary ammonium compounds and local anesthetics on the electrogenic component of the sodium pump in mammalian non-myelinated nerve fibers. *Eur. J. Pharmacol.* **6**, 138–142.
24. Erlanger J. and Gasser H. C. (1930) The action potential in fibers of slow conduction in spinal roots and somatic nerves. *Am. J. Physiol.* **92**, 43–82.
25. Feinstein M. B. (1964) Reaction of local anesthetics with phospholipids. A possible chemical basis for anesthesia. *J. Gen. Physiol.* **48**, 357–374.
26. Franz D. N. and Perry R. S. (1974) Mechanism for differential block among single myelinated and non-myelinated axons by procaine. *J. Physiol.* **236**, 193–210.
27. Frazier D. T., Narahashi T. and Yamada M. (1970) The site of action and active form of local anesthetics. II. Experiments with quaternary compounds. *J. Pharmacol. Exp. Ther.* **171**, 45–51.
28. Gasser H. S. and Erlanger J. (1929) The role of fiber size in the establishment of a nerve block by pressure or cocaine. *Am. J. Physiol.* 88, 581–591.
29. Gissen A. J., Gregus J. J. and Covino B. G. (1980) Relative sensitivity of myelinated and unmyelinated mammalian nerve fibers to various local anesthetic agents. *Anesthesiology*. In press.
30. Guidotti G. (1972) The composition of biological membranes. *Arch. Intern. Med.* **129**, 194–201.
31. Heavner J. E. and de Jong R. H. (1974) Lidocaine blocking concentration for B and C-nerve fibers. *Anesthesiology* **40**, 228–233.

32. Henderson R., Ritchie J. M. and Strichartz G. R. (1973) The binding of labelled saxitoxin to the sodium channels in nerve membranes. *J. Physiol.* **235**, 783–804.
33. Hendrickson H. S. (1976) The penetration of local anesthetics into phosphatidylcholine monolayers. *J. Lipid Res.* **17**, 393–398.
34. Hille B. (1966) The common mode of action of three agents that decrease the transient charge in sodium permeability in nerves. *Nature* **210**, 1220–1222.
35. Hille B. (1967) The selective inhibition of delayed potassium currents in nerve by tetraethylammonium ion. *J. Gen. Physiol.* **50**, 1287–1302.
36. Hille B. (1968) Pharmacological modifications of the sodium channels of frog nerve. *J. Gen. Physiol.* **51**, 199–219.
37. Hille B. (1971) The permeability of the sodium channel to organic cations in myelinated nerve. *J. Gen. Physiol.* **58**, 599–619.
38. Hille B. (1977) The pH-dependent rate of action of local anesthetics on the node of Ranvier. *J. Gen. Physiol.* **69**, 475–496.
39. Hille B. (1977) Local anesthetics: hydrophilic and hydrophobic pathways for the drug–receptor reaction. *J. Gen. Physiol.* **69**, 497–515.
40. Hodgkin A. L. (1964) The ionic basis of nervous conduction. *Science* **145**, 1148–1154.
41. Huxley A. F. (1964) Excitation and conduction in nerve: quantitative analysis. *Science* **145**, 1154–1159.
42. Johnson C. L., Goldstein M. A. and Schwartz A. (1973) On the molecular action of local anesthetics. I. The mitochondrion as a model membrane system for studying local anesthetic action. *Mol. Pharmacol.* **9**, 360–371.
43. Kao C. Y. (1966) Tetrodotoxin, saxitoxin and their significance in the study of excitation phenomena. *Pharmacol. Rev.* **18**, 997–1049.
44. Kendig J. J. and Cohen E. N. (1977) Pressure antagonism to nerve conduction block by anesthetic agents. *Anesthesiology* **47**, 6–10.
45. Kuperman A. S., Altura B. T. and Chezar J. A. (1968) Action of procaine on calcium efflux from frog nerve and muscle. *Nature* **217**, 673–675.
46. Kuperman A. J., Okamato M., Beyer A. M. et al. (1964) Procaine action: antagonism by adenosine triphosphate and other nucleotides. *Science* **144**, 1222–1223.
47. Lechat P., Deleau D. and Griffie R. A. (1964) Influence de l'ion potassium sur l'activite des anesthesiques locaux. *Med. Exp. (Basel)* **11**, 157–168.
48. Ling G. and Gerard R. W. (1949) The normal membrane potential of frog sartorius fibers. *J. Cell. Comp. Physiol.* **34**, 383–396.
49. McLaughlin S. (1975) Local anesthetics and the electrical properties of phospholipid bilayer membranes. *Mol. Mech. Anesth.* **1**, 193–220.
50. Mathews P. B. C. and Rushworth G. (1957) The relative sensitivity of muscle nerve fibers to procaine. *J. Physiol.* **135**, 263–269.
51. Meymaris E. (1975) Chemical anatomy of the nerve membrane. *Br. J. Anaesth.* **47** (Suppl.), 164–172.
52. Narahashi T., Anderson N. C. and Moore J. W. (1966) Tetrodotoxin does not block excitation from inside the nerve membrane. *Science* **153**, 765–767.
53. Narahashi T., Anderson N. C. and Moore J. W. (1967) Comparison of tetrodotoxin and procaine in internally perfused squid giant axons. *J. Gen. Physiol.* **50**, 1413–1428.
54. Narahashi T. and Frazier D. T. (1971) Site of action and active form of local anesthetics. *Neurosci. Res. Program Bull.* **4**, 65–99.
55. Narahashi T. and Frazier D. T. (1975) Site of action and active form of procaine in squid giant axons. *J. Pharmacol. Exp. Ther.* **194**, 506–513.
56. Narahashi T., Frazier D. T. and Takeno K. (1976) Effect of calcium on the local anesthetic suppression of ionic conductances in squid axon membranes. *J. Pharmacol. Exp. Ther.* **197**, 426–438.

57. Narahashi T., Frazier D. and Yamada M. (1970) The site of action and active form of local anesthetics. I. Theory and pH experiments with tertiary compounds. *J. Pharmacol. Exp. Ther.* **171**, 32–44.
58. Narahashi T., Yamada M. and Frazier D. T. (1969) Cationic forms of local anesthetics block action potentials from inside the nerve membrane. *Nature* **223**, 748–749.
59. Nathan P. W. and Sears T. A. (1961) Some factors concerned in differential nerve block by local anesthetics. *J. Physiol.* **157**, 565–580.
60. Papahadjopoulos D. (1920) Phospholipid model membranes. III. Antagonistic effects of Ca^{2+} and local anesthetics on the permeability of phosphatidylserine vesicles. *Biochim. Biophys. Acta* **211**, 467–477.
61. Ritchie J. M. and Greengard P. (1966) On the mode of action of local anesthetics. *Annu. Rev. Pharmacol.* **6**, 405–430.
62. Ritchie J. M., Ritchie B. and Greengard P. (1965) The active structure of local anesthetics. *J. Pharmacol. Exp. Ther.* **150**, 152–159.
63. Ritchie J. M., Ritchie B. and Greengard P. (1965) The effect of the nerve sheath on the action of local anesthetics. *J. Pharmacol. Exp. Ther.* **150**, 160–164.
64. Ritchie J. M., Rogart R. B. and Strichartz G. R. (1976) A new method for labelling saxitoxin and its binding to non-myelinated fibers of the rabbit vagus, lobster walking leg and garfish olfactory nerves. *J. Physiol.* **261**, 477–494.
65. Robertson J. D. (1959) The ultrastructure of cell membranes and their derivatives. *Biochem. Soc. Symp.* **16**, 3–43.
66. Roth S. H., Smith R. A. and Paton D. M. (1976) Pressure antagonism of anesthesia-induced conduction failure in frog peripheral nerve. *Br. J. Anaesth.* **48**, 621–628.
67. Sax M. and Pletcher J. (1969) Local anesthetics: significance of hydrogen bonding in mechanism of action. *Science* **166**, 1546–1548.
68. Scurlock J. E., Heavner J. E. and de Jong R. H. (1975) Differential B and C fiber block by an amide and an ester-linked local anaesthetic. *Br. J. Anaesth.* **47**, 1135–1139.
69. Seeman P. (1972) The membrane action of anesthetics and tranquilizers. *Pharmacol. Rev.* **24**, 583–655.
70. Shanes A. M. (1958) Electrochemical aspects of physiological and pharmacological action in excitable cells. Part II. The action potential and excitation. *Pharmacol. Rev.* **10**, 165–273.
71. Shanes A. M., Freygang W. H., Grundfest H. et al. (1959) Anesthetic and calcium action in the voltage clamped squid giant axon. *J. Gen. Physiol.* **42**, 793–802.
72. Shantz E. J. (1960) Biochemical studies of paralytic shellfish poisons. *Ann. N.Y. Acad. Sci.* **90**, 843–855.
73. Singer M. A. (1973) Interaction of local anesthetics and salicylate with phospholipid membranes. *Can. J. Physiol. Pharmacol.* **51**, 785–789.
74. Singer M. A. (1974) Effects of amiloride and dibucaine on a model phospholipid membrane: structure–activity relationships. *Biochem. Pharmacol.* **23**, 2939–2950.
75. Singer S. J. (1975) Architecture and topography of biologic membranes. In: Weissmann G. and Clarborne R. (ed.), *Cell Membranes.* New York, H. P. Publishing Co. Inc., pp. 35–44.
76. Singer S. J. and Nicholson G. L. (1972) The fluid mosaic model of the structure of cell membranes. *Science* **175**, 720–731.
77. Skou J. C. (1954) Local anesthetics. I. The blocking potencies of some local anesthetics and of butyl alcohol determined on peripheral nerves. *Acta Pharmacol. Toxicol. (Kbh)* **10**, 281–291.

78. Skou J. C. (1954) Local anesthetics. V. The action of local anesthetics on monomolecular layers of stearic acid. *Acta Pharmacol. Toxicol. (Kbh)* **10**, 317–324.
79. Skou J. C. (1954) Local anesthetics. VI. Relation between blocking potency and penetration of a monomolecular layer of lipoids from nerves. *Acta Pharmacol. Toxicol. (Kbh)* **10**, 325–337.
80. Smith S. M. and Rees V. L. (1948) Use of prolonged continuous spinal anesthesia to relieve vasospasm in peripheral embolism. *Anesthesiology* 9, 229–238.
81. Strichartz G. R. (1973) The inhibition of sodium currents in myelinated nerve by quaternary derivatives of lidocaine. *J. Gen. Physiol.* **62**, 37–57.
82. Strichartz G. (1975) Inhibition of ionic currents in myelinated nerves by quaternary derivatives of lidocaine. *Mol. Mech. Anesth.* **1**, 1–11.
83. Strichartz G. (1976) Molecular mechanisms of nerve block by local anesthetics. *Anesthesiology* **45**, 421–441.
84. Takman B. H. (1975) The chemistry of local anesthetic agents: classification of blocking agents. *Br. J. Anaesth.* **47** (Suppl.), 183–190.
85. Takman B. H., Boyes R. N. and Vassallo H. G. (1974) Local anesthetics. *Medicinal Chemistry*, 4th ed. New York, John Wiley and Sons, Inc.
86. Taylor R. E. (1959) Effect of procaine on electrical properties of squid axon membrane. *Am. J. Physiol.* **196**, 1071–1078.
87. Trevan J. W. and Boock E. (1927) The relation of hydrogen ion concentration to the action of the local anesthetics. *Br. J. Exp. Pathol.* 8, 307–315.
88. Truant A. P. and Takman B. (1959) Differential physical–chemical and neuropharmacologic properties of local anesthetic agents. *Anesth. Analg.* 38, 478–484.
89. Tucker G. T., Boyes R. N., Bridenbaugh P. O. et al. (1970) Binding of anilide-type local anesthetics in human plasma. I. Relationships between binding, physicochemical properties and anesthetic activity. *Anesthesiology* **33**, 287–303.
90. Ueda I., Tashiro C. and Arakawa K. (1977) Depression of phase-transition temperature in a model cell membrane by local anesthetics. *Anesthesiology* **46**, 327–332.
91. Watson P. J. (1960) The mode of action of local anaesthetics. *J. Pharm. Pharmacol.* **12**, 257–292.
92. Whitwam J. G. (1976) Classification of peripheral nerve fibers. *Anaesthesia* **31**, 494–503.

Felicity Reynolds

3 Transfer of Drugs Across Membranes

BIOLOGICAL MEMBRANES

The biological membrane of cardinal importance in the context of drug transfer is the plasma membrane, often called the cell membrane. The plasma membrane, and complex membranes derived from it, are often referred to as lipid membranes, or lipid barriers. The latter term is confusing as such membranes act as barriers only to non-lipids. The plasma membrane may form a continuous sheet surrounding each cell or bounding a syncytium, or when bounding cells joined by tight junctions. It may, on the other hand, form an effectively porous membrane as in certain types of capillary endothelium in which it bounds cells with gaps between them, is perforated by fenestrae or forms transport vesicles (*see* p. 149, Capillaries).

Most biological membranes are complex and consist of sheets of cells, together with their basement membrane. The latter forms a structural microskeleton which is made up of a network of mucopolysaccharides with some collagen fibres [88] and is generally highly permeable, except, for example, in the renal glomerulus (*see below*). Such complex membranes include

1. Capillary endothelium, of various types, one of which forms
2. the blood–brain barrier,
3. the renal tubule,
4. mucous membranes,
5. the placenta,

and all, except for the apparently more porous types of capillary endothelium, function as lipid membranes, that is lipid-soluble substances may diffuse across them with ease, while large or ionized hydrophilic molecules encounter a relative barrier, or cross by special transport processes.

DRUG CHEMISTRY

Drugs used by anaesthetists are, in the main, lipid-soluble foreign substances which cannot make use of specialized transport processes provided for compounds essential for metabolism.

NON-POLAR COMPOUNDS Inhalational anaesthetics are all non-polar (unable to ionize) lipid-soluble small molecules which readily diffuse across all biological membranes. Other non-polar compounds are Althesin (alphaxalone/alphadolone acetate) and propanidid, which are very poorly water soluble.

WEAK ACIDS Barbiturates are weak acids that are all around 50 per cent or less ionized at physiological pH. The non-ionized forms vary greatly in their lipid solubility from the hydrophilic phenobarbitone, on the one hand, to thiopentone and methohexitone, at the other end of the scale.

WEAK BASES include narcotics and local anaesthetics which are all more than 50 per cent ionized at physiological pH but which vary in their lipid solubility, and ketamine. Diazepam is such a very weak base that it ionizes only in very acid conditions and is not soluble in aqueous solution at or near physiological pH.

QUATERNARY AMMONIUM COMPOUNDS such as neuromuscular-blocking drugs are fully ionized and thus completely hydrophilic.

TYPES OF TRANSFER

Since the advent of the electron microscope, many assumptions that have been made relating drug transfer to membrane pore size have been hard to substantiate histologically [172]. In this section the modes of transfer that are theoretically available will be described.

Filtration and Bulk Flow

A solute may cross a semi-permeable membrane in the filtrate, provided the pores are large enough. The rate of transfer depends upon hydrostatic pressure. However, even for small water-soluble molecules, rate of transfer across most membranes appears to depend more upon concentration gradient than on perfusion pressure [63] arguing more for diffusion than for filtration. Certain capillaries, notably in the glomerulus where a huge volume of water is filtered, may be exceptions to this generalization.

Bulk flow takes place through arachnoid granulations, which have valves opening under hydrostatic pressure to allow passage of cerebrospinal fluid (CSF) into the venous sinuses [114], and out of liver sinusoids [65]. Bulk flow permits passage of water and solutes, quite irrespective of relative concentration in the media and of molecular size.

Diffusion

Diffusion, down an effective concentration or partial pressure gradient, is the principal means of transfer across membranes for respiratory gases and all drugs of cardinal importance to anaesthetists. The rules governing rate of diffusion will be outlined in a later section.

Facilitated Diffusion

This allows diffusion down a concentration gradient, but at a rate more rapid than would be predicted by simple physical laws. It is the means whereby sugars, which are purely hydrophilic, cross many membranes. One system involves a hypothetical diffusible carrier at the membrane surface, with affinity for the water-soluble molecule with which it forms a complex. This complex then diffuses across the membrane down a concentration gradient to the other face of the membrane where it is cleaved.

The gradient for the carrier alone is now in the reverse direction, so it returns to pick up more of the non-diffusible compound. Another theoretical system is the bucket brigade, whereby non-diffusible ligand is passed from hand to hand across a membrane by a system of acceptor–donor macromolecules. Carrier systems are saturatable and selective, in that D-glucose, for example, is transported more rapidly than L-glucose, while competition between sugars may be shown to delay diffusion. There appears to be no consumption of energy, however, and it is this characteristic principally that distinguishes it from the next type of transport. The system probably has little importance in drug transfer.

Active Transport

Such systems are generally specific for essential requirements of cells, use metabolic energy and can transport substances across membranes against a concentration gradient. Examples are the uptake of amino acids across the placenta and the blood–brain barrier [113] in which essential amino acids are taken up more rapidly than non-essential, and the sodium pump which transports sodium across cell membranes against a concentration gradient. The system involves Na^+- and K^+-dependent membrane-bound ATPase, a huge lipoprotein-enzyme, molecular weight 670 000, which extends the full thickness of the membrane. At the inner, cytoplasmic surface it is phosphorylated, in which state it has a high affinity for Na^+. The cation-binding sites are then translocated to the outer membrane surface and dephosphorylated. In this state they have a high affinity for K^+ and low for Na^+, thus releasing Na^+ and translocating K^+ to the interior of the cell. Other examples of active transport are secretion of H^+ in the stomach and uptake of iodine by the thyroid gland [63]. Penicillins and some other acidic drugs are actively secreted in the kidney tubule and taken up from the CSF by the choroid plexus [157], probably by a process normally transporting endogenous acids. Adrenergic neurone-blocking drugs, such as guanethidine, are actively taken up at sympathetic nerve endings by the noradrenaline uptake process, before they can act to prevent noradrenaline release. Their action is therefore inhibited by tricyclic antidepressant drugs, which block both noradrenaline and guanethidine uptake. Most drugs of primary importance to anaesthetists are very definitely alien substances and not actively transported.

Vesicular Transport

A plasma membrane can form invaginations which become pinocytotic vesicles. These tend to shrink within the cytoplasm of cells as the material within them is digested [88]. Studies of the amoeba, *Chaos chaos,* have shown that such gulps of the environment are not taken arbitrarily, but that desirable material, such as protein, first becomes concentrated on the cell surface, before being engulfed in this manner. In capillary endothelium, however, vesicles appear to be for transport across the meagre thickness of the cell cytoplasm, rather than for nutrition. The electron microscope marker, horseradish peroxidase, has been observed in vesicles in muscle capillary endothelium [172] and one might postulate such a route for the passage of neuromuscular drugs into muscle or their slow transfer across the placenta.

Exocytosis

In exocytosis the vesicular membrane becomes fused with the cell membrane, and then continuous with it, the contents being extruded: the reverse of pinocytosis or phagocytosis. Liver and pancreatic cells manufacture proteins which are extruded by exocytosis. Nerve terminals store neurotransmitters in vesicles, the entire contents of which are released from the interior of the cell by exocytosis.

PRINCIPLES GOVERNING DIFFUSION

Because diffusion is by far the most important mode of transfer of drugs across membranes, factors influencing the rate and extent of diffusion will be explored in detail.

Diffusion Rate

Expressed in simple terms, the *rate* of diffusion of a drug across a lipid membrane depends upon its concentration gradient and its molecular characteristics. Classically, the various factors have been related in the following formula [41, 109]:

$$\text{rate of diffusion} = \frac{K A (C_1 - C_2)}{X}$$

where K is the diffusion constant for the drug, and is related to molecular weight, shape, degree of ionization and lipid solubility, A is the area available for exchange, C_1 and C_2 are the concentrations on the two sides of the membrane and X is the thickness of the membrane. This formula needs interpreting with care.

Gradient

It is not necessarily the total concentration gradient of a drug which exerts the motive force for diffusion. For example:

1. A gas or vapour dissolved in a liquid diffuses down a gradient determined by its *partial pressure*, that is the pressure it would exert in the gas phase in equilibrium with the liquid. Absolute concentrations in different phases in equilibrium with one another vary depending upon the relative affinity of each phase for the gas. Thus it is a perfectly familiar concept that an inhalational anaesthetic diffuses down a pressure rather than a concentration gradient.

2. A weak acid or base is partially ionized in aqueous solution, and only that moeity which is non-ionized can diffuse readily across a lipid membrane. Only that fraction therefore can be expected to participate in a gradient for diffusion. Once the non-ionized form is in equilibrium on the two sides of the membrane no further net transfer takes place.
3. Many drugs are partly bound to plasma and also possibly to tissue protein. In the form of drug–protein complexes they do not readily diffuse across biological membranes, therefore only the *free* fraction of a drug can be said to exert a gradient for diffusion.

Thus only the *free non-ionized* fraction of total drug concentration is diffusible. This fraction alone therefore exerts the diffusion pressure. Rather than considering *total* drug concentration, as in the above equation, a more realistic figure might include only the diffusible concentration, or pressure concentration, equivalent to the partial pressure of a gas or vapour. This then removes the component, degree of ionization, from K, the constant for drug diffusion. This is obviously logical since degree of ionization is not a constant for the drug but varies with ambient pH. Nor would it be possible to replace degree of ionization with pK_a (that property of a molecule which determines its degree of ionization at a given pH, *see below* for derivation) in the equation since as pK_a rises diffusible concentration of an acid rises but that of a base falls. Moreover the equation totally ignores the effect of binding on diffusion rate.

Lipid Solubility

This term is used here to mean lipid/buffer partition coefficient (to the despair of the pure chemist, who regards it as meaning absolute solubility in lipid) since it is a less clumsy term, and only a little less correct than the loose and lengthy oil/water partition coefficient.

Lipid solubility is always quoted as an important characteristic determining diffusion rate across a lipid membrane. In fact, it has been shown to be more important than molecular radius in relation to permeability constants for lipid-soluble compounds [35]. Curry [41], however, predicts that too high a lipid partition coefficient will tend to trap drug within a lipid layer and so retard its diffusion. In practice such high solubility does not delay passage across a single, or even a double, layer of plasma membrane, such as capillary endothelium or the placental syncytiotrophoblast. A plasma membrane has such a tiny volume that it would readily become saturated and so allow drug to pass. Drug sequestration in lipid membranes may however delay *absorption* of a local anaesthetic from its site of action. The greater the lipid solubility of a local anaesthetic the more potent, and in general the longer its duration of *local* action [130]. Such a potent local anaesthetic may also yield a lower plasma concentration for a given locally administered dose [129]. High lipid solubility allows a local anaesthetic to pass in relatively high concentration to its site of action in the nerve cell membrane, leaving little in the aqueous phase in the extracellular fluid for absorption into the systemic circulation.

That lipid solubility is of prime importance in rate of transfer across membranes is admirably exemplified by the rate of passage of barbiturate across the blood–brain barrier [144]. Thus thiopentone, highly lipid soluble, can produce rapid onset of anaesthesia which is brief in duration because of redistribution, while pentobarbitone, for example, of intermediate lipid solubility, can only produce sleep of gradual onset and more prolonged duration, even when given by bolus [62], and the much less lipid-soluble phenobarbitone is even slower in onset no matter what the route of administration.

Amount of Drug Transfer

The total amount of drug crossing a membrane is the product of rate and duration of transfer. The length of time that net diffusion continues depends upon the maintenance of an effective diffusion gradient. This in turn depends on (*a*) flow rates and compartment volumes and (*b*) relative affinities.

Flow Rates and Compartment Volumes

During uptake of a drug, the blood supplying an organ or tissue carries the drug which tends to equilibrate at capillary level with the extracellular fluid. Equilibration does not occur immediately however, if the blood continues to import the drug. In this way a diffusion gradient is maintained until tissue equilibration has taken place. A high blood flow to a particular organ will therefore tend to promote passage of a drug into that organ provided the capillary endothelium and cell membranes are permeable to it. Hence the vessel-rich group of organs acquires a high concentration of a lipid-soluble drug more rapidly than does fat [62], which is poorly perfused.

Such highly lipid-soluble drugs as thiopentone and bupivacaine equilibrate in a single circulation with the brain [115]. Equilibration with other vessel-rich organs is rapid too. *Fig. 3.1* shows that from 2 min, bupivacaine concentration is falling in kidney, lung, heart and liver as well as brain [127]. Where then are such drugs going? Although the concentration of thiopentone in fat rises for an hour (*Fig. 3.2*), its early elimination from plasma and all the vessel-rich group is too rapid to be explained by localization in fat, as postulated by Brodie in 1952 (*see* [62]). It may be supposed that since muscle blood flow is relatively small at rest, skeletal muscle may be the next port of call after the vessel-rich group, and this is postulated for the inhalational anaesthetics [175]. The level of thiopentone, however, is falling in muscle over the same period of time as in brain (*Fig. 3.2*). Skin and bone marrow are relatively unexplored areas and may be the mystery tissues of intermediate equilibration rates [62].

A fluid flow on both sides of a complex membrane, for example at the placenta or in the renal tubule, may greatly enhance drug transfer, especially if a counter-current mechanism operates. In the placenta, the diffusion gradient is likely to be prolonged by umbilical blood flow, since the fetus represents a deeper compartment [82] than maternal tissues, and saturation is therefore delayed. For drugs which penetrate the blood–CSF barrier slowly, the gradient is maintained *for ever* by continuous CSF manufacture and bulk flow into the venous sinuses [42, 114]. These tissues are discussed individually below.

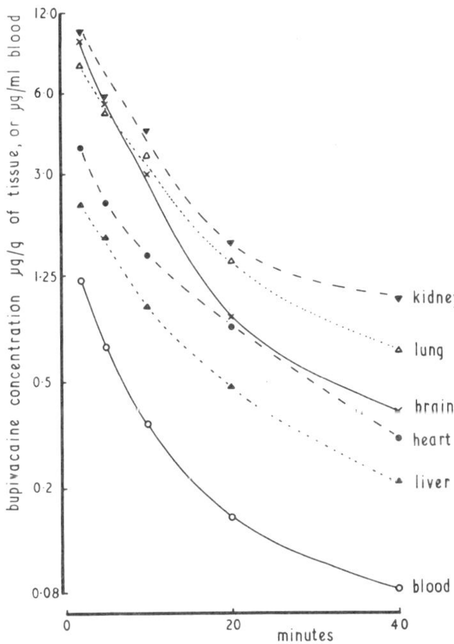

Fig. 3.1. Blood and tissue concentrations of bupivacaine in mice killed at 2, 5, 10, 20 and 40 min after intravenous injection of 0·12 mg. (*From Reynolds [127].*)

Relative Affinities (Equilibrium distribution coefficients)

The partition coefficients of drugs between two media separated by a membrane vary. If the affinity of the drug for the second medium is greater than for the first, more drug must cross the membrane to saturate the second medium and hence diffusion will continue for longer. This concept is familiar to anaesthetists in the context of uptake of inhalational anaesthetics. The uptake of an agent such as ether, with a high blood–gas partition coefficient, is prolonged if it is administered at a steady rate. This is a familiar example of a *concentration* gradient giving no clue to the direction of diffusion. Similarly halothane has high tissue–blood solubility coefficients and uptake into all tissues is more prolonged and extensive than with other agents in common use.

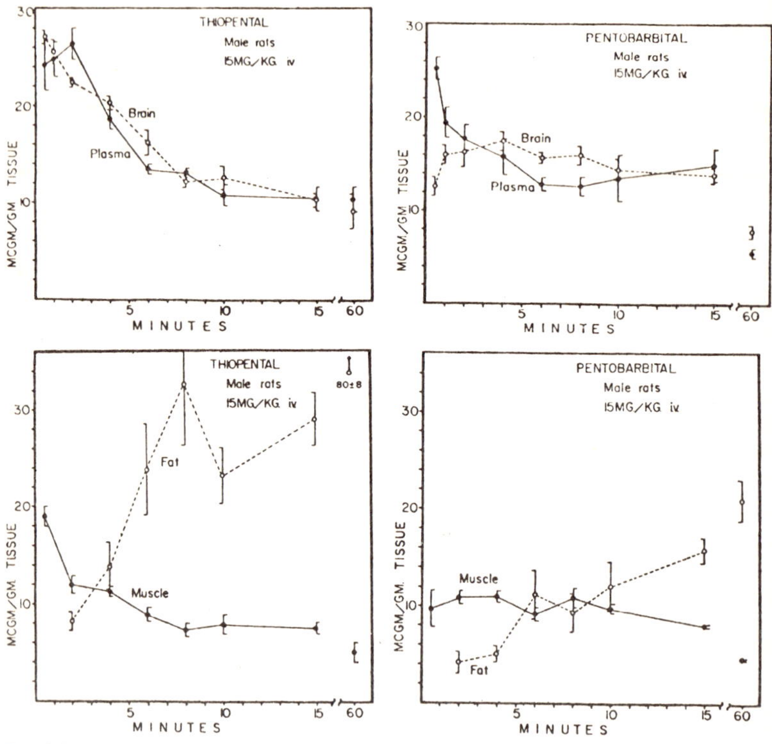

Fig. 3.2. Plasma and tissue concentrations of thiopentone (thiopental) and pentobarbitone (pentobarbital) after intravenous injection in rats. Each point represents the mean value for four rats, and vertical bars represent standard errors. (*Reproduced by kind permission of Goldstein and Aronow [62] and the* Journal of Pharmacology and Experimental Therapeutics.)

The same three factors determine the equilibrium distribution of non-volatile drugs as determine their rate of diffusion, namely: (*a*) lipid solubility, (*b*) pK_a and (*c*) protein binding.

Lipid Solubility

It is well recognized by anaesthetists that the affinity of adipose tissue for a lipid-soluble drug is such that it will continue to take up the drug long after other tissues which are better perfused, but have less capacity for the drug, are relatively saturated. This has been established for inhalational anaesthetics [175] and thiopentone [62].

pK_a

The ionization of a weak acid or base varies with the ambient pH, so as to minimize changes in $[H^+]$, the buffer action. The degree of ionization can be calculated from the Henderson–Hasselbalch equation, which is derived as follows.

By the law of mass action:

$$HA \rightleftharpoons H^+ + A^- \tag{1}$$

the relationship between the two sides of the equation being constant for a given acid. Thus:

$$\frac{[H^+]\ [A^-]}{[HA]} = K_a, \tag{2}$$

K_a being the acid dissociation constant. Taking the definition of an acid as a proton donor and of a base as a proton acceptor, equation (1) may be rewritten:

$$\text{acid} \rightleftharpoons H^+ + \text{base}.$$

In the case of an acidic drug, the acid is non-ionized (HA) and the base is an anion (A^-), while for a basic drug the base is non-ionized and the acid is the cation. Both an acid and a base can therefore have an acid dissociation constant K_a. Thus transposing equation (2):

$$[H^+] = K_a \frac{[\text{acid}]}{[\text{base}]} \tag{3}$$

and taking negative logarithms throughout:

$$pH = pK_a - \log \frac{[\text{acid}]}{[\text{base}]}. \tag{4}$$

The pH varies throughout the body from the plasma pH of 7·4 to that found in a less well-perfused intracellular environment of 7·0 or even less. More extreme changes than this are encountered in the urine, the pH of which may vary from 4 or 5 on the one hand to a postprandial alkaline tide more alkaline than plasma, and in the gastric lumen where gastric juice may have a pH value of 2 or less. Such overall pH variations affect the distribution of weak acids and bases.

Using the Henderson–Hasselbalch equation (4), one can calculate the distribution of a weak base such as bupivacaine with a pK_a of 8·2 across a hypothetical lipid membrane separating an extracellular fluid (ECF) pH 7·4 from one of 7·2 in intracellular fluid (ICF), supposing non-ionized base comes readily into equilibrium, while cation is barred.

ECF		ICF
pH 7·4	‖	pH 7·2
cation (6·3)	‖	cation (10)
$\rightleftharpoons$	‖	$\rightleftharpoons$
base (1)	‖	base (1)

Therefore $ICF_{7\cdot 2}$: ECF = 11 : 7·3 = 1·51.

Figures in brackets represent unit concentrations which, added together, go to make up the total concentration of drug free in solution, for calculating ICF : ECF ratio.

Making the same calculations for a pH gradient of 7·4–7·0, the ICF : ECF ratio is 2·31. The more acid the environment, the higher the concentration of base in solution at equilibrium. Carried to an absurd conclusion, since a basic drug will be about a million times more ionized than non-ionized in the gastric lumen, at equilibrium the gastric concentration for bupivacaine, for example, is 137-thousand times the ECF concentration. Fortunately such equilibrium is not achieved for parenterally administered basic drugs otherwise systemic concentrations would rapidly become undetectable. Basic drugs can, however, readily be detected in gastric contents, while, if given orally, gastric absorption is impossible. For a weaker base, concentration within cells is less than for a stronger base.

For an acid, such as for example phenobarbitone with a pK_a of 7·2, free concentration within cells is less than that in the ECF.

ECF		ICF
pH 7·4		pH 7·2
anion (1·58)		anion (1)
⇅		⇅
acid (1)		acid (1)

Therefore $ICF_{7\cdot2}$: ECF = 2 : 2·58 = 0·58.

Fig. 3.3 shows how the ICF : ECF concentration ratio at equilibrium varies with pK_a for acids and bases, at the relatively small pH gradient of 0·2. The weaker the acid or base, the nearer to unity is the ratio.

Altering pH gradients across lipid membranes can have important clinical implications in the distribution of drugs. For example, raising the $P\text{CO}_2$ can increase the brain and other tissue concentrations of barbiturates and deepen narcosis, while lowering the plasma level. Conversely, lowering the $P\text{CO}_2$ or administering bicarbonate has the reverse effect [63, 121]. By contrast, hyperventilation after administration of a basic narcotic analgesic such as morphine would increase the brain concentration and enhance the central nervous system effects [74]. Changing the ECF pH also alters renal excretion of weak acids and bases in such a way as to enhance the clinical effect of altered brain distribution (*see* the section on kidney *below*). Studies of *buccal absorption* (p. 159) of weak bases offer further evidence of the dominance of non-ionic diffusion in drug transfer across membranes.

The phenomenon which produces disparate concentrations of weak acids and bases in media of different pH values separated by a lipid membrane is known as diffusion trapping. A measured concentration gradient *less* than would be predicted on the grounds of non-ionic diffusion is usually ascribed to some degree of permeability of the membrane to the ionized fraction or to incomplete equilibration [96]. In practice, protein binding may be a more important factor than either of these. Across the placenta (*see later*), where the pH gradient is usually of a low order, its effect is often swamped by differences in protein binding in maternal and fetal blood.

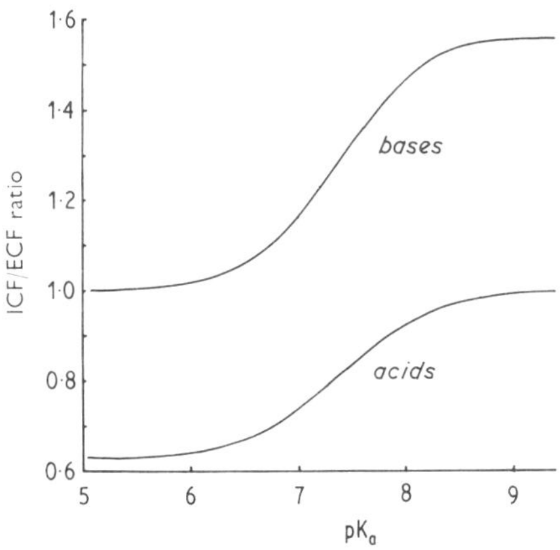

Fig. 3.3. Distribution of free drug across the cell membrane. ICF/ECF ratios (ordinate) calculated from the Henderson–Hasselbalch equation at each pK_a value, taking an ICF pH of 7·2 and ECF 7·4.

Protein Binding

Protein binding can reduce transfer of a ligand across a porous capillary membrane as well as across a lipid membrane. High plasma protein binding not only slows transfer by diffusion (*see above*) but also favours a high plasma concentration relative to that in ECF, CSF and glomerular filtrate, the concentration of protein in these three fluids being less than that in plasma [100, 121, 174]. The concentration of unbound phenytoin [69, 84], phenobarbitone and primidone [69] correlates well with, and is approximately equal to, CSF concentration in epileptic patients. Moreover, clinical signs of intoxication by phenytoin are more closely related to free than to total plasma concentration [16]. Saliva concentrations of certain drugs (p. 160) are also closely related to unbound plasma concentration.

Disparity in the abilities of maternal and fetal plasma proteins to bind drugs affects the equilibrium feto-maternal concentrations. For example, maternal plasma proteins bind local anaesthetics [127, 167, 168], phenobarbitone and phenytoin [49] more than do fetal, while they appear to bind salicylates less readily [83]. Moreover, cord albumin concentration is lower than maternal after Caesarian section but higher after vaginal delivery [93].

TISSUE DISTRIBUTION

Tissue concentrations of drugs are often higher than might be predicted from knowledge of their ionization and plasma protein binding characteristics. For example, for thiopentone, an acidic drug which is about 75 per cent ionized [155], one would predict tissue levels much lower than total plasma concentration. Lean tissue concentrations, however, are very similar to plasma, while fat concentration is higher [62].

Phenytoin is an acidic drug which is more than 90 per cent bound [135] and more frequently measured in steady-state conditions than is thiopentone. Brain concentrations of phenytoin, measured at temporal lobectomy in epileptic patients, are approximately equal to total plasma concentrations, while much higher than CSF concentrations [69]. Muscle concentrations, while correlating well with plasma concentrations, are slightly lower. Such relatively high lean tissue concentrations as are seen with thiopentone and phenytoin, may be explained in terms of high solubility in lipid elements in tissues, or binding to tissue proteins.

Tissue concentrations of basic drugs such as local anaesthetics would be predicted to be higher than free plasma concentrations on the grounds of their ionization, but plasma protein binding should offset the ion-trapping effect. Yet bupivacaine, highly lipid soluble and protein bound, and lignocaine, somewhat less so, are both taken up extensively by tissues. Two min after a bolus injection, brain, lung and kidney concentrations are 5–10 times those in plasma in rodents [127, 161]. The high affinity of lung tissue for drugs has been attributed to its content of surfactant [115]. Both drugs continue to be taken up by less well-perfused tissues for some hours [2, 127] (*Fig. 3.4*). Thus tissue binding is at least as extensive as plasma protein binding.

The extent of tissue uptake of a drug is generally measured in terms of its distribution volume (V_D) in litres per kilogram. This is that volume which the total body content of a drug would occupy if it were everywhere at a concentration equal to that in the plasma. Table 3.1 shows V_D values for a range of drugs. Bearing in mind that total body water is 0·5–0·6 l/kg, the uptake by spaces other than plasma of the upper three lipid-soluble drugs is clear. Thus nortriptyline, in common with other tricyclic antidepressants and many tranquillizers, is extensively concentrated in tissues. While plasma level is so low in relation to total body content, little drug is delivered to either liver or kidneys for elimination, and the half-life is proportionately long. Even for lignocaine and thiopentone, only a small proportion of drug is to be found in plasma after the first few seconds. Each must depend mainly upon metabolism to be eliminated, otherwise the half-life would be in the region of 100 years [25]. Tubocurarine, on the other hand, a totally hydrophilic drug, has a distribution volume less than the extracellular fluid, arguing some plasma protein binding [154], and its half-life, depending mainly on renal excretion, is relatively short.

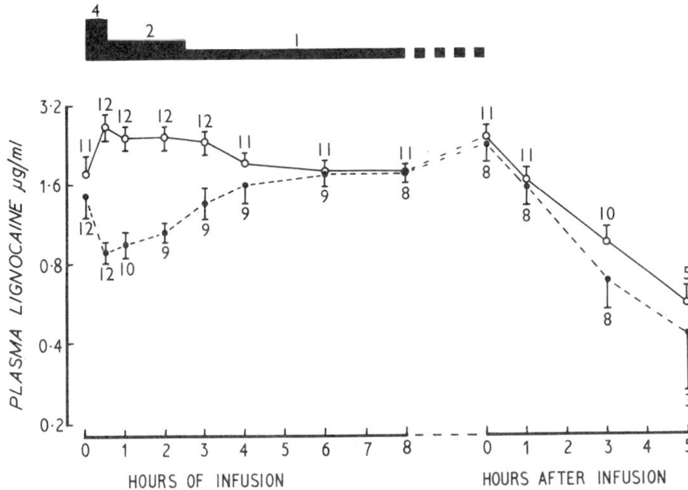

Fig. 3.4. Lignocaine infusions given to two groups of patients with arrhythmias following myocardial infarction. Each received a bolus (75 mg) at time 0, then one group (-- ● --) an infusion of 1 $mg.min^{-1}$ and the other (–○–) a declining rate shown in $mg.min^{-1}$ at the top: the 4–2–1 regime. Continuing tissue uptake of lignocaine makes the level in the first group rise slowly over 6 hr. The 4–2–1 regime is necessary to maintain adequate plasma levels during early tissue uptake (therapeutic range ≏ 7–17 μmol/l). Both groups show evidence of further tissue uptake between 8 hr and the end of the infusion. (*From Aps et al. [2]. Reproduced by kind permission of the* British Medical Journal.)

Table 3.1.

	V_D *(l/kg)*	*Half-life (hr)*
Nortriptyline [55]	22·1	34·2
Lignocaine [2]	1·5	2·4
Thiopentone [55]	1·2	4·0
Tubocurarine [55]	0·14	0·8

When assessing V_D it is important that steady-state conditions have first been attained [2]. This is difficult since true equilibrium never occurs with a drug which is extensively taken up by tissues. Deceptive results for V_D and half-life are obtained if they are measured while tissue distribution is incomplete: V_D will be too small and half-life too short.

When studying the transfer of drugs across membranes, it is desirable to establish first the equilibrium distribution. A steady-state ratio for distribution between two media is not always unity, which may cause confusion when studying transfer *rates.* This caution applies particularly to CSF: plasma [80] and fetal: maternal [131] ratios.

INDIVIDUAL MEMBRANE SYSTEMS

THE PLASMA MEMBRANE [94, 171]

The plasma membrane surrounds the cell and controls its internal environment by virtue of selective permeability. It carries specific surface receptors associated with the ability of the cell to specialize and to interact with other cells, with agonists and other chemicals.

The red cell membrane is the most frequently studied. It consists of about 50 per cent protein and 30 per cent or more of lipid, while less than 10 per cent is carbohydrate. The lipid content is much higher in the nerve cell membrane, providing an effective insulating layer. The protein content is mainly intrinsic, that is within the structure of the membrane, while a smaller proportion, surface protein, termed extrinsic, is easily removed on washing the membrane. Most of the lipid content of the cell membrane is phospholipid, which is amphipathetic in nature. The lipid is in two layers, with the molecules normally lying parallel to one another and arranged at right-angles to the plane of the membrane. It is assumed that the glycerol end of each molecule, which is hydrophilic, carrying as it does phosphate and other ionized groups, is to be found at the inner or outer surfaces of the membrane, while the lipophilic fatty acid chains are towards the centre. Large intrinsic protein molecules appear to float like icebergs protruding from this lipid bilayer and can move in the plane of the membrane, presumably with a hydrophilic pole protruding and hydrophobic pole concealed within the lipid. Many of the protein molecules are so large that, while coiled, they protrude from both surfaces of the membrane which is a mere 60–90 Å in thickness.

The plasma membrane is a simple biological lipid membrane, across which lipid-soluble compounds diffuse readily while water-soluble substances are more limited in their transfer. Water diffuses freely, though not as rapidly as lipid-soluble substances. Non-ionized water-soluble substances of low molecular weight ($<$60–100) are assumed to diffuse with water through hypothetical pores. The pores are probably formed by protein molecules. Ionized drugs diffuse only slowly [96], while ions such as Na^+ and K^+ are actively transported by ATPase (*see above* under Types of Transfer: Active Transport). Plasma membranes of excitable cells, such as nerve and muscle, are relatively impermeable to Na^+ in the resting state, but a large transient increase in permeability occurs on stimulation and is involved in propagation of an impulse. This increase in permeability is probably associated with an altered configuration in transport protein molecules, and may affect drug transfer. While it has generally been accepted that lignocaine diffuses to the interior aspect of the axonal membrane by non-ionic diffusion, its main action, that of occluding the Na^+ channels [136], is produced by the cation [137]. This action is shared by quaternary derivatives of local anaesthetics [111, 162], which are known to act only when applied to the axoplasmic aspect of the membrane. Hille [66] showed that highly lipid-soluble agents such as tetracaine (amethocaine) produced a rapid blocking effect on isolated single myelated nerve fibres while quaternary local anaesthetics applied internally required repeated depolarization to achieve their full effect. He suggested that such hydrophilic drugs can reach the receptors in the sodium channels only when the channels are open.

Carbon dioxide potentiates the stabilizing effect of local anaesthetics on axonal membranes [32]. There are several reasons for this [31]. When given in the form of lignocaine carbonate, the pH of the solution is higher than that of lignocaine hydrochloride, since it is the salt of a weaker acid. A higher concentration of uncharged base is therefore available for penetration. Once injected, carbon dioxide is released and, being a very rapid diffuser, reaches the interior of the axon sooner than does lignocaine. Within the axon it lowers the pH, thereby increasing the ionization of lignocaine. This has a twofold effect. Firstly the concentration of base is reduced, thereby increasing the diffusion gradient into the cell by ion trapping. Secondly, the concentration of active cation is increased. Finally carbon dioxide itself has a nerve-blocking effect on desheathed preparations.

The ability of drugs to cross cell membranes and consequently enter the intracellular compartment affects their distribution volume. This is discussed under Tissue Distribution (p. 146).

CAPILLARIES

Knowledge of capillary structure grew with the advent of the electron microscope. Hitherto, structure was surmised from the apparent permeability to molecules of different sizes. Thus brain capillaries on the grounds of their relative impermeability to hydrophilic compounds were assumed to be made up of endothelial cells that were continuously welded together; all other capillaries, classed together, were assumed to have intercellular clefts [115] and merely to be spot-welded [114]. Electron microscope studies do not endorse this generalization. Following his initial studies of the ultrastructure of vascular membranes however, Majno [88] classified capillaries into three types: type I, continuous; type II, fenestrated; type III, discontinuous – sinusoids.

I. *Continuous Capillaries*

Continuous capillaries have a continuous sheet of endothelium and a continuous basement membrane. Adjacent cells overlap one another, and the outer leaflets of adjacent membranes fuse along the luminal edge of each cleft: so-called 'tight junctions'. Capillary walls are 0·1–0·3 μm thick except at the nuclear bulge. Continuous capillaries are found in muscle (skeletal, cardiac and smooth), lung and central nervous system. In muscle, pinocytotic vesicles are numerous. In lung, capillary walls are very thin and vesicles fewer. Fewest vesicles are seen in central nervous system capillaries [122], in which the pericytes (isolated cells which surround capillaries) are embedded in a thick multiple-leaflet basement membrane, while glial cells ensheath 85 per cent of the outer layer.

II. *Fenestrated Capillaries*

Fenestrated capillaries also have a continuous basement membrane and tight junctions between cells. Endothelial cells are thinner (0·06–0·1 μm) and are pierced in places with windows about 0·1 μm in diameter through which the luminal cell membrane becomes continuous with the outer membrane. Fenestrae have been classified as either open or closed [88] ; in the latter a diaphragm of unknown composition is present [171] .

Fenestrated capillaries are found particularly in areas of fluid production implying a filtration function; thus they are present in the renal glomerulus, in which they are open [100] , in the choroid plexus, ciliary body, endocrine and exocrine glands [88] and in counter-current systems such as the renal medulla [146] .

III. *Discontinuous Capillaries*

In discontinuous capillaries or sinusoids there are intercellular gaps and the basement membrane is patchy or absent. Thus macromolecules and even whole cells can pass in and out. This type of capillary is found in the liver, spleen and bone marrow [88] .

There have been few direct studies of the transfer of drugs across capillary walls, though the generalization is often made that all molecules up to a molecular weight of 20–40 000 can escape from all capillaries except from those of the brain [115] , quite indiscriminately. This figure is an approximation which refers only to dextrans [125] . From this it would be inferred that all free drugs, whether ionized or not, would pass freely out of all non-CNS capillaries, though the protein-bound fraction would be retained to a large extent. Many studies have been made of the ability of various macromolecules to escape from the bloodstream at different sites.

Capillary permeability has been studied directly by electron microscopy using a marker such as horseradish peroxidase (molecular weight 40 000) which produces an electron-dense reaction product [15, 160, 172, 173] , with fluorescent dyes [65] , by measurement of the protein content of perivascular tissue [174] , in the limbs by measurement of lymph : plasma ratios [125] and in the glomerulus by measuring urine : plasma ratios [100, 124, 139] .

Measuring the protein content of perivascular tissue, in a site unspecified, Witte [174] found it to be about 20 per cent of that in plasma, the highest levels being found nearest the vessels, and in the region of the venules. Hauck [65] , studying the permeability of mesenteric microvasculature to fluorescent dyes and protein, confirmed the relatively high permeability of venules, while capillaries are intermediate and arterioles least permeable. Venules are said to have loose junctions, whose leakiness is labile and increased by histamine, 5-hydroxytryptamine (serotonin) and bradykinin [171]. Even in venules diffusion was mainly outwards in the mesentery, where lymphatics are numerous and connective tissue fibres appear to channel dyes towards the lymph capillaries [65]. The ultrastructure of mesenteric capillaries is similar to the continuous capillaries in cardiac and skeletal muscle [95]. Of continuous capillaries, those of the central nervous system have been said to show 'complete protein impermeability', and those of skeletal muscle 'small protein permeation', with fluid balance maintained by filtration and reabsorption while the contribution of lymph in muscle can be neglected. In contrast, in liver sinusoids there is complete protein permeability along the length of the capillary bed, with no gradient, and in this area lymph drainage is important [65].

Muscle

Physiologically, muscle capillaries behave as if they had large and small pores [172]. These have been supposed to represent cytoplasmic vesicles and intercellular junctions, respectively. Williams and Wissig [172] found that skeletal muscle capillary endothelium formed a substantial relative barrier to horseradish peroxidase, but was not impervious. Some marker was seen in vesicles, but they saw no evidence that loaded vesicles arrived at the contraluminal surface. They found no evidence that horseradish peroxidase penetrated the tight junctions, though they admitted passage could be occurring very slowly. The same workers previously [173] found evidence that microperoxidase crossed the capillary endothelium of the diaphragm. They felt justified in identifying the junction as the site of the small pore. It is not possible to deny this without knowing the nature of the material forming tight junctions. Studying myocardial capillary permeability to albumin, Na^+, K^+, glucose and sucrose, Bassingthwaighte and his colleagues [5] found evidence that such hydrophilic solutes penetrated 100 Å intercellular clefts.

Renkin and Garlick [125] studied the transcapillary exchange of large molecules between plasma and lymph in nephrectomized dogs. Sucrose or a range of dextrans were infused to maintain a steady plasma concentration, and lymph was collected from a hindlimb. They were thus principally studying muscle capillary permeability. The lymph : plasma ratio of sucrose reached a steady-state of 1 at 3–4 hr, while that for dextran was only 0·35 at 4–5 hr. They showed that capillary permeability to dextrans was considerably less than that to serum albumin, on a molecular weight basis: dextran at a molecular weight of 22 000 had a diffusion coefficient of the same order as serum albumin. The effective hydrodynamic radius of each in solution was similar at about 35 Å. They stated that the flexible chain configuration of the dextran molecule was looser than that of protein, and consequently the envelope was larger for a given molecular weight. They concluded that for the plasma–lymph barrier, molecular size was the discriminating characteristic, with permeability falling off sharply between 20 and 40 Å, coinciding with molecular weights of 10–30 000.

These limits on molecular radius coincide with those found by Robertson and his colleagues [139] for the fenestrated capillaries of the renal glomerulus, but do not bear out the prediction of Bassingthwaighte et al. [5] that there are pores of 100 Å radius, unless one allows for a water envelope for each molecule.

It would be interesting to know how the fully ionized neuromuscular-blocking drugs, for which there is indeed a blood–brain barrier, apparently reach the extracellular compartment in muscle with such rapidity. One cannot envisage that vesicular transport would be sufficiently quick to fit the known clinical facts, and it is clear that functionally if not structurally there must be adequate gaps.

Lung

Lung capillaries, like those of the central nervous system, have tight junctions [33] and few vesicles. They are, however, very thin walled [88] and are therefore tailor-made to allow rapid diffusion of respiratory and anaesthetic gases and vapours, which diffuse readily across lipid membranes. The uptake of anaesthetic gases will be the subject of a later review. The permeability of lung capillaries to hydrophilic molecules such as sucrose, glucose and sodium acetate, studied by Basset et al. [4] and to protein is not great. Permeability appeared to increase with flow, presumably because a larger number of capillaries filled, so increasing the extraction of marker substance into the scant lung parenchyma. It is clearly highly desirable that hydrophilic molecules such as protein should be unable to escape lung capillaries in normal circumstances because of the danger of pulmonary oedema. Extraction of blood-borne lipid-soluble non-volatile drugs by lung parenchyma is high, as discussed earlier (p. 146 and *Fig. 3.1*).

Drug transfer across central nervous system and renal capillaries is discussed in separate sections.

THE CENTRAL NERVOUS SYSTEM

In the past there have been several misconceptions about the blood supply to the brain. An early one was that the blood–brain barrier was absolute and that the brain received its nutrition solely from the CSF [42]. This clearly would be a very impractical way of reaching all parts of the brain rapidly. The view resulted from the observation that trypan blue injected systemically would stain all parts of the body except the CNS, yet injected into the CSF the brain was stained. The second misconception was that the CNS contained little or no extracellular fluid. In death, brain cells take up water by osmosis, but in life the ECF volume in the brain is of the same order as in other tissues: 10–15 per cent [114, 121]. The third was that the blood–brain barrier lay in the dense basement membrane and glial cells investing CNS capillaries [42, 80]. Electron microscope studies have shown that the principal barrier to diffusion is in the endothelial cells themselves [15, 42, 114].

Although structurally and functionally the nature of the blood–brain barrier and the blood–CSF barrier are very different, they show similar selective permeability, characteristic of a lipid membrane. Brain capillaries are continuous, with tight junctions, no fenestrae, few vesicles and a thick basement membrane which splits to enclose the pericytes. Glial cells invest 85 per cent of the outer layer [122]. Endothelial cells are united by tight junctions, preventing the passage of the electron microscope marker, horseradish peroxidase (molecular weight 40 000), everywhere except the area postrema, the median eminence and the pineal body [15], where the blood–brain barrier shows increased permeability to hydrophilic substances including non-lipid-soluble drugs. Capillaries of the choroid plexus are fenestrated, and perform the initial step in CSF production, that is filtration of fluid into the stromal space between capillary endothelium and ependymal epithelium. The ependymal lining of the ventricles forms specialized cells over the choroid surface, which are sealed laterally by tight junctions, and which allow more restricted filtration and perform active transport, in the final modification of the CSF [42]. Though brain capillaries are relatively impermeable to protein and to smaller hydrophilic molecules, choroid capillaries are not. Here protein passes into perivascular connective tissue, but enters CSF only slowly because of the impermeability of the ependymal epithelium [24]. Protein and peptides diffusing slowly through into the CSF are rapidly taken up again by cells of the choroid plexus. Elsewhere pia and ependymal membranes are more permeable because adjacent epithelial cells do not have occlusive tight junctions [42]. The CSF is in free communication with brain ECF, and tracers which cannot cross the blood–brain barrier diffuse readily into the brain when injected into the ventricles [24, 114]. Certain ependymal cells of the third ventricle, the tanycytes, are specialized to pinocytose macromolecules. They are believed to transport hormones from the CSF to particular areas of brain parenchyma [13, 21]. CSF drains into the venous sinuses via the arachnoid granulations. These contain valves which open under pressure and which have a pore size greater than 100 Å. Water plus all solutes irrespective of molecular size pass freely out of the CSF system by bulk flow. The CSF can therefore act as a sink for hydrophilic solutes such as metabolites in brain. It is clear therefore that tracer substances can pass freely from brain to CSF and vice versa, while in natural circumstances endogenous solutes pass from blood equally rapidly to brain and to CSF, and the two are in equilibrium.

Drug Penetration

We have seen earlier (p. 140) that highly lipid-soluble and diffusible substances such as thiopentone and inhalational anaesthetics pass readily into the brain at such a rate that brain and plasma concentrations are in equilibrium. For drugs of low lipid solubility penetration is slower.

Transfer of drugs across the blood–brain barrier may be studied by a single shot technique, such as that of Oldendorf, in which the uptake of a labelled drug is compared with that of tritiated water in what amounts to a single circulation [113, 114, 116]. This technique essentially studies rate of transfer and ignores steady-state brain : plasma or CSF : plasma ratios. If these are far from unity results of rate studies can be misleading [80].

Oldendorf et al. [116] studied single circulation penetration of narcotic analgesics in the rat. They found that morphine uptake was below the measurable level while codeine uptake was 24 per cent, methadone 42 per cent and heroin (diamorphine) 68 per cent of that of tritium. The contrast between heroin and morphine is associated with acetylation of the polar phenolic hydroxy groups of the latter drug and bears out what any junky can tell you, that main-lining heroin can give you a good kick. The steady-state brain : plasma ratios and rates of transfer of narcotics are likely to be reduced if the plasma pH falls and vice versa [72].

Oldendorf [114, 115] found that clearance by brain of nicotine, ethanol, imipramine, caffeine, procaine and antipyrine (phenazone) was virtually complete after bolus intravenous injection.

Hydrophilic compounds, such as inulin and ionized drugs, diffuse very much more slowly into CSF than does water, while they pass equally rapidly out at the arachnoid villi. The CSF : plasma ratio is therefore always low and never rises no matter how long is allowed for equilibration [121]. In addition to this sink action, prostaglandins, iodide, thiocyanate, 5-hydroxytryptamine, adrenaline, dyes, *p*-aminohippurate, metabolites and penicillin are actively taken up by cells of the choroid plexus and returned to the bloodstream against a concentration gradient [42, 80, 114, 121].

Certain amino acids, particularly essential ones, and sugars such as D-glucose are transported into brain by selective and saturatable carrier processes [113]. CSF levels are always lower than plasma, however, because of consumption by cells and because of active uptake by choroid plexus and brain [42]. Oldendorf [114] postulates that there are four carriers for transport across the blood–brain barrier: one for D-glucose and related hexoses, one for large neutral amino acids, one for basic amino acids and one for short-chain monocarboxylic acids. He suggests that amphetamine entry may be accelerated by one of these.

Neurotransmitters do not cross cerebral capillaries, the endothelial cells of which moreover contain dopa decarboxylase and monoamine oxidase [86]. The selective permeability of the blood–brain barrier is manipulated successfully in the treatment of Parkinsonism with levodopa. The blood–brain barrier is relatively impermeable to dopamine, the transmitter in short supply in Parkinsonism. It is, however, permeable to the precursor L-dopa, which is taken up by dopaminergic neurones in the CNS and converted to dopamine. The peripheral side effects of levodopa can be mitigated by giving a dopa decarboxylase inhibitor which cannot traverse the blood–brain barrier. Centrally induced nausea and vomiting are reduced because of increased permeability to the decarboxylase inhibitor of the capillaries supplying the chemoreceptor trigger zone in the area postrema. A lipid-soluble dopamine agonist such as bromocriptine is less specific than levodopa since it acts throughout the brain rather than just at dopaminergic nerve terminals [114]. It may be more successful than levodopa, however, if dopaminergic neurones have virtually degenerated and cannot decarboxylase dopa [118].

Penetration of the blood–brain barrier by the poorly lipid-soluble cytotoxic drugs is relevant to the treatment of cerebral leukaemia. Oldendorf [115] found that uptake by brain of methotrexate and cytosine arabinoside (cytarabine) was negligible. Bourke and co-workers [19] made a careful study of the penetration of 5-fluorouracil into brain after intravenous infusion in monkeys. Brain levels rose progressively over 60 min, suggesting slow penetration, but except in high perfusion areas such as the cerebral cortex did not approach arterial concentration. Uptake was better after ventriculo-cisternal perfusion which they suggest should be combined with systemic administration in leukaemia treatment. The metastases of solid tumours, however, acquire an abnormal vasculature with freely permeable capillaries.

The influence of lipid solubility, ionization and protein binding on the equilibrium distribution of drugs is discussed earlier (p. 141 *et seq.*).

Alteration of the Blood–Brain Barrier

Immutable though the tight junctions of the brain capillary endothelium may appear, the permeability of the blood–brain barrier does vary with circumstances.

Changes in temperature and pH alter partition coefficients of weak acids and bases [74], which will alter both their rate of transfer and their equilibrium distribution. Apart from this obvious factor, a reduction in $P\mathrm{a,co_2}$ reduces the entry to brain of hydrophilic compounds such as urea. This could be because of cerebral vasoconstriction [121] which could slow equilibration of many drugs. Forster and co-workers [58] studied the effect on the penetration of Evans blue into rabbit brains of thiopentone and halothane, combined with alterations in $P\mathrm{co_2}$. They state that while thiopentone causes cerebral vasoconstriction, halothane causes vasodilatation and blood–brain barrier permeability was maximum with halothane in the absence of hypokapnoea.

Electrically induced seizures have been found to increase blood–brain barrier permeability in patients [14] and in rats to horseradish peroxidase [15]. This change is probably secondary to an increase in arterial pressure. It has been postulated that acute hypertension widens the endothelial tight junctions [122], an explanation savouring of frozen pipes. Electron microscopy reveals increased pinocytosis in these circumstances [15] which would seem more plausible. Hyperosmolarity, induced by urea and electrolytes, similarly produces increased permeability which has been attributed to endothelial shrinkage opening intercellular clefts [123] but is again probably associated with an observed increase in pinocytosis [160].

The effects of noradrenaline on the cerebral circulation have been studied and are complex. Although noradrenaline cannot penetrate cerebral capillaries, levels in plasma and CSF have been found to be related [178]. Noradrenaline, like metaraminol, given systemically may cause hypertension and its associated changes [15]. Injected directly into the cerebral circulation it constricts cerebral vessels [86]. Given after urea which increases its penetration, there is an increase in cerebral blood flow which may be secondary to increased carbohydrate metabolism or increased synaptic activity in the brain [86].

THE KIDNEY

The capillaries of the renal glomerulus have open fenestrae and a continuous basement membrane [88]. They are designed to combine a high filtration rate with a high degree of impermeability to plasma proteins [100]. The impermeability to protein appears to come from the dense basement membrane, since both the fenestrae and the slits between the epithelial cells on the tubule side of the basement membrane are too wide to offer any resistance [124]. Water and small molecular weight solutes are filtered into the tubule at a rate governed by hydrostatic minus colloid osmotic pressure [139]. The protein concentration in the Bowman's capsule space is small, and it diminishes further as protein is taken up by pinocytosis by the cells of the proximal tubule [171].

To assess glomerular capillary permeability on a molecular weight basis, Mogensen [100] studied renal clearance in normal and diabetic subjects of a range of dextrans, which are neither secreted nor reabsorbed in the tubule [139]. He found clearance to be related to glomerular filtration and to decline exponentially with molecular weight to reach a clearance near zero at a molecular weight of 55 000. This approximates to a molecular radius of about 52 Å. In diabetics both glomerular filtration rate and dextran clearance were high. Professor Robertson and his colleagues [139] showed that dextran clearance was inversely related to molecular radius between 20 and 40 Å (*Fig. 3.5*). Below this level permeation was as free as that of water. Considering proteins, the same range of behaviour could be observed between inulin, on the one hand, which is cleared at the glomerular filtration rate, and albumin at the other, which is virtually barred. Clearance of albumin cannot however be assessed in the usual way, since it is reabsorbed in the proximal tubule.

As glomerular filtration rate increases, urine clearance of dextrans decreases [100, 139]. It appears therefore that macromolecules traverse glomerular capillaries by a combination of bulk flow, in which they are filtered less rapidly than water, and diffusion, down the gradient so created.

Renkin [124] pointed out that in the glomerulus, molecular radius does not appear to govern transfer of different molecular types as it does in limb capillaries [125] and that the glomerulus is relatively *less* permeable to protein than to dextran.

It is well established that unbound drugs, which have molecular weights in the hundreds rather than the thousands, are filtered freely in the glomerulus, whether ionized or not.

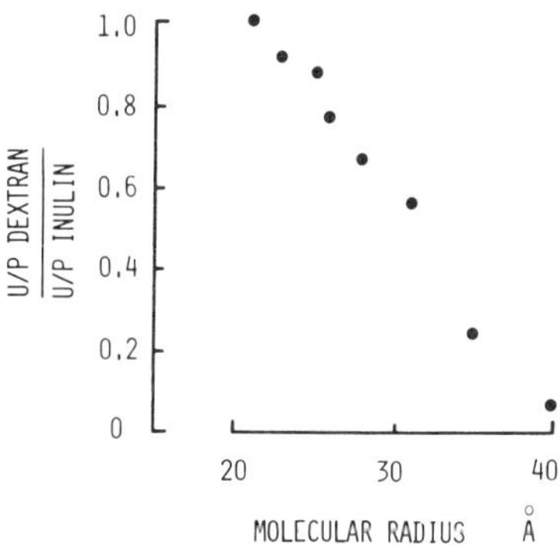

Fig. 3.5. Renal clearance ratio (ordinate) of a range of dextrans, related to molecular radius (abscissa). Clearance ratio (dextran/inulin) is used to compensate for the effect of glomerular filtration rate in dextran clearance. (*Data reproduced by kind permission of Professor Robertson [139].*)

The renal tubule acts as a lipid membrane since the cells which form it are bound together by tight junctions and complex interdigitations [171]. Peritubular capillaries are fenestrated, highly permeable to macromolecules and designed to absorb large volumes of fluid [146]. The reabsorption of over 99 per cent of the glomerular filtrate volume creates a concentration gradient for the reabsorption by diffusion of all drugs that are lipid soluble. Such reabsorption may be modified or even reversed by altering urinary pH. Eriksson [53] compared the clearances of prilocaine and lignocaine with that of inulin in human subjects. Clearances of both drugs exceeded that of inulin in an acid urine, while in alkaline urine they were less. His findings suggested free permeability of tubule cells to the non-ionized fraction and complete impermeability to cations, while it appeared that fractions protein-bound and taken up in red cells could rapidly be liberated to take part in non-ionic diffusion processes, as predicted by Milne et al. [96]. Even when the urine is acid, however, the overall percentage excretion of unchanged local anaesthetics is not great [6, 128]. Excretion of amphetamine, on the other hand, can be increased to a clinically important extent by acidifying urine with ammonium chloride [9].

The excretion of weak acids such as barbiturates (pK_a range 7·2–8·2) is favoured by alkalinizing the urine with sodium bicarbonate which will increase their ionization from say 50 per cent at pH 7·4 to 91 per cent at pH 8·4. Salicylate is a stronger acid (pK_a 3), which is actively transported in the renal tubule (*see below*), yet increasing the urinary pH from 5 to 8 (increasing the ionized fraction from 99 per cent to 99·999 per cent) can increase urinary excretion threefold (*Fig. 3.6*), such is the force of the ion-trapping effect on the gradient of non-ionized salicylate.

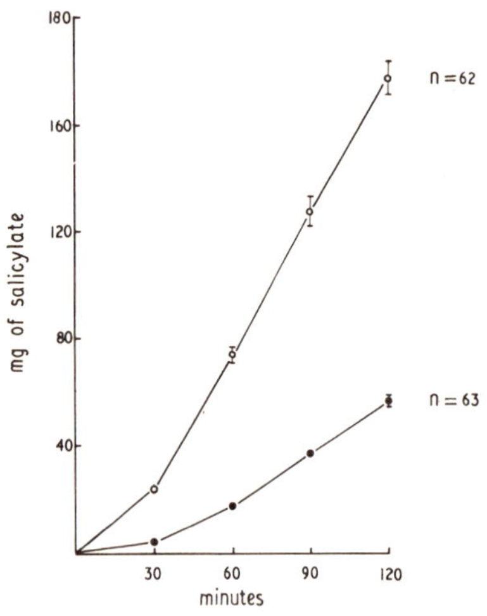

Fig. 3.6. Cumulative excretion of salicylate in 125 medical students after 856 mg orally (1 g of sodium salicylate). Mean total excretion ± standard error is shown at each half-hour period. One group (–○–) received sodium bicarbonate, 10 g at –60 min which maintained urine pH at 7·5–9. The other group (–●–) received ammonium chloride, 7 g, urine pH 4–5·5.

In addition to non-ionic diffusion, acidic drugs may be actively transported in the renal tubule. In the proximal tubule there are special mechanisms for the reabsorption and secretion of organic acids [22] involving a carrier substance. Penicillin is actively secreted at such a rate that its clearance approximates to the renal plasma flow. Such transport may be inhibited by probenicid, which competes for the carrier, so as to reduce penicillin clearance to that of the glomerular filtration rate. Aspirin, phenylbutazone, thiazide diuretics and frusemide are all actively secreted in the proximal tubule and tend to inhibit urate excretion. Urate is actively transported in both directions, the secretion pathway being more readily inhibited but the reabsorption being the larger component. Small doses of uricosurics therefore may increase plasma urate, whereas large doses reduce it.

MUCOUS MEMBRANES

Mucous membranes behave as lipid membranes, across which drugs diffuse at a rate largely dependent upon their lipid solubility.

The Eye

The potency of atropine-like drugs in producing midriasis when applied to the conjunctival sac is in part determined by their degree of ionization [153]. The corneal epithelium is the greatest barrier to diffusion in this circumstance since it is composed of tightly packed layers of cells. A highly lipid-soluble β-blocker such as pindolol has systemic β-blocking effects when applied to the conjuctival sac [156]. This effect is attributed to absorption after passing down the nasolacrimal duct.

The Nose

Drugs are occasionally administered via nasal mucous membrane, usually for a local effect, for example nasal decongestants, but also for their systemic effect, as snuff. Vasopressin may be given by this route. Being a peptide, it is digested if swallowed but, although hydrophilic, manages to diffuse slowly into the systemic circulation

The Mouth

Drugs, which if swallowed would be inactivated in the gastrointestinal tract or the liver may be absorbed directly into the systemic circulation from the buccal and oral cavities. Glyceryl trinitrate is chewed and sucked in the treatment of angina, to avoid its high hepatic first pass clearance. Oxytocin, another peptide hormone, may be given by the buccal route to accelerate labour. Because of its hydrophilic nature, absorption of oxytocin by this route is slow and therefore sustained.

Buccal Absorption

Evidence of the prevalence of non-ionic diffusion in drug transfer across membranes is provided by studies of so-called 'buccal absorption' [7, 9, 127]. Weakly acidic or basic drugs dissolved in buffer at varying pH values are held and agitated in the mouth for a period of time after which the contents of the mouth are expelled and residual drug measured. The mucous membrane of oral and buccal cavities acts as a lipid membrane across which drug diffuses. Absorption of basic drugs is maximum from buffer at high pH, it is greater at high pH for drugs of greater lipid solubility, and the rate of increase of absorption with rise in pH depends on the pK_a of the drug. In *Fig. 3.7,* bupivacaine, which has a higher pK_a than lignocaine and mepivacaine, is not absorbed at all from a buffer pH less than 5, while at higher pH values its absorption exceeds that of the other

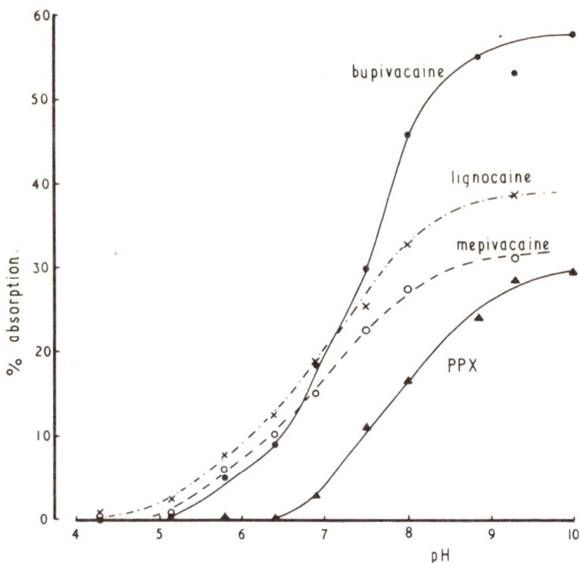

Fig. 3.7. Absorption from the oral mucosa of local anaesthetics and pipecolylxylidine (PPX), a more hydrophilic metabolite of mepivacaine and bupivacaine. The mixture of drugs was dissolved in a range of buffers. (*See* text p. 159)

two because of its higher lipid solubility. Such changes in buccal absorption very nicely predict alterations in renal excretion that can be achieved by varying urinary pH [9].

Saliva

Drugs may pass *into* saliva *from* the circulation. Saliva drug measurements are used in routine drug monitoring (for drugs such as anticonvulsants) because they reflect free drug concentration [36, 110, 135]. The relationship holds good for a drug such as phenytoin, which is poorly ionized at physiological pH, irrespective of saliva pH or flow [135]. Saliva concentration of phenobarbitone is lower than free plasma concentration, and the correlation less perfect, as the drug is more ionized than phenytoin and saliva pH varies and is less than plasma [132]. With drugs that are more strongly ionized still (propranolol, pethidine) the relationship is random [110].

Trachea and Bronchi

Local anaesthetics applied to the upper air passages are rapidly absorbed across the mucous membrane into the bloodstream [3, 26, 44]. Absorption of lignocaine may be less rapid when it is applied by spray to the larynx and pharynx rather than to the trachea [40] where more reaches the greater surface area of the lower bronchial tree. Bupivacaine and lignocaine, inhaled as aerosols of particle size 7–11 μm, can suppress respiratory reflexes such as the stretch reflex and the cough reflex, mediated by receptors in the submucosa [39, 71]. In this respect the more lipid-soluble bupivacaine produces the more profound and predictable effect.

Gastrointestinal Tract

Drugs that are swallowed may be destroyed by gastric acid (penicillin), broken down enzymatically (peptide hormones), conjugated in the gut wall (morphine) or metabolized by the liver (lignocaine). Apart from these minor mishaps, absorption of drugs in the gastrointestinal tract follows the same rules for non-ionic diffusion as apply to other lipid membranes, while certain drugs such as orally active penicillins may be actively transported. This vast subject will not be covered further here as it is not of prime importance to anaesthetists.

THE PLACENTA

The ultrastructure of the placenta varies with species and with gestation time. The human placenta in late gestation is of the haemomonochorial type, i.e. a single layer of fetal chorionic tissue separates the maternal blood from fetal capillary endothelium. Early in gestation chorionic tissue erodes the uterine spiral arteries, and thereafter maternal blood enters the maternal sinuses, which have no lining of maternal tissue, from jet-like open ends of these arteries. Fetal chorionic tissue is arranged in about 100 cotyledons, each one of which is made up of numerous complex chorionic villi, of which the total surface area amounts to about 7 m^2 at term [59]. Each villus is covered with a single continuous trophoblastic layer, the syncytiotrophoblast, enclosing a core of chorionic connective tissue, in which lie the fetal capillaries. Beneath the syncytiotrophoblast are islands of cells, the cytotrophoblast, which do not form a barrier between maternal and fetal blood. The syncytiotrophoblast is the business part of the placenta and regions are differentiated to perform separate functions.

Secretion

The surface of most of the syncytiotrophoblast is covered with microvilli, which become shorter and more dense during gestation, to increase placental surface area. They are rich in ATPase and at their bases form pinocytotic vesicles, which transport protein. Hormone production and transfer, and specialized transport processes, appear to take place in these areas.

Transfer by Diffusion

In certain areas microvilli are absent, the syncytiotrophoblast is thinner and becomes fused or closely applied to the capillary endothelium beneath, to form vasculo-syncytial membranes. These bulge into intervillous spaces and are specialized primarily for rapid transfer by diffusion of respiratory gases.

A similar range of processes transfer substances across the placenta as is available in other membranes [90] (*see* Types of Transfer, p. 136). Again, all the evidence suggests that lipid-soluble drugs cross the placenta by passive diffusion, and in this respect the placenta behaves similarly to other lipid membranes. Transfer presumably takes place mainly across vasculo-syncytial membranes. There is some evidence that in the intact placenta there are theoretical stomata which only open at fetal perfusion pressures in excess of 100–160 mmHg [79]. Although the placenta is apparently leakier than the blood–brain barrier, quaternary ammonium compounds crossing it slowly, this difference could be explained not by the superior impermeability of the blood–brain barrier, but by the sink effect of the CSF (p. 154).

All drugs cross the placenta, and with prolonged maternal administration, the dose received by the fetus is appreciable. The rate and extent of transfer are important only when a drug is used acutely near delivery. Given at this time it may affect the ability of the neonate to survive, and the dose received transplacentally is an important determinant of its effect. This review is therefore mainly concerned with drugs used in labour. Placental transfer of drugs is generally assessed by measuring fetal : maternal concentration ratios. These need careful interpretation because they are influenced by all the following factors: (*a*) the site of sampling from maternal and fetal blood, (*b*) the rate of transfer of drug across the placenta, (*c*) the relative affinity of maternal and fetal plasma for the drug and (*d*) the extent of equilibration.

Sampling Site

On the maternal side, blood is commonly sampled from a cubital vein. The drug concentration will not necessarily equal that in the uterine vein, since the fetus is a deeper compartment than the maternal forearm, and during uptake of the drug he extracts more from the maternal circulation. Arterial blood will tell us only what arrived at the placental bed, not what equilibrated with it. Uterine venous sampling is revealing [158] but rarely feasible. On the fetal side the situation is more complex. Umbilical venous (UV) blood is commonly sampled, yet this is a pre-mixed site containing blood before its dilution with the rest of the venous return (*see Fig. 3.8*). Sampling here is analogous to sampling from the maternal cubital vein proximal to the site of injection. Even fetal arterial blood is not homogeneous, and umbilical arterial concentration does not necessarily reflect that going to the brain. Because of the peculiarities of the fetal circulation with little mixing in the right atrium, when large amounts of drug cross the placenta, carotid concentration is higher than that in the umbilical artery. All these strictures are particularly applicable when drug concentrations are changing rapidly.

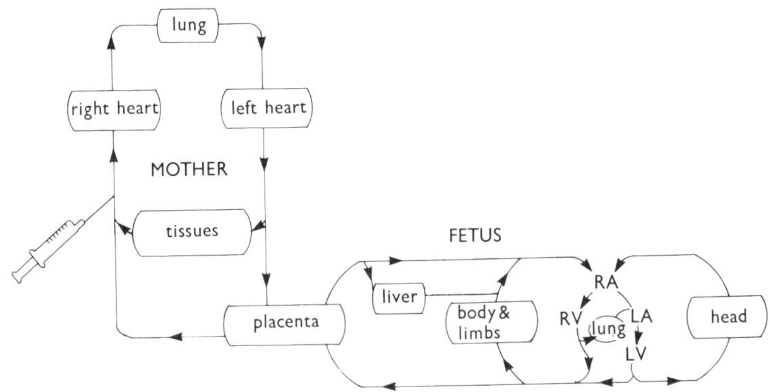

Fig. 3.8. Diagram of the maternal and fetal circulations. An intravenous bolus to the mother is diluted by her own venous return and taken up to some extent by her lungs before reaching her own tissues and the placenta. There are further dilutions before the drug reaches fetal brain: (*a*) the placenta may take up a small proportion, (*b*) a variable proportion (around half) of the UV flow goes to the liver where drug is extracted and partly metabolized, (*c*) the remainder goes via the ductus venosus to the IVC where it is diluted by the venous return from the fetal body and limbs, (*d*) there may be some mixing in the right atrium (RA) with SVC blood and (*e*) mixing with the small volume of blood perfusing the lung antenatally. (*Reproduced from Reynolds [131] by kind permission of Pitman Medical Publishing Company.*)

Rate of Placental Transfer

The same drug factors govern this as govern rate of diffusion elsewhere (p. 138). There are, however, factors peculiar to the placenta.

DIFFUSION CAPACITY The placenta has a great reserve capacity for diffusion. Fibrin deposition in the maternal intervillous spaces does not apparently impair materno-fetal exchange [59]. It is usually accompanied by fibrosis of the associated fetal villi and up to 30 per cent of exchange area may be lost without detriment to the fetus. Not so placental infarction, which may be associated with intrauterine death and eclampsia. The major cause of placental insufficiency is a reduction in maternal blood supply.

Lipid-soluble drugs diffuse rapidly across the placenta. There is a good reason to suppose that uterine venous and umbilical venous concentrations are in equilibrium for drugs such as nitrous oxide [158], thiopentone [57], and bupivacaine [133, 134]. The rate-limiting step in equilibration of the whole fetus is therefore not placental diffusion but blood flow [147]. Drugs of intermediate lipid solubility appear to cross the placenta by non-ionic diffusion at a rate proportional to their lipid solubilities [18, 109]. Fully ionized drugs such as quaternary ammonium compounds do cross the placenta but much more slowly [17, 45, 75, 76, 117, 165, 177]. In such cases transfer is diffusion-limited, and the term placental 'barrier' is appropriate.

MATERNAL AND FETAL BLOOD FLOW tend to maintain the supply of drug and its gradient across the placenta. High maternal blood flow accelerates total drug transfer and hence full fetal equilibration. Thus theoretically a baby not jeopardized by placental insufficiency is more likely to suffer prolonged drug effects. Uterine contraction temporarily reduces maternal placental blood flow and therefore reduces transfer of a suitably timed bolus injection [64]. Similarly at vaginal delivery, cord compression and consequently reduced fetal flow in the placenta may limit placental transfer of a thiopentone bolus [55]. The actual effect that a bolus of thiopentone, for example, has on the baby is well recognized to be much less than that on the mother. This has nothing to do with any placental 'barrier'. The explanation can be found in the nature and relationship of the maternal and fetal circulations, as represented in *Fig. 3.8*. The bolus, injected into the maternal forearm, is diluted once by the rest of the maternal venous return before reaching both the maternal tissues and the placenta. Given complete placental equilibration the same bolus therefore reaches both UV and maternal brain. Across the placenta, however, the bolus meets not a single organ but a whole new world. Initially there may be some placental uptake and even metabolism of the drug [78] though the capacities of both are quickly saturated. About 50 per cent of the UV blood passes to the liver and the remainder to the inferior vena cava via the ductus venosus. The fetal liver has a considerable capacity to concentrate drugs [56, 60] and some to metabolize them [68]. What remains of the drug bolus in the ductus venosus is diluted by the rest of the venous return from the lower half of the body and passes to the right atrium. Here it may be mixed to some extent with superior vena caval blood, before the majority passes to the left atrium, left ventricle, aorta and carotid artery to the brain. It is thus easy to see how a bolus to the mother is decimated before reaching fetal brain.

Relative Affinity of Maternal and Fetal Plasma for the Drug

When UV blood is sampled at birth, the fetal : maternal ratio is rarely 1; it is not necessarily related to sampling time, but is rather a characteristic of the particular drug. This is because, for weak acids and bases and non-polar compounds given in labour, though UV blood may be in equilibrium with maternal blood leaving the placental bed, maternal and fetal blood differ in their affinities for the drug. As described earlier (p. 145), the pH gradient across the placenta has a small effect, which tends in many cases to be swamped by a difference in protein-binding affinities. This effect is illustrated in *Fig. 3.9* for bupivacaine. Gibb et al. [61] showed that inhalational anaesthetics were not all equally soluble in maternal and fetal blood.

The Extent of Equilibration

Theoretical considerations governing the rate of equilibration of drug in fetal tissues have been ably analysed by Professor Dawes [43] and Pro-

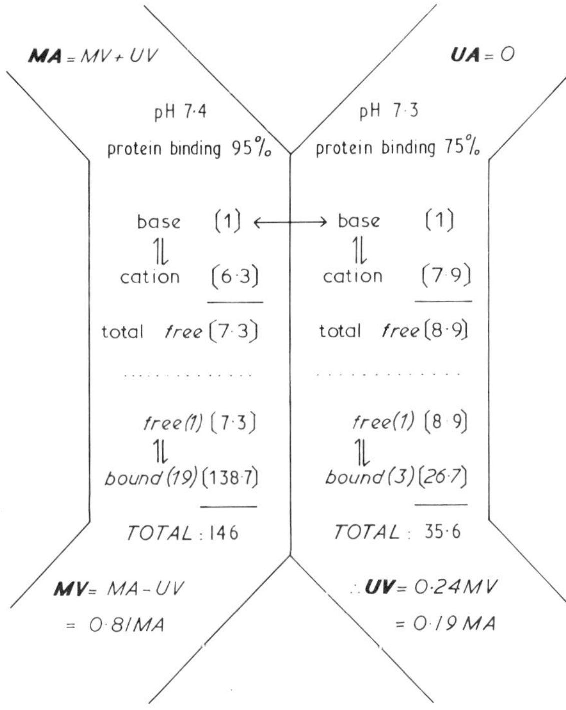

Fig. 3.9. Placental transfer of bupivacaine: the effect of ion trapping and protein binding. The left-hand channel represents the maternal placental flow and the right the fetal. They are assumed to be equal. When the drug first enters the maternal artery (MA) none is present in the umbilical artery (UA). The free non-ionized base equilibrates, but because of different affinities UV concentration is only 0·24 × MV. Because so little is extracted from maternal blood, 80 per cent equilibration (MV = 0·81 × MA) takes place immediately. This is analogous to the rapid initial rise in partial pressure of nitrous oxide in arterial blood, because of its low blood–gas partition coefficient. In this example parallel flow is assumed rather than cross current or counter current. (*Reproduced from Reynolds [131] by kind permission of Pitman Medical Publishing Company.*)

fessors Goldstein, Aronow and Kalman [63] and will be summarized here. Making certain assumptions about the fetal circulation, and neglecting elimination, these authorities calculated that while oxygen, with a small distribution volume, would be 90 per cent equilibrated in 6–8 min, for antipyrine, distributed in the total body water the equivalent time would be 30–40 min. For drugs actually concentrated in tissues as are some central nervous depressants and allied drugs, equilibration would take even longer. These calculations assumed instantaneous placental diffusion (valid for thiopentone and nitrous oxide for example) and homogeneous fetal tissues. Thus equilibration will be even slower for more water-soluble drugs and for poorly perfused tissues.

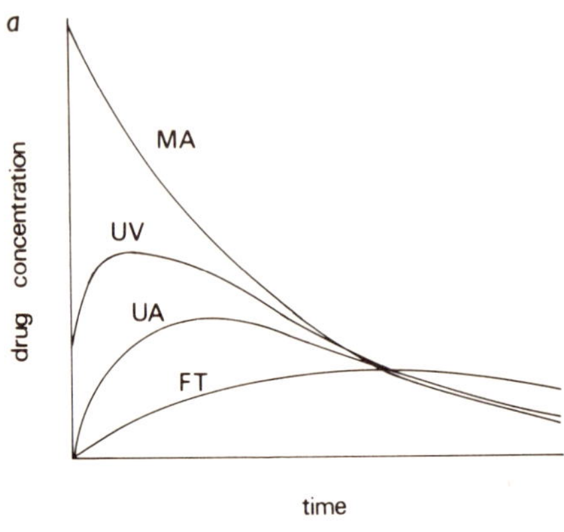

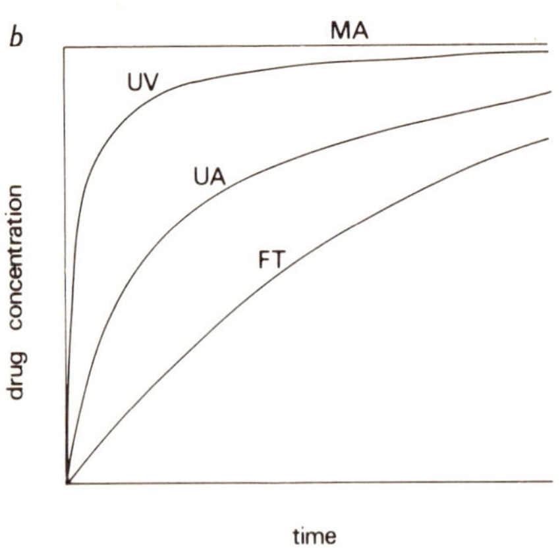

Fig. 3.10. Kinetics of materno-fetal equilibration. *a*, Hypothetical concentrations after a maternal intravenous bolus of a drug with a short half-life in the maternal circulation, which crosses the placenta with ease and is distributed throughout the fetal body water. *b*, If material concentration remains constant, fetal levels rise higher than in *a*, but only reach maternal concentration at infinity. MA = maternal artery; UV = umbilical vein; UA = umbilical artery; FT = fetal tissues. (*Reproduced from Reynolds [131] by kind permission of Pitman Medical Publishing Company.*)

In *Fig. 3.10* two theoretical situations are represented, in which effects of metabolism are neglected. In the upper graph, the mother has been given a bolus intravenous injection of a drug, the concentration of which then declines rapidly as it is distributed in the maternal tissues. The more quickly the maternal concentration falls, the more rapidly will UV concentration approach, or in some cases even exceed it. The lag in UA concentration reflects tissue uptake. Fetal tissue levels rise the most slowly and will remain high the longest. In the lower graph, the maternal arterial concentration is steady and theoretically equilibrium between maternal and fetal circulations will only be attained at infinite time. Thus although equilibration is slower, fetal tissue levels are potentially higher than in the upper graph. Indeed, detrimental effects from prolonged general anaesthesia and prolonged high maternal levels of other CNS depressant drugs are well documented [23].

For a drug with a short half-life in the maternal circulation, it is clear that fetal tissue levels are but a fraction of the initial maternal concentration. The bolus effect on the baby is therefore small (*see above*), but a full systemic dose given by intravenous bolus to the mother may have a more marked effect on the baby than the same dose given slowly or intramuscularly. Crawford and Rudofsky [38] showed that more pethidine reaches the baby after an intravenous bolus than after an intramuscular injection to the mother. In the latter, maternal arterial concentration is never very high. Umbilical venous concentrations of pethidine rapidly exceeded maternal in a study in sheep [149] after intravenous injection, though after intramuscular injection in clinical practice fetal : maternal ratios exceed 1 only after about 140 min [29] by which time maternal concentrations are very low.

Drugs used in labour rarely behave as predictably as in *Fig. 3.10*, and maternal and fetal concentrations fluctuate continually, upsetting the equilibrium.

Drug Elimination

Differences in drug elimination between fetus and mother mean that there must be a two-way passage of unchanged drug and metabolites. Nitrous oxide can be rapidly taken up by maternal inhalation, and almost as rapidly eliminated in her expired air. This route however is not available to the fetus who must pass inhalational anaesthetics back to the mother. Indeed the placenta is the most important route of elimination of all drugs for the fetus, who may survive doses lethal to the neonate. Since lipid-soluble drugs diffuse most readily, it is important that the fetus should *not* be able to form hydrophilic metabolites, so he passes chloramphenicol, for example, back to the mother for conjugation. Such metabolites would otherwise become trapped in the fetal environment, and accumulate particularly in amniotic fluid, as do hydrophilic drugs given to the mother over a long period [177]. There is evidence that the fetus can *N*-dealkylate drugs [50, 67, 89, 148], primary and secondary amines then returning to the mother, but that hydroxylation and conjugation processes are sluggish or absent [89, 92, 97, 112, 141].

Placental Transfer of Individual Drugs

Inhalational Anaesthetics

Inhalational anaesthetics diffuse rapidly across the placenta and the affinities of maternal and fetal blood for the agents are similar, the greatest disparity being for halothane which is 1·3 times as soluble in maternal as in fetal blood [61]. Distribution volumes however are high, so full fetal equilibration is not rapid [91]. During prolonged anaesthesia for Caesarian section, Stenger et al. [158] showed that uterine venous nitrous oxide rose more slowly than maternal arterial concentration to reach about 90 per cent of it at 35 min, and that uterine venous and UV concentrations at delivery were equal. In much other work, only UV and maternal arterial or brachial venous (MV) concentrations at delivery are measured. At Caesarian section UV : MV ratios have been found to be 0·66 for halothane and 1·0 for ether [169] and 0·7 for methoxyflurane [34, 152], though less than this for short operations. When anaesthesia followed analgesia with methoxyflurane, UV : MV ratios were similar though absolute levels higher [34].

Uptake of inhalational anaesthetics is therefore analogous to that shown in the lower graph in *Fig. 3.10*, and it is not surprising that the longer the period of maternal anaesthesia before delivery, the greater the detriment to the fetus.

Barbiturates

These drugs diffuse across the placenta at a rate dependent upon their lipid solubility [30]. Mirkin [99] states that many barbiturates cross the placenta 'with ease . . . as a consequence, equilibrium . . . is often established within minutes'. This is a non-sequetor. Thiopentone equilibrates *across the placenta* in a single circulation, yet because of its high V_D, full fetal equilibration is a long process [56]. Because thiopentone is given by bolus, its transfer is subject to placental blood-flow changes (p. 164). Fetal concentrations of barbiturates rarely exceed maternal [46, 55, 57, 81], which is compatible with a small ion-trapping effect in the mother, and negligible disparity in protein binding.

Ketamine

Ketamine crosses the placenta rapidly, UV concentration exceeding maternal 1½ min after injection [51]. There is evidence that it may impair placental function either by augmenting uterine contractions or by vasconstriction.

Narcotic Analgesics

Narcotic analgesics are more than 95 per cent ionized at physiological pH. Nevertheless even pethidine, not one of the most lipid soluble, crosses the placenta so rapidly that when injected intravenously in ewes, UV concentrations exceeded maternal within a minute of the end of the infusion [149]. In clinical practice, UV : maternal ratios of about 1 are commonly observed [8, 103] and they have been found to rise with time [29]. UV : maternal ratios are higher than those of pentazocine [8, 103], the latter drug being much less lipid soluble. Methadone ratios are generally lower: about 0·1 after a single dose [1] and 0·5 after chronic administration [140]. This drug is highly lipid soluble, so used chronically placental distribution is likely to be near equilibrium, and disparities must be accounted for by high maternal protein binding.

The effects of pethidine and pentazocine on the neonate at birth may be slight and indistinguishable [48, 102]. Only pethidine has been extensively scrutinized for later effects on the neonate. Even small doses produce evidence of depression of respiration [138, 163], of suckling and of other neurobehavioural responses [20]. Neonatal depression is greatest when pethidine has been given 3 hr or more before delivery [108, 150] and may be due to fetal accumulation of pethidine or its metabolites [107, 159].

Tranquillizers

Phenothiazines, such as promethazine and promazine, are widely used in labour, yet their placental transfer has been little studied. Since they are weak bases which affect the central nervous system, they inevitably cross the placenta in appreciable quantities in the non-ionized form [170]. Promazine has been shown to cross rapidly, but fetal levels have been found to be lower than maternal [37].

Benzodiazepines have been extensively studied. Diazepam, when used acutely in labour, crosses the placenta rapidly; within a few minutes the fetal : maternal ratio is about 1 [54, 64, 89] and rises to 2 within a few hours [54, 70, 89, 148]. Diazepam is about 95 per cent bound in adults, and a very small increase in binding on the fetal side could account for this high equilibrium ratio. The placental transfer of a maternal bolus can be reduced slightly by synchronizing injection with a contraction [64], but long term use of diazepam is associated with loss of fetal autonomic control of heart rate [148], neonatal hypothermia, hypotonia and raised serum bilirubin [47]. Nitrazepam, given 12 hr before delivery, produces approximately equal fetal and maternal concentrations [73].

Autonomic Drugs

The placental transfer of catecholamines is negligible [12, 119] though synthetic β-stimulants and blockers cross the placenta slowly [119, 145]. Atropine, a weak base, crosses rapidly, the UV : MV ratio attaining 0·93 at 5 min, when the UA : UV ratio was 0·5 [77]. Neostigmine, which possesses a quaternary ammonium group, would be likely to cross slowly, and indeed when given to the mother it fails to reduce atropine tachycardia in the fetus [98].

Neuromuscular-blocking Drugs

Neuromuscular-blocking drugs are fully ionized, and diffuse only very slowly across the placenta. Clearly there is familiar clinical evidence, as well as circumstantial laboratory evidence [28, 176], of an effective placental barrier to these drugs. Sensitive assay techniques can detect small and slowly increasing concentrations of alcuronium [166], dimethyltubocurarine (metocurine) [76] and pancuronium [17] in cord blood in obstetrics, and of suxamethonium in monkeys [45]. True neuromuscular blockade is only likely to occur in the neonate after prolonged and generous maternal administration, and indeed such a case has been reported after 245 mg of tubocurarine had been given to a mother in status epilepticus [117].

Diazoxide

Diazoxide is a weak acid used in labour as an antihypertensive or to inhibit uterine contractions [105]. In combination with chlormethiazole, its use may be associated with neonatal hypotonia and hypoventilation [72], and it may also cause neonatal hypotension [105] and diabetes in animals [126]. Fetal arterial concentrations reach maternal arterial concentrations in 1–2 hr [105].

Local Anaesthetics

Local anaesthetics are weak bases that are mostly more lipid-soluble than narcotic analgesics. They cross the placenta rapidly and fetal : maternal ratios reflect the protein-binding characteristics of the individual drugs rather than the sampling times. UV : maternal ratios range from 0·24 to 0·3 for bupivacaine [10, 11, 87, 133, 134, 167] and etidocaine [85, 104, 120], about 0·55 for lignocaine [52, 133, 164, 165], 0·7 mepivacaine [27, 101, 106] and >1 for prilocaine [52]. Local anaesthetics are less bound in fetal than in maternal blood [127, 167, 168], such disparity having most effect in the most highly bound (*Fig. 3.9*).

The greater safety for the baby of bupivacaine [143] over lignocaine and mepivacaine [106, 142, 151] lies not in its lower fetal : maternal ratios, since *free* concentration (that fraction related to pharmacological effectiveness) is equal in mother and fetus [167]. Rather it lies in its long duration of action and consequent greatly reduced tendency to accumulate in the systemic circulation [127, 133].

REFERENCES

1. Aps C. (1978) Personal communication.
2. Aps C., Bell J. A., Jenkins B. S. et al. (1976) Logical approach to lignocaine therapy. *Br. Med. J.* **1**, 13–15.
3. Aström A. (1966) The pharmacological action of local anesthetics. *Acta Anaesthesiol. Scand.* Suppl. 25, 19–22.
4. Basset G., Fulla Y., Moreau F. et al. (1975) Lung capillaries permeability to small molecules. *Bibl. Anat.* **13**, 17–20.
5. Bassingthwaighte J. B., Yipintsoi T. and Grabowski E. F. (1975) Myocardial capillary permeability: hydrophilic solutes penetrate 100 Å intercellular clefts. *Bibl. Anat.* **13**, 24–27.
6. Beckett A. H., Boyes R. N. and Appleton P. J. (1966) The metabolism of excretion of lignocaine in man. *J. Pharm. Pharmacol.* **18**, 76S–81S.

7. Beckett A. H., Boyes R. N. and Triggs E. J. (1968) Kinetics of buccal absorption of amphetamines. *J. Pharm. Pharmacol.* **20**, 92–97.
8. Beckett A. H. and Taylor J. F. (1967) Blood concentrations of pethidine and pentazocine in mother and infant at time of birth. *J. Pharm. Pharmacol.* **19**, 50S–52S.
9. Beckett A. H. and Triggs E. J. (1967) Buccal absorption of basic drugs and its application as an *in vivo* model of passive drug transfer through lipid membranes. *J. Pharm. Pharmacol.* **19**, 31S–41S.
10. Belfrage P., Berlin A., Raabe N. et al. (1975) Lumbar epidural analgesia with bupivacaine in labor. Drug concentration in maternal and neonatal blood at birth and during the first day of life. *Am. J. Obstet. Gynecol.* **123**, 839–844.
11. Belfrage P., Raabe N., Thalme B. et al. (1975) Lumbar epidural analgesia with bupivacaine in labor. Determination of drug concentration and pH in fetal scalp blood, and continuous fetal heart rate monitoring. *Am. J. Obstet. Gynecol.* **121**, 360–365.
12. Berg D., Schulz J., Wernicke K. et al. (1973) The effect of experimental acute decrease of uterine perfusion and maternal hypoxia on the fetus. *J. Perinat. Med.* **1**, 36–52.
13. Bleier R. (1970) The relations of ependyma to neurons and capillaries in the hypothalamus: a Golgi–Cox study. *J. Comp. Neurol.* **142**, 439–463.
14. Bolwig T. G., Hertz M. M., Paulson O. B. et al. (1977) The permeability of the blood–brain barrier during electrically induced seizures in man. *Eur. J. Clin. Invest.* **7**, 87–93.
15. Bolwig T. G., Hertz M. M. and Westergaard E. (1977) Acute hypertension causing blood–brain barrier breakdown during epileptic seizures. *Acta Neurol. Scand.* **56**, 335–342.
16. Booker H. E. and Darcey B. (1973) Serum concentrations of free diphenylhydantoin and their relationship to clinical intoxication. *Epilepsia* **14**, 177–184.
17. Booth P. N., Watson M. J. and McLeod K. (1977) Pancuronium and the placental barrier. *Anaesthesia* **32**, 320–323.
18. Boulos B. M., Davis L. E., Larks L. S. et al. (1971) Placental transfer of drugs iv. Placental transfer of chlorpromazine, pentobarbital phenylbutazone with fetal electrocardiographic changes as determined by direct lead tracing. *Arch. Int. Pharmacodyn.* **194**, 403–414.
19. Bourke R. S., West C. R., Chheda G. et al. (1973) Kinetics of entry and distribution of 5-fluorouracil in cerebrospinal fluid and brain following intravenous injection in a primate. *Cancer Res.* **33**, 1735–1746.
20. Brackbill Y., Kane J., Manniello R. L. et al. (1974) Obstetric premedication and infant outcome. *Am. J. Obstet. Gynecol.* **118**, 377–384.
21. Brawer J. R. (1972) The fine structure of the ependymal tanycytes at the level of the arcuate nucleus. *J. Comp. Neurol.* **145**, 25–41.
22. Brazeau P. (1975) Inhibitors of tubular transport of organic compounds. In: Goodman L. S. and Gilman A. (ed.), *The Pharmacological Basis of Therapeutics.* New York, Macmillan, pp. 860–866.
23. Brazelton T. B. (1961) Psychophysiological reactions in the neonate. II. Effect of maternal medication on the neonate and his behaviour. *J. Pediatr.* **58**, 513–518.
24. Brightman M. W. (1967) The intracerebral movement of proteins injected into blood and cerebrospinal fluid of mice. *Prog. Brain Res.* **29**, 19–37.
25. Brodie B. B. (1964) Distribution and fate of drugs; therapeutic implications. In: Binns T. B. (ed.), *Absorption and Distribution of Drugs.* London, E. & S. Livingstone, pp. 199–251.
26. Bromage P. R. and Robson J. G. (1961) Concentrations of lignocaine in blood after intravenous, intramuscular, epidural and endotracheal administration. *Anaesthesia* **16**, 461–478.

27. Brown W. U., Bell G. C., Lurie A. O. et al. (1975) Newborn blood levels of lidocaine and mepivacaine in the first postnatal day following maternal epidural anesthesia. *Anesthesiology* **42**, 698–707.
28. Buller A. J. and Young I. M. (1949) The action of *d*-tubocurarine chloride on foetal neuromuscular transmission and the placental transfer of this drug in the rabbit. *J. Physiol.* **109**, 412–420.
29. Caldwell J., Wakile L. A., Notarianni L. J. et al. (1977) Transplacental passage and neonatal elimination of pethidine given to mothers in childbirth. *Br. J. Clin. Pharmacol.* **4**, 715P–716P.
30. Cassano G. B., Ghetti B., Gliozzi E. et al. (1967) Autoradiographic distribution study of 'short acting' and 'long acting' barbiturates: ^{35}S-thiopentone and ^{14}C-phenobarbitone. *Br. J. Anaesth.* **39**, 11–20.
31. Catchlove R. F. H. (1972) The influence of CO_2 and pH on local anesthetic action. *J. Pharmacol. Exp. Ther.* **181**, 298–309.
32. Catchlove R. F. H. (1973) Potentiation of two different local anaesthetics by carbon dioxide. *Br. J. Anaesth.* **45**, 471–474.
33. Chinard F. P. (1970) Permeability of the pulmonary blood–gas barrier. In: Crone C. and Lassan N. A. (ed.), *Capillary Permeability*. Copenhagen, Monksgaard, pp. 605–613.
34. Clark R. B., Cooper J. O., Brown W. E. et al. (1970) The effect of methoxyflurane on the foetus. *Br. J. Anaesth.* **42**, 286–294.
35. Collander R. and Bärlund H. (1933) Permeabilitätsstudien an *Chara ceratophylla:* II. Die Permeabilität für Nichtelektrolyte. *Acta Bot. Fenn.* **11**, 1.
36. Cook C. E., Amerson E., Poole W. K. et al. (1975) Phenytoin and phenobarbital concentrations in saliva and plasma measured by radioimmunoassay. *Clin. Pharmacol. Ther.* **18**, 742–747.
37. Crawford J. S. and Rudofsky S. (1965) Placental transmission and neonatal metabolism of promazine. *Br. J. Anaesth.* **37**, 303–313.
38. Crawford J. S. and Rudofsky S. (1965) The placental transmission of pethidine. *Br. J. Anaesth.* **37**, 929–933.
39. Cross B. A., Guz A., Jain S. K. et al. (1976) The effect of anaesthesia of the airway in dog and man: a study of respiratory reflexes, sensations and lung mechanics. *Clin. Sci.* **50**, 439–454.
40. Curran J., Hamilton C. and Taylor T. (1975) Topical analgesia before tracheal intubation. *Anaesthesia* **30**, 765–768.
41. Curry S. H. (1974) *Drug Disposition and Pharmacokinetics.* Oxford, Blackwell.
42. Davson H. (1976) The blood–brain barrier. *J. Physiol.* **255**, 1–28.
43. Dawes G. S. (1973) Theory of fetal drug equilibration. In: Boreus L. (ed.), *Fetal Pharmacology*. New York, Raven Press, pp. 381–397.
44. Deacock A. R. and Simpson W. T. (1964) Fatal reactions to lignocaine. *Anaesthesia* **19**, 217–221.
45. Drabkova J., Crul J. F. and van der Kleijn E. (1973) Placental transfer of ^{14}C labelled succinylcholine in near-term *Macaca mulatta* monkeys. *Br. J. Anaesth.* **45**, 1087–1096.
46. Draffan G. H., Dollery C. T., Davies D. S. et al. (1976) Maternal and neonatal elimination of amobarbital after treatment of the mother with barbiturates during late pregnancy. *Clin. Pharmacol. Ther.* **19**, 271–275.
47. Drew J. H. and Kitchen W. H. (1976) The effect of maternally administered drugs on bilirubin concentration in the newborn infant. *J. Pediatr.* **89**, 657–661.
48. Duncan S. L. B., Ginsburg J. and Morris N. F. (1969) Comparison of pentazocine and pethidine in normal labor. *Am. J. Obstet. Gynecol.* **105**, 197–202.
49. Ehrnebo M., Agurell S., Jalling B. et al. (1971) Age differences in drug binding by plasma proteins: studies on human foetuses, neonates and adults. *Eur. J. Clin. Pharmacol.* **3**, 189–193.

50. Eliot B. W., Hill J. G. and Cole A. P. (1975) Continuous pethidine/diazepam infusion during labour and its effects on the newborn. *Br. J. Obstet. Gynaecol.* **82**, 126–131.
51. Ellingson A., Haram K., Sagen N. et al. (1977) Transplacental passage of ketamine after intravenous administration. *Acta Anaesthesiol. Scand.* **21**, 41–44.
52. Epstein B. S., Banerjee S. G. and Coakley C. S. (1968) Passage of lidocaine and prilocaine across the placenta. *Anesth. Analg. (Cleve.)* **47**, 223–227.
53. Eriksson E. (1966) Prilocaine: an experimental study in man of a new local anaesthetic with special regards to efficiency, toxicity and excretion. *Acta Chir. Scand.* Suppl. 358.
54. Erkkola R., Kangas L. and Pekkarinen A. (1973) The transfer of diazepam across the placenta during labour. *Acta Obstet. Gynecol. Scand.* **52**, 167–170.
55. Finster M., Mark L. C., Morishima H. O. et al. (1966) Plasma thiopental concentrations in the newborn following delivery under thiopental–nitrous oxide anesthesia. *Am. J. Obstet. Gynecol.* **95**, 621–629.
56. Finster M., Morishima H. O., Mark L. C. et al. (1972) Tissue thiopental concentrations in the fetus and newborn. *Anesthesiology* **36**, 155–158.
57. Flowers C. E. (1959) The placental transmission of barbiturates and their pharmacological action on the mother and the infant. *Am. J. Obstet. Gynecol.* **78**, 730–742.
58. Forster A., Van Horn K., Marshall L. F. et al. (1977) Influence of anesthetic agents on blood–brain barrier function during acute hypertension. *Acta Neurol. Scand.* Suppl. 56, 60–61.
59. Fox H. (1979) The correlation of placental structure and function. In: Chamberlain G. and Wilkinson A. (ed.), *Placental Transfer.* Tunbridge Wells, Pitman Medical, pp. 15–30.
60. Geddes I. C., Brand L., Finster M. et al. (1972) Distribution of halothane–^{82}Br in maternal and foetal guinea pig tissues. *Br. J. Anaesth.* **44**, 542–547.
61. Gibb C. P., Munson E. S. and Tham M. K. (1975) Anesthetic solubility coefficients for maternal and fetal blood. *Anesthesiology* **43**, 100–103
62. Goldstein A. and Aronow L. (1960) The durations of action of thiopental and pentobarbital. *J. Pharmacol. Exp. Ther.* **128**, 1–6.
63. Goldstein A., Aronow L. and Kalman S. M. (1974) *Principles of Drug Action,* 2nd ed. New York, John Wiley & Sons.
64. Haram K., Bakke O. M., Johannessen K. H. et al. (1978) Transplacental passage of diazepam during labor: influence of uterine contractions. *Clin. Pharmacol. Ther.* **24**, 590–599.
65. Hauck G. (1975) Permeability of the mesenteric microvasculature – tissue specificity and importance for basic research. *Bibl. Anat.* **13**, 9–12.
66. Hille B. (1977) Local anesthetics: hydrophilic and hydrophobic pathways for the drug–receptor reaction. *J. Gen. Physiol.* **69**, 497–515.
67. Hogg M. I. J., Wiener P. C., Rosen M. et al. (1977) Urinary excretion and metabolism of pethidine and norpethidine in the newborn. *Br. J. Anaesth.* **49**, 891–899.
68. Horning M. G., Butler C. M., Nowlin J. et al. (1975) Drug metabolism in the human neonate. *Life Sci.* **16**, 651–672.
69. Houghton G. W., Richens A., Toseland P. A. et al. (1975) Brain concentrations of phenytoin, phenobarbitone and primidone in epileptic patients. *Eur. J. Clin. Pharmacol.* **9**, 73–78.
70. Idänpään-Heikkilä J. E., Jouppila P. I., Poulakka J. O. et al. (1971) Placental transfer and fetal metabolism of diazepam in early human pregnancy. *Am. J. Obstet. Gynecol.* **109**, 1011–1016.
71. Jain S. K., Trenchard D., Reynolds F. et al. (1973) The effect of local anaesthesia of the airway on respiratory reflexes in the rabbit. *Clin. Sci.* **44**, 519–538.

72. Johnson R. (1976) Adverse neonatal reaction to maternal administration of intravenous chlormethiazole and diazoxide. *Br. Med. J.* **1**, 943.
73. Kangas L., Kanto J. and Erkkola R. (1977) Transfer of nitrazepam across the human placenta. *Eur. J. Clin. Pharmacol.* **12**, 355–357.
74. Kaufman J. J., Koski W. S. and Benson D. W. (1977) Temperature and pH sensitivity of the partition coefficient as related to the blood–brain barrier to drugs. *Exp. Eye Res.* **25**, 201–203.
75. Kivalo I. and Saarikoski S. (1972) Placental transmission and foetal uptake of ^{14}C-dimethyltubocurarine. *Br. J. Anaesth.* **44**, 557–561.
76. Kivalo I. and Saarikoski S. (1976) Placental transfer of ^{14}C-dimethyltubocurarine during Caesarian section. *Br. J. Anaesth.* **48**, 239–242.
77. Kivalo I. and Saarikoski S. (1977) Placental transmission of atropine at full term pregnancy. *Br. J. Anaesth.* **49**, 1017–1021.
78. Kyegombe D., Franklin C. and Turner P. (1973) Drug-metabolising enzymes in the human placenta, their induction and repression. *Lancet* **1**, 405–406.
79. Lemtis H. and Kirchner H. (1974) A rapid procedure for testing the integrity of the maternal–fetal barrier in spontaneously delivered placentas. *J. Perinat. Med.* **2**, 130–134.
80. Levin E. (1977) Are the terms blood–brain barrier and brain capillary permeability synonymous? *Exp. Eye Res.* **25** (Suppl.), 191–199.
81. Levy C. J. and Owen G. (1964) Thiopentone transmission through the placenta. *Anaesthesia* **19**, 511–523.
82. Levy G. and Hayton W. L. (1973) Pharmacokinetic aspects of placental drug transfer. In: Boreus L. (ed.), *Fetal Pharmacology.* New York, Raven Press, pp. 29–39.
83. Levy G., Procknal J. A. and Garrettson L. K. (1975) Distribution of salicylate between neonatal and maternal serum at diffusion equilibrium. *Clin. Pharmacol. Ther.* **18**, 210–214.
84. Lund L., Berlin A. and Lunde P. K. M. (1972) Plasma protein binding of diphenylhydantoin in patients with epilepsy. *Clin. Pharmacol. Ther.* **13**, 196–200.
85. Lund P. C., Cwik J. C., Gannon R. T. et al. (1977) Etidocaine for Caesarian section – effects on mother and baby. *Br. J. Anaesth.* **49**, 457–460.
86. MacKenzie E. T., McCulloch J., O'Keane M. et al. (1976) Cerebral circulation and norepinephrine: relevance of the blood–brain barrier. *Am. J. Physiol.* **231**, 483–488.
87. Magno R., Berlin A., Karlsson K. et al. (1976) Anaesthesia for Caesarian section IV: placental transfer and neonatal elimination of bupivacaine following epidural analgesia for elective Caesarian section. *Acta Anaesthesiol. Scand.* **20**, 141–146.
88. Majno G. (1965) Ultrastructure of the vascular membrane. In: Hamilton W. F. (ed.), *Handbook of Physiology,* Section 2. *Circulation,* vol. III, pp. 2293–2375.
89. Mandelli M., Morselli P. L., Nordio S. et al. (1975) Placental transfer of diazepam and its disposition in the newborn. *Clin. Pharmacol. Ther.* **17**, 564–572.
90. Marx G. F. (1961) Placental transfer and drugs used in anesthesia. *Anesthesiology* **22**, 294–313.
91. Marx G. F., Joshi C. W. and Orkin L. R. (1970) Placental transmission of nitrous oxide. *Anesthesiology* **32**, 429–432.
92. Meffin P., Long G. J. and Thomas J. (1973) Clearance and metabolism of mepivacaine in the human neonate. *Clin. Pharmacol. Ther.* **14**, 218–225.
93. Mendenhall H. W. (1970) Serum protein concentrations in pregnancy. III Analysis of maternal–cord serum pairs. *Am. J. Obstet. Gynecol.* **106**, 718–720.
94. Meymaris E. (1975) Chemical anatomy of the nerve membrane. *Br. J. Anaesth.* **47**, 164–172.

95. Michel C. C., Curry F. E., Mason J. C. et al. (1975) Permeability and selectivity of capillaries in the mesentery of the frog. *Bibl. Anat.* **13**, 6–8.
96. Milne M. D., Scribner B. H. and Crawford M. A. (1958) Non-ionic diffusion and the excretion of weak acids and bases. *Am. J. Med.* **24**, 709–729.
97. Mirkin B. L. (1970) Developmental pharmacology. *Annu. Rev. Pharmacol.* **10**, 255–272.
98. Mirkin B. L. (1973) Drug distribution in pregnancy. In: Boreus L. (ed.), *Fetal Pharmacology.* New York, Raven Press, pp. 1–26.
99. Mirkin B. L. (1976) In: *Perinatal Pharmacology and Therapeutics.* New York, Academic Press, p. 44.
100. Mogensen C. E. (1970) The permeability of the glomerular capillaries as studied by renal dextran clearance in normal and diabetic subjects. In: Crone C. and Lassen N. A. (ed.), *Capillary Permeability.* Copenhagen, Munksgaard, pp. 531–543.
101. Moore D. C., Bridenbaugh L. D., Bagdi P. A. et al. (1968) Accumulation of mepivacaine hydrochloride during caudal block. *Anesthesiology* **29**, 585–588.
102. Moore J., Carson R. M. and Hunter R. J. (1970) A comparison of the effects of pentazocine and pethidine administered during labour. *J. Obstet. Gynecol. Br. Commonw.* 77, 830–836.
103. Moore J., McNabb T. G. and Glynn J. P. (1973) The placental transfer of pentazocine and pethidine. *Br. J. Anaesth.* **45**, 798–801.
104. Morgan D. J., Cousins M. J., McQuillan D. et al. (1977) Disposition and placental transfer of etidocaine in pregnancy. *Eur. J. Clin. Pharmacol.* **12**, 359–365.
105. Morishima H. O., Cohen H., Brown W. U. et al. (1973) The inhibitory action of diazoxide on uterine activity in the subhuman primate: placental transfer and effect on the fetus. *J. Perinat. Med.* **1**, 13–23.
106. Morishima H. O., Daniel S. S., Finster M. et al. (1966) Transmission of mepivacaine across the human placenta. *Anesthesiology* **27**, 147–154.
107. Morrison J. C., Whybrew W. D., Rosser S. I. et al. (1976) Metabolites of meperidine in the fetal and maternal serum. *Am. J. Obstet. Gynecol.* **126**, 997–1002.
108. Morrison J. C., Wiser W. L., Rosser S. I. et al. (1973) Metabolites of meperidine related to fetal depression. *Am. J. Obstet. Gynecol.* **115**, 1132–1137.
109. Moya F. and Thorndike V. (1962) Passage of drugs across the placenta. *Am. J. Obstet. Gynecol.* **84**, 1778–1798.
110. Mucklow J. C., Bending M. R., Kahn G. C. et al. (1978) Drug concentration in saliva. *Clin. Pharmacol. Ther.* **24**, 563–570.
111. Narahashi T., Frazier D. T. and Yamada M. (1970) The site of action and active form of local anesthetics. I. Theory and pH experiments with tertiary compounds. *J. Pharmacol. Exp. Ther.* **171**, 32–44.
112. O'Donoghue S. E. F. (1971) Distribution of pethidine and chlorpromazine in maternal, foetal and neonatal biological fluids. *Nature* **229**, 124–125.
113. Oldendorf W. H. (1971) Brain uptake of radiolabelled amino acids, amines and hexoses after arterial injection. *Am. J. Physiol.* **221**, 1629–1639.
114. Oldendorf W. H. (1974) Blood–brain barrier permeability to drugs. *Annu. Rev. Pharmacol.* **14**, 239–248.
115. Oldendorf W. H. (1976) Certain aspects of drug distribution to brain. *Adv. Exp. Med. Biol.* **69**, 103–109.
116. Oldendorf W. H., Hyman S., Braun L. et al. (1972) Blood–brain barrier: penetration of morphine, codeine, heroin, and methadone after carotid injection. *Science* **178**, 984–986.
117. Older P. O. and Harris J. M. (1968) Placental transfer of tubocurarine. *Br. J. Anaesth.* **40**, 459–463.
118. Pearce I. and Pearce J. M. S. (1978) Bromocriptine in Parkinsonism. *Br. Med. J.* **1**, 1402–1404.

119. Van Petten G. R. and Willes R. F. (1970) β-adrenoceptive responses in the unanaesthetised ovine foetus. *Br. J. Pharmacol.* **38**, 572–582.
120. Poppers P., Covino B. and Boyes N. (1975) Epidural block with etidocaine for labour and delivery. *Acta Anaesthesiol. Scand.* Suppl. 60, 89–93.
121. Rall D. P. and Zubrod C. G. (1962) Mechanisms of drug absorption and excretion – passage of drugs in and out of the central nervous system. *Annu. Rev. Pharmacol.* **2**, 109–128.
122. Rapoport S. I. (1976) Opening of the blood–brain barrier by acute hypertension. *Exp. Neurol.* **52**, 467–479.
123. Rapoport S. I., Hori M. and Klatzo I. (1972) Testing of a hypothesis for osmotic opening of the blood–brain barrier. *Am. J. Physiol.* **223**, 323–331.
124. Renkin E. M. (1970) Permeability and molecular size in peripheral and glomerular capillaries. In: Crone C. and Lassan N. A. (ed.), *Capillary Permeability.* Copenhagen, Munksgaard, pp. 544–547 and discussion.
125. Renkin E. M. and Garlick D. G. (1970) Transcapillary exchange of large molecules between plasma and lymph. In: Crone C. and Lassan N. A. (ed.), *Capillary Permeability.* Copenhagen, Munksgaard, pp. 553–559.
126. Report (1970) Studies show diazoxide crosses the placenta. *JAMA* **212**, 720.
127. Reynolds F. (1970) Systemic toxicity of local analgesic drugs with special reference to bupivacaine. M.D. Thesis, University of London.
128. Reynolds F. (1971) Metabolism and excretion of bupivacaine in man – a comparison with mepivacaine. *Br. J. Anaesth.* **43**, 33–37.
129. Reynolds F. (1971) A comparison of the potential toxicity of bupivacaine, lignocaine and mepivacaine during epidural blockade for surgery. *Br. J. Anaesth.* **43**, 567–572.
130. Reynolds F. (1978) The pharmacology of local anaesthetic drugs. In: Churchill-Davidson H. C. (ed.), *A Practice of Anaesthesia.* London, Lloyd-Luke, pp. 1096–1126.
131. Reynolds F. (1979) Drug transfer across the placenta. In: Chamberlain G. and Wilkinson A. (ed.), *Placental Transfer.* Tunbridge Wells, Pitman Medical, pp. 166–181.
132. Reynolds F. (1978) Personal observation.
133. Reynolds F. and Taylor G. (1970) Maternal and neonatal concentrations of bupivacaine: a comparison with lignocaine during continuous extradural analgesia. *Anaesthesia* **25**, 14–23.
134. Reynolds F. and Taylor G. (1971) Plasma concentrations of bupivacaine during continuous epidural analgesia in labour: the effect of adrenaline. *Br. J. Anaesth.* **43**, 436–440.
135. Reynolds F., Ziroyanis P. N., Jones N. F. et al. (1976) Salivary phenytoin concentrations in epilepsy and in chronic renal failure. *Lancet* **2**, 384–389.
136. Ritchie J. M. (1975) Mechanism of action of local anaesthetic agents and biotoxins. *Br. J. Anaesth.* **47**, 191–198.
137. Ritchie J. M., Ritchie B. and Greengard P. (1965) The effect of the nerve sheath on the action of local anesthetics. *J. Pharmacol. Exp. Ther.* **150**, 160–164.
138. Roberts H., Kane K. M., Percival N. et al. (1957) Effects of some analgesic drugs used in childbirth with special reference to variation in respiratory minute volume of the newborn. *Lancet* **1**, 128–132.
139. Robertson C. R., Deen W. M., Chang R. L. S. et al. (1975) Determinants of fluid and solute transport across capillary walls of the renal glomerulus. *Bibl. Anat.* **13**, 32–35.
140. Rosen T. S. and Pippenger C. E. (1975) Disposition of methadone and its relationship to severity of withdrawal in the newborn. *Addict. Dis.* **2**, 169–178.
141. Sanner J. H. and Woods L. A. (1965) Comparative distribution of tritium-labelled dihydromorphine between maternal and fetal rats. *J. Pharmacol. Exp. Ther.* **148**, 176–184.

142. Scanlon J. W., Brown W. U., Weiss J. B. et al. (1974) Neurobehavioral responses of newborn infants after maternal epidural anesthesia. *Anesthesiology* **40,** 121–128.
143. Scanlon J. W., Ostheimer G. W., Lurie A. O. et al. (1976) Neurobehavioral responses and drug concentrations in newborns after maternal epidural anesthesia with bupivacaine. *Anesthesiology* **45,** 400–406.
144. Schanker L. S. (1961) Mechanisms of drug absorption and distribution. *Annu. Rev. Pharmacol.* **1,** 29–44.
145. Schifferli P.-Y. and Caldeyro-Barcia R. (1973) Effects of atropine and beta-adrenergic drugs on the heart rate of the human fetus. In: Boreus L. (ed.), *Fetal Pharmacology*. New York, Raven Press, pp. 259–278.
146. Schnermann J. (1975) Transcapillary fluid flow in the peritubular microvasculature of the kidney. *Bibl. Anat.* **13,** 36–39.
147. Seeds A. E., Stolee A. and Eichhorst C. (1976) Permeability of human chorion laeve to diazepam and meperidine. *Obstet. Gynecol.* **47,** 28–30.
148. Sereni F. (1973) The need for further data. *Clin. Pharmacol. Ther.* **14,** 662–665.
149. Shier R. W., Sprague A. D. and Dilts P. V. (1973) Placental transfer of meperidine HCl. Part II. *Am. J. Obstet. Gynecol.* **115,** 556–559.
150. Shnider S. M and Moya F. (1964) Effects of meperidine on the newborn infant. *Am. J. Obstet. Gynecol.* **89,** 1009–1015.
151. Shnider S. M. and Way E. L. (1968) Plasma levels of lidocaine (Xylocaine) in mother and newborn following obstetrical conduction anesthesia. *Anesthesiology* **29,** 951–958.
152. Siker E. S., Wolfson B., Dubnansky J. et al. (1968) Placental transfer of methoxyflurane. *Br. J. Anaesth.* **40,** 588–592.
153. Smith S. A. (1976) Factors determining the potency of mydriatric drugs in man. *Br. J. Clin. Pharmacol.* **3,** 503–507.
154. Smith S. E. (1976) Neuromuscular blocking drugs in man. In: Zaimis E. (ed.), *Handbook of Experimental Pharmacology*, vol. 42. Berlin, Springer Verlag, pp. 593–660.
155. Smith S. E. and Rawlins M. D. (1973) *Variability in Human Drug Response.* London, Butterworths.
156. Smith S. E., Smith S. A., Reynolds F. et al. (1979) Ocular and cardiovascular effects of local and systemic pinodol. *Br. J. Ophthalmol.* **63,** 63–69.
157. Spector R. and Lorenzo A. V. (1974) The effects of salicylate and probenecid on the cerebrospinal fluid transport of penicillin, aminosalicylic acid and iodine. *J. Pharmacol. Exp. Ther.* **188,** 55–65.
158. Stenger V. G., Blechner J. N. and Prystowsky H. (1969) A study of prolongation of obstetric anesthesia. *Am. J. Obstet. Gynecol.* **103,** 901–907.
159. Stephen G. W. and Cooper L. V. (1977) The role of analgesics in respiratory depression: a rabbit model. *Anaesthesia* **32,** 324–327.
160. Sterrett P. R., Thompson A. M., Chapman A. L. et al. (1974) The effects of hyperosmolarity on the blood–brain barrier. A morphological and physiological correlation. *Brain Res.* **77,** 281–295.
161. Sung C. Y. and Truant A. P. (1954) The physiological disposition of lidocaine and its comparison in some respects with procaine. *J. Pharmacol. Exp. Ther.* **112,** 432–443.
162. Takman B. (1975) The chemistry of local anaesthetic agents: classification of blocking agents. *Br. J. Anaesth.* **47,** 183–190.
163. Thalme B., Belfrage P. and Raabe N. (1974) Lumbar epidural analgesia in labour. I. Acid–base balance and clinical condition of mother, fetus and newborn child. *Acta Obstet. Gynecol. Scand.* **53,** 27–35.
164. Thomas J., Climie C. R., Long G. et al. (1969) The influence of adrenaline on the maternal plasma levels and placental transfer of lignocaine following lumbar epidural administration. *Br. J. Anaesth.* **41,** 1029–1034.

165. Thomas J., Climie C. R. and Mather L. E. (1968) Placental transfer of lignocaine following lumbar epidural administration. *Br. J. Anaesth.* **40**, 965–971.

166. Thomas J., Climie C. R. and Mather L. E. (1969) The placental transfer of alcuronium. *Br. J. Anaesth.* **41**, 297–302.

167. Thomas J., Long G., Moore G. et al. (1976) Plasma protein binding and placental transfer of bupivacaine. *Clin. Pharmacol. Ther.* **19**, 426–434.

168. Tucker G. T., Boyes R. N., Bridenbaugh P. O. et al. (1970) Binding of anilide-type local anesthetics in human plasma: II. Implications *in vivo*, with special reference to transplacental distribution. *Anesthesiology* **33**, 304–314.

169. Uchman G. and Guzikowska E. (1975) A method to assess the passage of diethyl ether and halothane across the placenta during anaesthesia for Caesarian section. *Anaesth. Resusc. Intensive Ther.* 3, 213–220.

170. Ullberg S. (1973) Autoradiography in fetal pharmacology. In: Boreus L. (ed.), *Fetal Pharmacology.* New York, Raven Press, pp. 55–69.

171. Weiss L. and Greep R. O. (1977) *Histology*, 4th ed. New York, McGraw-Hill.

172. Williams M. C. and Wissig S. L. (1975) The permeability of muscle capillaries to horseradish peroxidase. *J. Cell. Biol.* **66**, 531–555.

173. Wissig S. L. and Williams M. C. (1974) Passage of microperoxidase across the endothelium of capillaries of the diaphragm. *J. Cell. Biol.* **63**, 375a.

174. Witte S. (1975) Measurement of plasma protein in the perivascular tissue. *Bibl. Anat.* **13**, 72–73.

175. Wollman H. and Smith T. C. (1975) Uptake, distribution, elimination and administration of inhalational anesthetics. In: Goodman L. S. and Gilman A. (ed.), *The Pharmacological Basis of Therapeutics.* New York, Macmillan, pp. 71–80.

176. Young I. M. (1949) Abdominal relaxation with decamethonium iodide (C10) during Caesarian section. *Lancet* **1**, 1052.

177. Young I. M. (1953) The placental transfer of hexamethonium bromide and the origin of amniotic fluid in the rabbit. *J. Physiol.* **122**, 93–101.

178. Zeigler M. G., Lake C. R., Wood J. H. et al. (1977) Relationship between norepinephrine in blood and cerebrospinal fluid in the presence of a blood–cerebrospinal fluid barrier for norepinephrine. *J. Neurochem.* **28**, 677–679.

J. M. Manners

4 Anaesthesia for Cardiac Surgery

INTRODUCTION

The first planned operation on the heart in man in 1924 [94] heralded the development of a specialty where an estimated 100 000 operations are anticipated each year in the USA [362] and perhaps 10 000 in the United Kingdom [129]. Most of this surgery is now carried out as an open operation with the aid of cardiopulmonary bypass, first introduced in 1954 [154]. A certain number of closed cardiac procedures and palliative operations in infants with congenital heart disease are also performed. The Wessex Cardiac Unit, serving a population of three million, performs about 400 open heart operations and 40 non-bypass operations each year. This is less than the estimated incidence of coronary artery disease alone, for which surgery would be beneficial [245]. With an increase in resources further expansion would therefore be expected.

A survey of anaesthesia for cardiac surgery in any unit must take into account the end result in terms of hospital mortality, long term survival and quality of life. This review of the present practice in the Wessex Cardiac Unit is made against such a background [311, 368, 369].

Cardiac surgery has become a well-established and repetitive exercise. This lends itself to a team organization. In the operating and recovery rooms the team is composed of surgeons, anaesthetists, technicians and nurses, with additional laboratory technical aid and the normal acute hospital services. The role of the various personnel has evolved in a number of ways. In general it seems that surgeons and anaesthetists have been able, under their supervision, to delegate the management of the heart–lung machine to technicians and the care of patients requiring mechanical and pharmacological support in the recovery room, to nurses. Further evolution in some centres, with the aid of systems analysis and protocols has seen the application of computers, and the introduction of biomedical instrumentation technicians [387]. The use of non-medical assistants for the well-defined surgical techniques of heart surgery is now established [253], but the use of anaesthetic nurses or technicians as anaesthetic assistants in the same way, has not yet been accepted in the United Kingdom.

Anaesthesia for cardiac surgery provides an outstanding illustration of the application of pharmacology and physiology to the practice of medicine. There is a wide selection of anaesthetic agents. Perhaps as important as their principal anaesthetic action is their effect on the cardiovascular system. Clinical anaesthetic management also involves a detailed appreciation of the effects of disease and surgery, and the use of mechanical and pharmacological support on the cardiovascular and respiratory systems. Thus a review of cardiac anaesthesia must include some aspects of the physiology of the heart and circulation, and some principles of cardiopulmonary bypass. Cardiovascular monitoring and support are also within the anaesthetist's sphere, as well as certain aspects of postoperative care.

PHYSIOLOGICAL CONSIDERATIONS

The Circulation

The application of cardiovascular physiology to the problems of cardiac surgery has led to its appreciation in the fields of anaesthesia and intensive care. Particular developments include more widespread use of the concept of preload and afterload in relation to stroke volume, an increased awareness of myocardial oxygen supply and demand, and further discrimination in the interpretation of both central venous and pulmonary capillary wedge pressures.

Oxygen Flux

The quantity of oxygen delivered to the tissues each minute has been described as the oxygen flux [326]. The determinants of oxygen flux are the cardiac output, haemoglobin, haemoglobin saturation and dissolved oxygen. There is no adequate compensatory mechanism for an acute and profound reduction in cardiac output. A fundamental and rational approach to therapy for a low cardiac output requires an appreciation that stroke volume is influenced by three factors: the preload which decides the myocardial fibre end-diastolic length, the contractile state of the myocardium augmented by sympathetic stimulation, and the afterload [54, 55]. The afterload is the myocardial systolic wall tension which is a function of intraventricular pressure and volume and will be altered by such factors as vascular impedance and ventricular wall compliance.

An increase in preload increases stroke volume, but when cardiac function is severely impaired it may not affect the cardiac output to any great extent (*Fig. 4.1a*). It may however, by increasing ventricular volume, increase ventricular wall tension with adverse consequences. Conversely, a reduction in preload (venous unloading) in the failing heart may not reduce stroke volume but may reduce afterload even without a fall in vascular resistance.

Reduction of afterload by systemic arteriolar dilatation when the left ventricle is normal does not greatly augment ventricular stroke volume. The more abnormal the function of the ventricle, the greater the rise in stroke volume as arterial impedance is lowered [81] (*Fig. 4.1b*).

These essential features of the failing heart have now been recognized therapeutically when intravascular volume is increased, myocardial con-

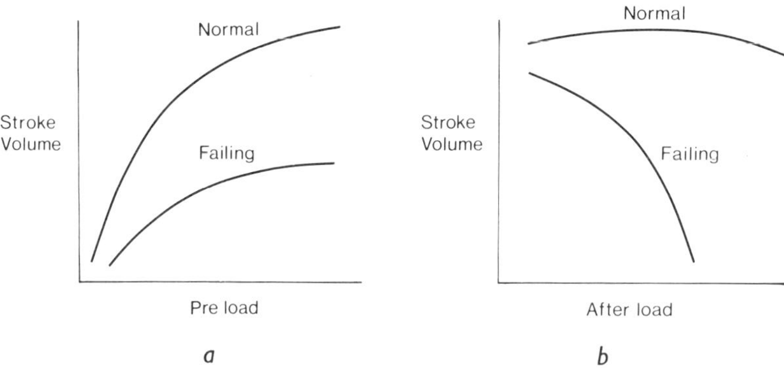

Fig. 4.1. a, Stroke volume increases as the preload increases. Stroke volume increases less for the same incremental increase in preload when the myocardium is failing. Stroke volume falls less with a reduction in preload, when the myocardium is failing. *b,* Stroke volume changes little with an increase in afterload in the normal heart. Stroke volume falls with an increase in afterload in the failing heart. Stroke volume rises with reduction in afterload only when the heart is failing.

tractility is augmented or vascular resistance is altered to improve cardiac output and thus oxygen flux.

Metabolic Demands of the Myocardium

The metabolic demands of the myocardium have become most evident with the development of surgery for coronary artery disease. An awareness of the balance between myocardial oxygen supply and demand has become important, particularly with the recognition that subendocardial ischaemia may occur even when the coronary arteries are normal. Hoffman and Buckberg [197] have described the pathophysiology of subendocardial ischaemia. In the presence of maximally dilated coronary arteries, perfusion of the left ventricular subendocardial layer depends upon the difference between aortic diastolic and left ventricular diastolic or coronary sinus pressure, and the duration of diastole. Blood flow to the subendocardium can therefore be represented by the area between the aortic and left ventricular pressures in diastole, the diastolic pressure time index (DPTI) (*Fig. 4.2*).

The needs of the left ventricle for oxygen are roughly proportional to the area of the left ventricular pressure curve in systole [277, 380], the systolic pressure time index (SPTI). The flow through the subendocardial layer is about the same as the subepicardial flow. It is suggested that a fall in the ratio of DPTI to SPTI to less than 0·5 would indicate subendocardial ischaemia. The presence of anaemia or hypoxaemia would increase the possibility of subendocardial ischaemia even with a normal ratio [56].

In the absence of a pressure gradient from left ventricle to aorta, an

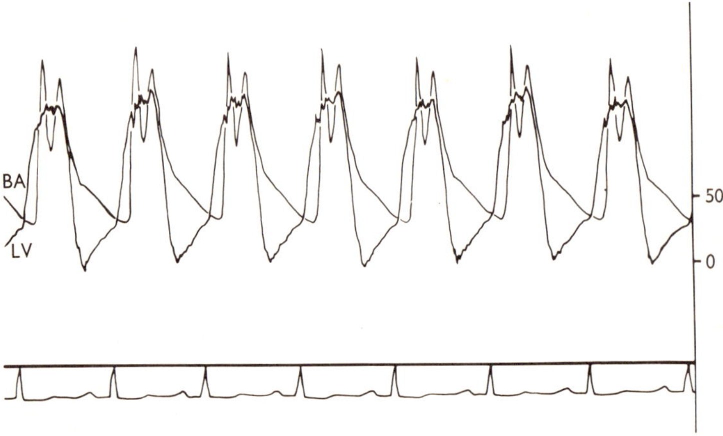

Fig. 4.2. Dynamic recording of brachial artery pressure superimposed on left ventricular pressure (mmHg) in a patient with aortic regurgitation. The diastolic pressure time index is small compared with the systolic pressure time index, indicating subendocardial ischaemia.

endocardial viability ratio (EVR) has been calculated from the equation [307]:

$$\text{EVR} = \frac{\text{MDP} - \text{MLAP}.\,T1}{\text{MSP}.\,T2}\,.$$

MDP = mean aortic diastolic pressure.
MLAP = mean left atrial pressure.
MSP = mean aortic systolic pressure.
$T1$ = diastolic time interval.
$T2$ = systolic time interval.

The implications of this working hypothesis relating to the use of anaesthetic agents and pharmacological support to the circulation are considerable, but with some reservations [150]. In general terms it would seem advisable to avoid shortening the diastolic time and avoid increasing the systolic blood pressure above normal if subendocardial ischaemia is to be minimized.

An additional and simple indicator of left ventricular myocardial oxygen consumption is given by the product of heart rate and systemic systolic pressure [319]. A number of derived variables are commonly used to attempt to express the work and contractility of the heart.

Left ventricular work = cardiac index × (mean aortic pressure – left atrial pressure) × 0·0136.

Time tension index = mean aortic pressure × heart rate × duration of systole.

Mean systolic ejection rate = stroke index/duration of systole.

Venous Pressure

One of the earlier accounts of the use of central venous pressure in cardiac surgery specifically described it as an indicator of the adequacy of transfusion [416]. Since then papers have appeared describing the lack of correlation between central venous pressure and left atrial pressure [147], cardiac output [23], blood volume [144] and fluid requirements [372]. It is therefore remarkable that even now overhydration has been attributed to absence of monitoring by measurement of central venous pressure (CVP) [179]. The CVP merely indicates the ability of the right ventricle to pump additional blood being presented to it [175, 449]. Even so, the interpretation of the CVP is by no means simple [172, 373]. It may be altered by the volume presented to the right atrium, but also by right ventricular factors, factors beyond the right ventricle and by external pressure on the right atrium. Qvist [347], for instance, has shown that the CVP rises with intermittent positive-pressure ventilation (IPPV) and positive end expiratory pressure (PEEP) due to a raised intrathoracic pressure. Since this pressure is also exerted on the right ventricle, the pressure which causes the right ventricle to fill is the difference between CVP and mean intrathoracic pressure (the transmural pressure). Thus the CVP may rise but the filling pressure fall when IPPV and especially PEEP are applied.

Left Atrial Pressure

In normal dogs a correlation between right atrial pressure (RAP) and left atrial pressure (LAP) shows that LAP = (RAP × 2) + 2 [174]. However, in heart disease the lack of correlation between LAP and RAP [40, 379] has led to direct or indirect monitoring of LAP [415]. Direct LAP measurement can easily be obtained during cardiac surgery and continued afterwards by insertion of a catheter when the chest has been opened. Indirect methods must be used if an LAP measurement is regarded as mandatory before this. The use of the Swan Ganz catheter for this purpose has been recently reviewed [120, 328]. Even when properly placed this catheter may not give an accurate indication of LAP. When pulmonary wedge pressure (PWP) was more than 15 mmHg the 95 per cent confidence interval for predicting LAP was at least ± 5 mmHg [444], while a discrepancy between PWP and LAP occurred during IPPV with PEEP [196, 271]. Even when the indirect measurement correlates with LAP the reliability of this in estimating left ventricular end-diastolic pressure (LVEDP) has been questioned, since the left atrial 'a' wave, not mean LAP, correlates with LVEDP [139].

Cardiopulmonary Bypass

Although the real time manipulation of the extracorporeal circulation is rightly undertaken by perfusion technicians, the equipment and techniques used have a direct bearing on anaesthetic management. Clearly the goal is a well-perfused viable patient at the end of perfusion, and an uncomplicated period of cardiopulmonary bypass (CPB) is less likely to require anaesthetic measures to deal with inadequate function of heart, lungs, kidneys or brain. The degree of haemodilution and fluid load are important, as are electrolyte and acid–base balance. Adequate heparinization and the least possible damage to blood constituents are also relevant to the postperfusion period.

The current techniques for extracorporeal circulation have recently been brought together [211]. The Wessex Unit use a variety of disposable bubble oxygenators including the Harvey, Galen and Bentley Temptrol and Spiraflo BOS-10. In due course membrane oxygenators may demonstrate sufficient superiority to replace bubble oxygenators for routine open heart surgery, as well as fulfilling their present role for more prolonged cardiorespiratory support [473].

Pulsatile Flow

A consideration of the pumps used during bypass and the possibility once again of producing a pulsatile flow have been discussed [31, 78, 363]. The merits of using pulsatile CPB may in one respect relate to its maintenance of the normal hypothalamic pituitary response to stress which does not occur during smooth non-pulsatile flow [422]. However, the short term diminution of the stress response by hypothermia, morphine, neuroleptanalgesia and epidural analgesia has been regarded as a possible advantage by some writers. Perhaps any clinical advantages of a pulsatile flow producing for instance plasma stress levels of thyroid and adrenal hormones, will become more apparent with prolonged supportive bypass. Even equipment which provides a pulsatile flow may not produce a pressure waveform beyond the aortic cannula which simulates normal arterial perfusion [471].

Priming

The extracorporeal circuit is usually filled with a clear fluid prime except in infants and other patients where because of their small size or low haemoglobin, a non-blood prime would reduce the packed cell volume below 20 per cent. The advantages of non-blood primes have been established and the metabolic changes reviewed [115]. A variety of clear fluids have been advocated including 5 per cent dextrose [86], balanced electrolyte solution [363], Ringer's lactate [320] and Ringer's acetate solutions [263]. This Unit uses 2 l of Ringer's lactate solution with the addition of 60 mg heparin for adults. When it is necessary to add blood during priming, citrate-phosphate-dextrose (CPD) or acid-citrate-dextrose (ACD) preserved blood with 15 mg heparin and 0·5 g calcium gluconate for each 500 ml is used. Ten to 15 mM sodium bicarbonate for each 500 ml of relatively fresh bank-blood adequately corrects any base deficit. When additional volume is required in the oxygenator during bypass, Ringer's lactate solution is added if the packed cell volume is greater than 20 per cent, and bank-blood, with heparin and calcium, if less than 20 per cent. The lactate load of 29 mM/l compares with a production of 55 mM/hr in a 70 kg man [80]. This does not produce a persisting lactic acidosis, presumably because the liver and kidneys are capable of removing it even when there is a decrease in blood flow. On the contrary, the alkalinizing effect could contribute to the alkalaemia and hypokalaemia which frequently occur after cardiac surgery [242] – and the plasma glucose concentration may rise, particularly in diabetics [424]. Some cardiac units add albumin [374], mannitol [376] or rheodextran [201] to maintain plasma oncotic pressure and thus diminish the loss of crystalloid solution to the functional interstitial space during and after bypass.

Filters

All the aspirate from the operating field which is not discarded is passed through a 40 μm filter before being returned to the oxygenator, and bank-blood added to the oxygenator is also filtered. An on-line arterial filter will also remove aggregates and is also an efficient microbubble trap, although air trapped in this way can give rise to large emboli [272]. An improved state of the central nervous system after bypass has been attributed to the inclusion of an arterial filter [194]. However, there is not absolute agreement that arterial line filters are essential [31, 258]. For instance, the passage of platelet aggregates to the patient may not necessarily be detrimental since these may break down into individual platelet components after passage through the reticulo-endothelial system [190].

Hypothermia

Hypothermia reduces metabolic demands in the curarized patient and therefore provides an additional safety factor if perfusion is not optimal for any reason. It can also be a useful therapeutic tool postoperatively if cardiac output or arterial oxygen tension remains unacceptably low despite conventional support. During CPB it is usual to cool the patient, using the oxygenator heat exchanger, to an oesophageal temperature of 30 °C in this Unit. Any disadvantages of increased systemic resistance are offset by haemodilution. The muscle mass may still be cold at the end of CPB despite restoration of oesophageal and nasopharyngeal temperatures to normal. A circulating water blanket continues the rewarming in the post-bypass period. Muscle relaxants which are not generally reversed at the end of the operation, and vasodilator drugs included in the anaesthetic technique both contribute towards the avoidance of adverse effects of residual cold [365]. The influence of cold on the activity of non-depolarizing muscle relaxants is of no clinical consequence in our practice.

When coronary perfusion is maintained during CPB hypothermia is limited so that the heart continues to beat. This avoids the disruption of coronary perfusion which takes place during ventricular fibrillation. However, this technique of myocardial preservation has largely been replaced by the use of cardioplegia solutions.

Cardioplegia

The current method in this Unit for the preservation of the myocardium during intracardiac procedures utilizes the cold cardioplegia solution developed by the St Thomas's Hospital Group [185] (Table 4.1). This

Table 4.1. St Thomas's Hospital Cardioplegia Injection and Cardioplegia Solution

mM	*Cardioplegia injection 20 ml*	*Ringer's solution 1000 ml*	*Cardioplegia solution*
Sodium		147·5	147·5
Potassium	16	4	20
Calcium		2	2
Magnesium	16		16
Chloride	48	156	204
Procaine	273 mg		273 mg

solution rapidly induces diastolic cardiac arrest and so facilitates surgery. It prevents rapid exhaustion of high energy substrates which are therefore available as soon as the cardioplegia solution is washed out by warm blood. It also prevents the accumulation of metabolites during the absence of coronary perfusion which would otherwise cause cell destruction [143].

Several techniques have been used to produce suitable conditions for cardiac surgery, with varying degrees of myocardial preservation. Aortic cross-clamping with ischaemic arrest was fundamentally damaging. Intermittent or continuous coronary perfusion at normal or hypothermic temperatures, while sustaining a more viable heart, did not provide still, relaxed conditions and sometimes caused technical difficulties. Topical profound hypothermia confined to the heart and pericardium has been used for many years [208]. An additional contribution to myocardial preservation has been an awareness that the left ventricular endocardium is poorly perfused during ventricular fibrillation or low coronary perfusion pressure. The administration of methyl prednisolone [262] or beta-blockers [355] before aortic cross-clamping has been thought to be beneficial.

Several cardioplegia solutions have recently been developed, including the Bretschneider [354], Kirsh [235] and St Thomas's Hospital [185] infusates. These solutions are cold when they are administered. Under controlled laboratory conditions using isolated rat hearts, the St Thomas's Hospital solution provided substantially more protection than other infusates [228]. There may still be some doubt regarding the need for a cardioplegia solution when simple profound local hypothermia of the heart, using normal saline appears to suffice in the short term for ischaemic periods of 90 min [171, 453]. It might seem that more protection is afforded, the lower the heart temperature, since for instance, the metabolic rate at 10 °C is 10 per cent of that at 37 °C [151]. Tyers [435] has shown in rats that selective myocardial hypothermia by the intracoronary injection of a solution at 10–15 °C gave better functional and metabolic results than injections at 4 °C or 20 °C. Even with solutions administered at 4 °C in man, myocardial temperature may be in the 16–24 °C range [364]. Hence further studies are required to define the optimum temperature with metabolic arrest [186] and measurement of infusate and myocardial temperature may be desirable.

When the patient has been rewarmed and the aortic cross-clamp removed, vigorous ventricular activity is evident within minutes and spontaneous reversion to rhythmic contractions occurs in many patients [140, 364]. Otherwise coarse ventricular fibrillation is easily converted into an organized ventricular contraction.

Profound Hypothermia

The various techniques of profound hypothermia with circulatory standstill provide a still, dry operating field and no anxieties regarding interference with perfusion cannulas and bypass during the cardiac correction. Drew [108] employed CPB alone to induce profound hypothermia, while Barratt-Boyes [28] has popularized the Kyoto technique [191] of surface cooling infants followed by a limited period of CPB. We use this method in infants less than 10 kg in weight and usually less than 1 year, to cool to a nasopharyngeal temperature of 18–20 °C. The Seattle group [104] described surface cooling only to achieve the same degree of hypothermia and so avoid CPB altogether. This would seem to be disadvantageous in that rewarming is slow and manual cardiac massage is required during the early stages of surface rewarming.

The advantages of the Kyoto technique are attributed to a reduced period of CPB and uniform cooling of the whole body, including the muscle mass. This results in a lower oxygen consumption at the pre-arrest temperature of 18–20 °C than when CPB alone is used. Perhaps circulatory arrest may then be more prolonged and safer than when core cooling is used. Abbott [2] has recently analysed the oxygen consumption and reserve in profoundly cooled infants. Oxygen consumption at 20 °C may be about 25 per cent of the basal rate, or perhaps 10 ml/min in a 5 kg infant of 0·3 m^2 surface area. Haemoglobin would be fully saturated at this temperature and there is an increase in dissolved oxygen (31 ml l^{-1}

$100\,kPa^{-1}$) throughout the total body water. Despite this increased oxygen reserve and low metabolic rate, an oxygen debt must accumulate after more than 17 min of circulatory arrest at 20 °C. However, the rate of anaerobic metabolism is also low, and perhaps varies from organ to organ, at this temperature. Periods of 60 min of no circulation at 20 °C have not produced evident brain damage [375, 404]. Other methods of preserving the brain for even longer periods will no doubt be developed using barbiturate [393] or piracetam [357], for instance. On resumption of bypass at 20 °C the dissolved oxygen content of the body is restored in 5–10 min [176]. Core rewarming has the advantage of speed and rapid restoration of the heart and liver towards normal function.

PATIENT MONITORING

Monitoring in relation to cardiac surgery and postoperative care continues to expand in capability, while critical evaluation points the way to future developments [234]. The cost–effectiveness of monitoring [250], and indeed of all surgical treatment [311], is a dilemma which becomes increasingly evident as the average hospital cost for each patient–day continues to rise. It would therefore seem that before more expensive methods of monitoring are established in cardiac anaesthetic practice, it is necessary to have some material conviction that the results of surgery will be improved. Only by the collection and analysis of data will improvements in individual patient care, or effectiveness of particular operations be demonstrated.

Almost all the monitoring recently described by Saidman and Ty Smith [377] could be applied with some justification to cardiac anaesthesia and postoperative care. Sophisticated cardiovascular monitoring and computer calculation of a number of variables [387], or respiratory monitoring with computation of compliance and work of breathing [463], may be considered a research approach by some, although the information generated often influences those without such complicated measuring devices. However, anaesthetic care of patients during and after cardiac surgery, even in the most simple way, includes on-line monitoring of the cardiovascular system, and intermittent blood sampling for blood gas, electrolyte and haematological measurements.

Electrocardiograph

The standard limb leads and V5 electrodes are commonly used to provide an oscilloscope display. The limb leads are employed primarily for diagnosis of rhythm disturbances and V5 for detection of anterolateral ischaemia. An intravenous catheter containing an electrocardiogram (ECG) lead is available for the analysis of supraventricular rhythms which are not obvious from other leads. The CM5 configuration suggested by Prys-Roberts [344] is inconvenient during surgery but could be used in the postoperative period. A variety of ECG pads which can be simply placed underneath the chest during surgery has not been found to be sufficiently reliable and discriminatory in our experience.

Central Venous Pressure

Internal jugular cannulation preferably on the right side using the method of English [128] is now commonly practised and is the technique of choice in this Unit. Contraindications to this technique include local infection and tumours. Particular care is exercised in the presence of ascending aortic aneurysms, aortic dissection, aortic regurgitation, coarctation of the aorta, transposition, previous right Blalock anastomosis, and in patients already anticoagulated. The patient is usually anaesthetized and controlled ventilation commenced before introduction of the venous catheter; and ECG monitoring is established even if the patient is awake.

If there is doubt about the site of the vein, it is first sought with a 21 g 1¼ in needle attached to a syringe. Confirmation that the catheter has been correctly placed requires the easy aspiration of venous blood, the demonstration of both a venous and respiratory oscillation of pressure, and an appropriate venous pressure. The surface marking of the right atrium lies between the second and sixth costal cartilages so that a measure on the front of the chest and against the catheter emerging from the neck will allow the tip to be placed correctly. A second venous catheter is often placed in the same internal jugular vein, anticipating the need for catecholamine support which is given in a venous line independent of measurement of venous pressure.

The lower approach to the jugular vein [128, 352] is used in infants and small children using 20 g or 18 g Medicut or Cathlon cannulas. A towel, or assistant's fist, placed beneath the shoulders provides suitable extension of the neck, while the operating table is in a steep Trendelenberg position. The cannula is inserted at the apex of the supraclavicular triangle in a direction which is caudal, posterior and slightly medial, just deep to the sternoclavicular joint. When the vein has been entered the cannula can be gently advanced as blood flows freely from it. The cannula is then attached to an Abbott T connection, and to a water manometer, or transducer system. Again the vein can be sought using a fine needle attached to an aspirating syringe before insertion of the larger diameter cannula [340]. If an artery is inadvertently entered, it may be possible to stopper the cannula and leave it *in situ* while the vein is found. The arterial cannula can then be removed and firm pressure applied. There is an advantage in having a venous pressure cannula above the superior vena caval perfusion cannula in children particularly. It is then a simple matter to detect obstruction to venous drainage either before or during bypass. Cannulation of the left internal jugular vein is useful in this respect, in the presence of a left superior vena cava.

Alternative approaches to the superior vena cava include supraclavicular and infraclavicular puncture, or an antecubital or external jugular approach. The certainty of introducing the catheter into the superior vena cava is less with all these methods, although even the external jugular approach will succeed using a blunt-ended flexible catheter with side holes [134]. Catheters introduced through cannulas have now taken the place of catheters through needles [384], and the many varieties have been reviewed [135]. In adults our preference is for a 24 in catheter so that at least half of it lies outside the vein and provides an easily accessible injection site during surgery.

Arterial Blood Pressure

An invasive method is necessary to provide a continuous dynamic display on an oscilloscope, a trend recording during anaesthetic and surgical events and access to an artery for blood samples. Improved Doppler methods of blood pressure measurement and the development of multipurpose cutaneous monitors for blood gases may perhaps displace the invasive method in less complicated types of surgery.

Current literature still describes 18 g or 20 g cannulas for invasive arterial monitoring [39]. Our present technique employs a 22 g Angiocath cannula for all patients, from infants to adults. Since the right arm has often been used for previous cardiac catheterization, the left radial artery is cannulated if possible. The right radial artery is selected however, in the presence of aortic coarctation, persistent ductus arteriosus, traumatic thoracic aortic rupture and any other situation where interruption of the patency of the left subclavian artery is anticipated.

Adult patients are almost invariably calm and sedated on arrival in the anaesthetic room so that arterial puncture may be carried out without local analgesia and without patient discomfort. Infants and children are anaesthetized before the procedure. Once the line of the artery has been appreciated by palpation of the extended wrist it is usually possible to insert the cannula into the artery at a shallow angle without transfixing it. The skin is preferably pierced at the level of the radial styloid rather than more proximally where the artery is at a greater depth. The cannula is attached to a T-connector, manometer tubing and pressure transducer. A pressure gauge can alternatively be used to display a mean pressure in the anaesthetic room [475]. Great care is taken to avoid the injection of air or particulate matter into the system, in view of its retrograde passage to the vertebral artery [270] as well as to the hand. If the left radial artery has not been successfully cannulated it is almost always possible to introduce a cannula percutaneously into the right radial, the brachial [27], the axillary [10], the dorsalis pedis [225] or the femoral artery [85]. It would be unwise to use the ulnar artery if the radial has already been damaged. A longer cannula such as an 18 g Cathlon would be suitable for brachial artery cannulation in adults or femoral artery in small children. The potential for serious infection is generally thought to be greater when the femoral site is used.

Despite recommendations to carry out the Allen test [13] or its modifications [61] before radial cannulation, we have not adopted this procedure. There have been no recognizable complications which could be attributed to this approach in 2000 patients. Significant impairment of hand perfusion would be expected to produce colour, temperature or sensory changes in the hand, thenar pain perhaps or thenar wasting. It is reassuring to know that compression of the radial artery never reduced thumb arterial pressure to a level associated with symptoms of inadequate blood supply [209].

Some Units still prefer to cut down onto a peripheral artery to introduce a cannula, and there is some merit in this as a quick routine technique while other anaesthetic procedures are taking place.

Left Atrial Pressure

Left atrial pressure monitoring is usually effected by the introduction of a catheter by the surgeon, into the left atrium or via the right superior pulmonary vein at the end of bypass. Indirect measurement by the use of a flow-directed catheter is sometimes advocated. There may be some advantage in having this information during induction of anaesthesia and before or during bypass. At induction a considerable increase in pulmonary capillary wedge pressure has been demonstrated [345] with an implied danger of pulmonary oedema if it exceeds 25–30 mmHg. It may be considered advisable to treat such a transient change. During CPB, indirect left atrial monitoring allows recognition of back pressure on the lungs due to left ventricular distension [69]. This will enable measures to be taken to prevent left ventricular damage or pulmonary interstitial oedema. Each Unit has its own methods for avoiding this problem, usually by venting the left ventricle directly or through the left atrium. During coronary artery bypass grafting, left ventricular venting is usually avoided so that left atrial monitoring may then be particularly useful. The disadvantages of using a flow-direction catheter in adults include the failure rate [415], the complications relating to it [62] and its presence in the tricuspid valve.

If a 5 gauge Swan Ganz catheter is selected it may usually be introduced through a 12 g cannula inserted percutaneously into the jugular vein. If a 7 gauge catheter is introduced by this route a cardiac catheter introducer is required. Alternatively, the catheter may be inserted into a median cubital vein. The precise techniques for floating the catheter through the right atrium, right ventricle and pulmonary artery have been well described [62, 474].

It is difficult to see this relatively expensive, sometimes time-consuming technique, which is not without its failures and complications, becoming a routine means of monitoring the left atrial pressure for cardiac surgical patients.

Cardiac Output

It would seem self-evident that measurement of cardiac output was required if proper control of the blood pressure, cardiac output and vascular resistance were to be maintained. Because this measurement is still not a simple, non-invasive and accurate bedside technique, it has not become an accepted routine measurement in all cardiac units. The flow-direction catheter and uncomplicated instrumentation has made the thermodilution method popular, giving rapid serial bedside measurements [148]. Other methods include dye dilution, impedance plethysmography [243], analysis of aortic pressure contour [346], electromagnetic flow [136] and echocardiography [26, 337, 353]. Radionuclide imaging of the heart [452] allows assessment of the fraction of the left ventricular contents which is ejected with each beat, and perhaps it will be possible to to use this non-invasive and repeatable method at the bedside.

Indirect assessment of stroke volume and cardiac output is made in a number of ways. Direct display of the blood pressure on an oscilloscope gives some impression of the stroke volume from the pressure pulse contour, the systemic resistance from the diastolic pressure and myocardial contractility from the rate of rise of aortic pressure. A low venous oxygen saturation has been regarded as a possible indication of low cardiac output [50, 241], although Kirklin [233] has demonstrated that it is an unreliable guide. Nevertheless, a low venous oxygen tension or a low cardiac output has been associated with acute cardiac surgical deaths in children [330]. Paradoxically, during bypass a low mixed venous oxygen tension and a high arterio-venous oxygen content difference was associated with better tissue oxygenation [177]. Cool extremities but a normal or raised core temperature [57] and low urine output have been clinical guides that cardiac output may be less than optimal. An increasing or persisting non-respiratory acidaemia is also an indirect indicator that tissue hypoxia is occurring and may be due to a low cardiac output.

Temperature

The patient's temperature is measured during surgery principally because patients are electively or inadvertently cooled. Postoperatively core and peripheral temperatures may be monitored. A low temperature often indicates residual hypothermia following bypass, but may point to a low cardiac output.

During anaesthesia oesophageal and nasopharyngeal thermometers, and in some Units rectal or muscle probes are employed. *Oesophageal temperature* reflects the temperature of the heart and descending thoracic aorta and therefore gives a guide to the input temperature from the heart–lung machine, or the temperature of the posterior region of the heart. The probe should be placed so that the tip lies in the lowest quarter of the oesophagus [454]. *Nasopharyngeal temperature* is thought to reflect brain temperature less inaccurately than oesophageal temperature, although in non-bypass patients it is less reliable than the lower oesophagus in estimating cerebral temperature [455]. It is of special importance when using the profound hypothermia technique for surgery in infants. The probe should be inserted towards the superior meatus, excluded from the room air, and not introduced so far that it passes into the oropharynx. *Rectal temperature* is of little value during surface cooling when it may reflect the environmental rather than the patient's core temperature. Muscle temperatures were measured during the early evolution of CPB. It is still evident that despite normal nasopharyngeal and oesophageal temperatures at the termination of bypass, patients are often hypothermic at the end of operation. This has a significant influence on the immediate postoperative management. Monitoring of *myocardial temperature* has been proposed when the cold cardioplegic method of myocardial preservation is used. The presence of needle probes might be considered inconvenient and their placement in any region of conducting tissue, harmful. *Big toe temperature* has been measured postoperatively as a guide to the degree of peripheral dilatation, bearing in mind the core temperature [295]. In infants, in a thermally neutral environment, a fall in toe temperature when the abdominal skin temperature is an optimal 36 °C is taken to indicate that the cardiovascular status has declined.

The Brain

Electroencephalographic monitoring, at one time routine during open heart surgery, has fallen into disuse. It has been revived with the development of the cerebral function monitor [52]. This detects cortical disturbances but focal lesions may not be apparent. Its main purpose would seem to be an assurance that the cerebral cortex is adequately perfused during bypass. Haemodynamic events at this time, such as interruption of the circulation, misplacement of the aortic cannula, low perfusion pressure or obstructed venous drainage should be self-evident. The monitor might be an aid in avoiding awareness during bypass, especially when intravenous anaesthetic agents are being used [111, 341].

Blood Gas and Acid–Base Status

These measurements are routinely available during and after surgery. At present intermittent measurements using automated gas analysers [48, 309] may be made from samples easily obtained from the radial artery cannula. On-line measurement [20, 162] using intravascular electrodes is possible, but the cost and diameter of the probes may be considered disadvantageous. Measurement using cutaneous electrodes [204, 205] is possible, but this technique has not been sufficiently assessed to displace established methods. Blood gas measurements are made at 37 °C and can be corrected to the patient's oesophageal or nasopharyngeal temperature if this is thought to be helpful. The appreciation that the haemoglobin dissociation curve shifts as the 2,3-diphosphoglyceric acid (2,3-DPG) content of red cells changes, has brought dubious benefits in patient management. The *P*50 which characterizes the oxygen affinity for haemoglobin can simply be calculated from the equation [450]:

$$P50 = 3{\cdot}55 \times \frac{P\text{O}_2\,\text{C}}{P\text{O}_2\,\text{S}}\ \text{kPa.}$$

$P\text{O}_2$ C is the measured $P\text{O}_2$ corrected for measured pH and temperature to pH 7·4 and temperature 37 °C. $P\text{O}_2$ S is the $P\text{O}_2$ corresponding to the measured SO_2 on the standard oxygen–haemoglobin equilibration curve.

Serum Electrolytes

Sodium and potassium measurements are made at regular intervals during the perioperative period. Ionized calcium and magnesium levels will probably seem essential when they can be estimated easily.

Variations in sodium level requiring consideration are uncommon. It can be unduly raised by the addition of sodium bicarbonate to the small acid blood prime used for children, or if used in large quantities to correct recurring non-respiratory acidaemia. A low serum sodium is not uncommon in the presence of heart failure but does not usually require specific treatment.

Potassium has received most attention because of the relationship between heart failure, hypokalaemia, digitalis and arrhythmias [116]. Fluctuations in serum potassium always occur during heart surgery. These are due to preoperative heart failure and diuretic therapy, and to the operative variables of ventilation and acid–base balance, increased renin and aldosterone levels [214], perfusion prime and cardioplegia solution, administration of diuretics and the urine output. Curiously, a large diuresis during bypass without the aid of diuretics may consist of urine with electrolyte concentrations close to those of plasma. A large diuresis is not necessarily an indication for giving potassium supplements in this instance. A rise in serum potassium is not commonly seen during surgery unless the cardioplegia solution drains into the oxygenator. A rapid rise postoperatively may be an early indicator of an inadequate cardiac performance in infants with complex congenital abnormalities.

A persistently low ionized calcium level has been shown in seriously ill patients [109]. The needs of stressed infants for calcium is well established [371] and postoperative calcium therapy has been aided by the development of the means of measuring ionized calcium levels.

Hypomagnesaemia may develop in patients with heart failure because of secondary aldosteronism [202] or due to diuretics [110]. It also persists in patients who have undergone CPB for congenital or acquired defects [350, 451]. The addition of magnesium to a clear fluid oxygenator prime reduces the incidence and duration of a low serum magnesium [70, 333]. The presence of magnesium in the St Thomas's cardioplegia solution may have the added advantage of avoiding such a deficiency. Since administered magnesium contributes to an increase in intracellular potassium [114, 390], it may be a factor in the restoration of a stable normal rhythm after bypass. Magnesium has also been shown to be effective in terminating ventricular fibrillation when the heart is cold [64]. Routine magnesium supplements have been advocated after open heart surgery [224, 232]. There are therefore good reasons for thinking that magnesium monitoring may be important.

Haemoglobin and Coagulation

The haemodilution technique of CPB requires the packed cell volume (PCV) to be measured at regular intervals, so that if it falls below 20 per cent, blood can be added to the oxygenator. After bypass, a low PCV is managed by increasing the excretion of water and electrolytes with diuretics, and giving whole blood or red cell concentrates if the patient can tolerate blood volume expansion. Despite the rheological advantages of a low PCV, restoration of haemoglobin level towards normality would seem to benefit the oxygen flux.

There is a three–fourfold variation in heparin sensitivity and half-life among patients [65]. Large standard doses of heparin and protamine neutralization, based on body weight or surface area may therefore be excessive in some patients. To achieve more accurate control, some cardiac Units have advocated using the Activated Clotting Time [24, 66]. Less heparin, less protamine and less blood loss were reported than in patients given 3 mg heparin/kg initially, and 1·5 mg/kg every 45 min, neutralized by protamine sulphate in the ratio of 1·5 : 1. It should not be forgotten, however, that the dose of protamine to exactly neutralize heparin immediately following bypass is less than the dose to prevent heparin rebound [127]. This Unit still compares a thrombin time after protamine has been given, to a control sample of blood taken from the patient before heparinization. Should bleeding continue after heparin has been neutralized, it is customary to carry out a platelet count. A count of less than 40 000 mm^3 may be contributing to a coagulation defect soon after bypass [279]. The concentration of platelets is higher with a haemodilution technique than when donor blood is added to the oxygenator [263], but their function is depressed [187]. The ability of platelets to aggregate and adhere is not normally measured, but these functions may be more important than the actual count. The role of anaesthetic agents which produce inhibition of platelet aggregation is not clear [29]. The use of drugs such as dipyridamole [38] during bypass causing a transitory inhibition of platelet aggregation and an increased count afterwards has yet to be explored clinically. The substitution of prostacyclin for heparin may also result in better platelet preservation [470]. Further coagulation studies are rarely carried out in the Unit since the present management of non-surgical bleeding always includes the administration of fresh blood, fresh frozen plasma and platelets, and the removal if possible of the precipitating factors.

Plasma Glucose

Hyperglycaemia is to be expected during CPB [33, 193], although in our experience profound hypoglycaemia has occasionally been found in patients presenting for emergency cardiac surgery. The blood sugar may also fall to hypoglycaemic levels in infants and small children at induction of anaesthesia or in the immediate postoperative period [447]. The plasma glucose level is therefore measured during anaesthesia in all neonates and small children, in all seriously ill patients and in diabetics. After operation it is measured in all patients in the course of the first 24 hr, in the previous groups subsequently, and in all patients receiving intravenous or nasogastric nutrition.

Osmolality and Oncotic Pressure

The clinical usefulness of serum osmometry has been apparent for many years [7, 327]. Low serum osmolality is due to hyponatraemia and a high osmolality to hypernatraemia, hyperglycaemia, uraemia or other solutes [290]. It is therefore an additional means of monitoring the water, electrolyte and other metabolic disturbances associated with heart disease and cardiac surgery.

The partition of water between the plasma and interstitial space is influenced by the colloid osmotic pressure. The use of haemodilution perfusion techniques, with crystalloid solution primes for the extracorporeal circuit will reduce this oncotic pressure [130]. There will be a tendency for the interstitial fluid to increase and plasma volume to decrease during and after bypass [37]. Pulmonary oedema may appear at a lower left atrial pressure than anticipated when the oncotic pressure is low [401, 402]. Nevertheless, a lack of correlation between oncotic pressure minus pulmonary capillary wedge pressure and interstitial pulmonary oedema has been shown [440]. It has been suggested that there is an increase in pulmonary lymph removal in this circumstance, and that albumin administration to increase oncotic pressure may not be necessary. Howland [203] concluded that the use of an oncometer provided a rational approach when giving plasma products for oncotic purposes during the perioperative period.

Urine

A bladder catheter is inserted in all patients for open heart surgery except in the most simple and short procedures. This allows monitoring of hourly urine output and quality of urine if necessary. At least 0·5 ml kg^{-1} hr^{-1} in adults and 1 ml kg^{-1} hr^{-1} in children is expected. Urine output is also closely monitored to follow water balance, so that the operative fluid load is seen to be eliminated during and after surgery. If renal insufficiency is suspected, the quality of urine is measured even if the quantity is more than optimum. The urine osmolality [45], sodium and urea [256] content are useful guides to renal performance, and osmolality is one essential monitor of the state of hydration of infants. Estimations of urine quantity and quality are also obligatory when intravenous or nasogastric feeding is instituted postoperatively, to provide additional information regarding nitrogen balance and carbohydrate control.

CARDIOVASCULAR SUPPORT

Volume

Before considering pharmacological or mechanical support for the heart, it is absolutely necessary to be sure that the filling pressures of the left and right ventricle are optimal. The central venous pressure as an indicator of filling pressure may not reflect left atrial pressure, nor vice versa. It is therefore usual to measure both pressures after CPB and at least correlate the preload with both pressures before relying on central venous pressure alone. When there is doubt about the contractility of the left ventricle, monitoring of both central venous and left atrial pressures is continued into the postoperative period.

It would be ideal to have an on-line measurement of cardiac output as the preload is increased. In practice an indirect assessment of the cardiac output is made. This includes observation of the oscillocope display of blood pressure and ECG, skin colour and temperature, arterial and venous blood gas and acid–base status, urine output, and during surgery, direct observation of the heart.

If there are clinical indications of reduced perfusion and the LAP or if appropriate, CVP is below the upper limit of normal (12 mmHg and 5 mmHg) [166], then the patient's blood volume is increased. Further transfusion may be undertaken cautiously in patients with impaired myocardial function to an LAP of 18 mmHg. It is most important to consider all the technical and physiological factors which may alter the venous pressure readings to be certain that they are not giving misleading information and that the preload is optimal.

Contractility

The relationship between force and velocity of myocardial performance, without the influence of preload and afterload describes the contractile state of the myocardium [53] although there have been some recent objections to this basic concept [221]. The contractility of the heart, and hence the cardiac output due to this factor, is adversely affected by a number of circumstances. Arrhythmias and heart rate influence the degree of filling of the ventricle and its coordination in ejecting its contents. The quantity of coronary flow may be inadequate due to coronary artery disease and coronary emboli, particularly of air or calcium debris. The quality of coronary blood also affects contractility so that hypoxia, hypercarbia, non-respiratory acid–base changes, electrolyte abnormalities and cold may all be relevant to poor cardiac performance at some stage during cardiac surgery. The effect of drugs, particularly anaesthetic agents, beta-adrenoceptor blockers and protamine may be pertinent. All these causes of poor cardiac function must be remembered as well as inadequate preload and excessive afterload, before recourse is made to agents which increase myocardial contractility.

Sodium Bicarbonate

Sodium bicarbonate is administered to correct a non-respiratory acidaemia. It may be given to the patient when the measured acid–base balance shows a base excess of −5 mM or more. An assessment of the patient and correction of the cause of the disturbance is more effective than correcting this number alone [322]. It is also given empirically while awaiting blood gas measurements, when the circulation is arrested for more than a brief time at normothermia or there is a period of low perfusion before or after bypass. The usual dose in this situation is 1 mM/kg and repeated once if necessary pending laboratory results. Alternatively, the formulae of base deficity × body weight/5 and duration of cardiac arrest (min) × body weight/10 [155] could be used to calculate the dose of bicarbonate in mM. The solution used in adults is 8·4 per cent while in infants, where solutions of very high osmolality can be damaging, it is 4·2 per cent (0·5 mM/ml).

Hydrogen Ion

Hydrogen ion infusions to treat non-respiratory alkalaemia [462], are virtually never required, since potassium chloride will correct this abnormality adequately..

Calcium

Calcium was recognized as a positive inotrope by Ringer in 1883. Repeated administration of calcium, like any other electrolyte, would be expected to cause a cumulative rise in serum level. Westhorpe [451] has confirmed a high ionized calcium level after CPB when calcium has been given routinely. Nevertheless, prolonged hypocalcaemia has been reported in some critically ill patients [109].

Intravenous calcium is also effective in reversing the fall in ionized calcium and cardiac output due to citrate contained in blood and blood products [67]. There is considerable doubt about the need for routine calcium administration during blood transfusion. Bunker [68] considered that an empirical dose of calcium with each unit of blood was not without its own dangers and reported a level of 18·8 mg/100 ml in one patient. Denlinger [99] has shown that the total serum calcium does not change and the fall in ionized calcium is a transient phenomenon during citrated blood transfusion.

Calcium is now given sparingly in various anaesthetic circumstances during cardiac resuscitation for its inotropic effect, and its protection against the negative inotropic effects of bicarbonate given during this procedure [383]; if the venous pressures are at the upper limit of normal and the systemic blood pressure is rather less than considered desirable; routinely only with a very fast blood transfusion when both blood pressure and venous pressure may be unavoidably low. In this Unit, calcium is given as gluconate 1 g in 10 ml in a dose of 0·5 g in adults and 10 mg/kg in infants and children. The suggestion has been made that calcium gluconate is unsuitable for resuscitation because the release of physiologically active ionized calcium may depend on the rate of metabolism of the gluconate radical [158]. White [456] found that 10 ml of 10 per cent calcium chloride increased the plasma ionized calcium level by an average of 15·2 mg/100 ml, while 30 ml of 10 per cent calcium gluconate increased it by 12·3 mg/100 ml. The ratio of total to ionized calcium was more predictable when chloride was given.

The Catecholamines (Table 4.2)

Adrenaline

Adrenaline stimulates both alpha- and beta-adrenoceptors, increasing myocardial contractility in a most decided and effective way [79]. Large doses produce a marked tachycardia and ventricular irritability. Its peripheral effects are mixed and there may be a fall in systemic resistance with

Table 4.2. Summary of Principal Haemodynamic Effects of Catecholamines

	Adrenaline	*Dopamine*	*Dobutamine*	*Isoprenaline*	*Noradrenaline*
Beta 1 stimulation	+++	+++	+++	+++	+++
Alpha stimulation	+	+ to +++	+	0	+++
Cardiac output	++	++	++	++	0
Heart rate	+	++	+	+++	– to 0
Systemic resistance	0 to ++	0 to +++	0 to +	– to 0	+++
Pulmonary resistance	++	0 to +++	– to +	– to 0	+++

low doses and a rise at higher levels. It is certainly temporarily effective in all but the most irretrievable situation of low cardiac output and low blood pressure so that it is the favoured initial pressor in this instance. As an infusion 1–5 μg/min are given to adults. The more recently introduced and more specific pressors together with other therapy can usually be substituted for it after initial support. Adrenaline is also a first choice pressor as a bolus for cardiac arrest, commencing with 0·1–0·5 mg in adults and 2 μg/kg in infants, in a solution containing 1 mg adrenaline in 10 ml.

Dopamine

This naturally occuring precursor of noradrenaline has both alpha- and beta-receptor stimulating properties. It increases cardiac output without usually producing the marked tachycardia found with isoprenaline, although an undesirable increase in heart rate and ventricular irritability may occur [74]. It is not a powerful vasopressor at low doses of 2–4 $\mu g\,kg^{-1}\,min^{-1}$, when the systemic and pulmonary vascular resistances may fall [198]. Renal and mesenteric blood flow may rise due to dopaminergic vasodilatation as well as an increase in cardiac output, leading to increased urine production. At a high dosage of 50 $\mu g\,kg^{-1}\,min^{-1}$, systemic and pulmonary resistance rise (coronary vasoconstriction has been described) and urine flow decreases due to the more prominent alpha-adrenergic activity. Stephenson [403] found that the urine flow response to dopamine was its only clinical advantage over adrenaline in adults. Dopamine at present is our first choice catecholamine for infants and children and the substitute for adrenaline as it is being reduced in adults. Daenan [95] has published a table of concentrations of dopamine for an infusion so that 1 microdrop (1/60 ml) contains the same number of μg of dopamine as the weight of the child in kg. This can more simply be achieved by adding an amount of dopamine in mg which is six times the patient's weight in kg to 100 ml of infusate [72].

Dobutamine

Dobutamine, the most recently introduced inotrope, is principally a β_1-adrenoceptor agonist, increasing cardiac output, and myocardial contractility with a fall in LVEDP. The differences between dobutamine and dopamine have been discussed by Tuttle [433], Yates [472] and Goldberg [164]. Dobutamine has comparatively little effect on heart rate and aortic pressure [222, 410], two determinants of myocardial oxygen consumption. The systemic and pulmonary vascular resistance fell when it was administered to patients in severe heart failure [257], by virtue of an increase in cardiac output. When dobutamine was compared with isoprenaline during emergence from CPB, it increased the cardiac output more and the heart rate less than isoprenaline [427]. It does not appear to have been compared with adrenaline at this phase of cardiac surgery, when a short term pressor response as well as an increase in contractility sometimes seems desirable. Such a situation can arise when the aorta has been unclamped and air has inadvertently embolized into the coronary arteries. The clinical benefit of having catecholamines with improved specificity is self-evident, and the combination of dobutamine with peripheral vasodilators would seem to be an appropriate combination for the present approach to the management of the failing heart. An infusion of dobutamine is usually commenced at 5–10 $\mu g\,kg^{-1}\,min^{-1}$.

Isoprenaline

Isoprenaline, a beta-adrenergic agonist produces both an increase in myocardial contractility and heart rate. In view of its adverse effects of tachycardia and diastolic hypotension on subendocardial perfusion [63], increased myocardial oxygen consumption and incidence of arrhythmias, this drug is less commonly used nowadays. An infusion is begun at 0·5–1 μg/min in adults.

Noradrenaline

Noradrenaline is not often considered as a necessary drug for cardiovascular support with its predominantly alpha-adrenergic stimulating effect, and rise in systemic and pulmonary vascular resistance. In low dosage it increases cardiac output, but with more than 3 μg/min the increase in afterload is not accompanied by a rise in output. It has been proposed as an agent which limits myocardial necrosis following coronary occlusion [314], but other therapeutic considerations have led to this application being superseded.

All these catecholamines with the exception of dobutamine will produce tissue necrosis if they become extravasated. Therefore they must be administered through a central venous line. Pressors are always given using a minidrop drip set (60 drops = 1 ml) and metered using a drip controller. A variety of apparatus has been described for this purpose [359], but our choice is a drop counter, despite variations in drop size and some irregularity of drop rate.

Table 4.3. Quantities of Catecholamines Added to a Volume of 500 ml to Provide an Infusion for Cardiovascular Support, Administered Through a Minidrip Set (60 Drops = 1 ml)

	Quantity (mg)	*μg/ml*	*μg/minidrop*
Adrenaline	10	20	0·3
	2	4	0·06
Dopamine	400	800	13
	200	400	6·6
	100	200	3·3
Dobutamine	500	1000	16
Isoprenaline	5	10	0·16
	1	2	0·03

All pressors are diluted before administration as an infusion (Table 4.3). The prescribing literature describes the appropriate dose in terms of $\mu g\ kg^{-1}\ min^{-1}$ but in practice it is simpler to describe the administration as drops/min. It is customary to commence the chosen pressor drip rate in adults at 5–10 drops/min and titrate the infusion against the responses of the patient.

Selection of Pressors

Pressors are selected in preparation for cardiovascular crises which may arise at any time. They are also used to provide a sustained stimulus, usually after CPB, but occasionally before institution of bypass or indeed preceding the induction of anaesthesia. Adrenaline is the most commonly used inotrope as an infusion in the Unit. It is consistently effective in its action, there are many years of experience in its use, and it is cheap to discard if only required for a short period. Dopamine is currently used for infants if necessary. In low dosage it is suitable for adults with pulmonary hypertension. It is also given postoperatively to succeed adrenaline if the patient is oliguric, with cold blue skin, and only requires a moderate pressor effect. Dobutamine is selected particularly in those adults who have been shown to have poor myocardial function preoperatively, although it could become the catecholamine of choice as more clinical experience is gained. However, even these patients may benefit from an initial stimulus from adrenaline at the termination of bypass, before progressing to dobutamine. An appreciation of the effectiveness of reducing afterload may also indicate that a peripheral vasodilator should be administered concurrently with an inotrope infusion provided that the mean arterial pressure is 80 mmHg [406]. Isoprenaline may now be selected when the heart rate is less than 60/min and myocardial contractility appears to be less than optimal. Ventricular or atrial pacing are sometimes more appropriate for a low heart rate and low blood pressure. Isoprenaline has been favoured for patients with pulmonary hypertension [299]. The suggestion has also been made that its specific beta-agonist activity makes it the drug of choice to antagonize beta-adrenoceptor blocking drugs if required [332].

Steroids

The possible benefits to the heart and circulation of steroids given in pharmacological doses may be related to their effect on myocardial compliance and systemic resistance. Toyama [428] has shown that when dogs have been subjected to aortic cross-clamping for 30 min, the administration of hydrocortisone 150 mg/kg either before clamping or after unclamping, failed to improve myocardial contractility. However, the decrease in diastolic left ventricular compliance of the steroid-treated dogs was significantly less, and on this basis its use might be considered following ischaemic cardioplegia. Large doses of steroids have certainly been shown to reduce systemic and pulmonary vascular resistance [103] so that this effect together with a diminution of fall in left ventricular compliance may be of benefit in the immediate post-bypass period.

The suggestion that steroids stabilize the lysosomal membrane [261] and may reduce infarct size has not been confirmed [360]. Attempts to clarify their effect on lysosomal enzyme release during CPB have been published [161]. The conventional pharmacological dose of methylprednisolone is 30 mg/kg.

Glucagon

Glucagon has been commended as an effective drug for increasing cardiac output, without inducing arrhythmias [396]. Its inotropic action is not blocked by propranolol [159]. Smith noted that the increase in cardiac output was still evident after half an hour, while Williams [460] found that its cardiovascular action was short-lived and varied considerably among patients. Abbott [1] described rises in blood pressure in 5 children with 'low cardiac output failure' when glucagon was administered half-hourly from 14 to 40 hr after open heart surgery. No problems relating to a high blood glucose or low serum potassium caused by glucagon have been reported. The dose suggested for adults is 3–5 mg [460] or 10 mg [396]. Children have been given between 50 μg [1] and 150 μg/kg [215] repeated every 30 min.

Glucose, Insulin and Potassium

Glucose, insulin and potassium (GIK) have been shown to be beneficial in the treatment of heart failure due to coronary heart disease [280]. Improved contractility at the termination of bypass in one patient has been ascribed to a single dose of 25 ml of 50 per cent glucose, 25 units of insulin and 5 mM potassium chloride [153]. No improvement in cardiac function was found by Bradley [51] in 10 patients given glucose, insulin and potassium following valve surgery. A GIK regime was probably responsible for the severe hypophosphataemia following open heart surgery which has recently been reported [414]. Despite this low phosphate level, there was only a small effect on red cell 2,3-DPG and calculated haemoglobin *P*50.

Aminophylline

Aminophylline by its direct inotropic effect and release of catecholamines increases cardiac output. It also produces smooth muscle relaxation so that venous pressure falls, and there is vasodilatation of coronary, pulmonary and systemic vessels [165]. Its diuretic effect is short-lived. It has not been adopted as an infusion to be given for cardiovascular support but is sometimes administered as a slow bolus injection of 250 mg in 10 ml to adults.

Arrhythmias

Clinical aspects and mechanics of arrhythmias causing perioperative cardiac dysfunction have been reviewed recently [248]. The most common abnormalities requiring treatment during anaesthesia are ventricular fibrillation, tachycardia and premature beats. Various degrees of heart block are also encountered, while supraventricular changes of rate and rhythm do not always demand therapy. It is always therefore essential before, during and after anaesthesia to have available a defibrillator with internal and external paddles and a pacemaker box with suitable connections. Hypoxaemia, acidaemia, hypokalaemia and hypothermia must be corrected while considering drug therapy for arrhythmias.

A number of drugs are commonly used and can be classified according to Vaughan Williams (Table 4.4) [437].

Table 4.4. Antiarrhythmic Drugs – Vaughan Williams Classification

Class I	*Class II*	*Class III*	*Class IV*
Reduced rate of diastolic depolarization	*Sympathetic activity diminished*	*Prolonged action potential and refractory period*	*Calcium movement blocked*
Lignocaine	Beta blockers	Sotalol	Verapamil
Disopyramide	Bretylium	Disopyramide	(Disopyramide)
Mexiletine			
Phenytoin			
Quinidine			
Procainamide			

Lignocaine

Lignocaine is effective in the treatment of ventricular premature beats and ventricular tachycardia. It is given as a bolus injection of 1 mg/kg which has an effective half-life of 12–15 min [178]. It is given as an infusion for recurrence of ventricular arrhythmias. The metabolism of lignocaine is abnormal in patients with heart failure and its half-life after an infusion of 1·4 mg/min for 36 hr was increased from 1·4 to 4·3 hr [339]. With circulatory or hepatic dysfunction, a lignocaine infusion soon reaches therapeutic levels and there is an increased risk of toxicity with prolonged administration [18]. An infusion should therefore commence at 1 mg/min in adults after cardiac surgery.

Disopyramide

Disopyramide is an antiarrhythmic agent likely to influence a wide variety of electrophysiological disorders [117]. It has a potent local anaesthetic action like lignocaine. It delays atrioventricular node conduction and has a slight negative inotropic effect. It should be avoided in patients where heart block might be exaggerated, and given over 5–10 min when administered intravenously. It has been shown to reduce the incidence of ventricular arrhythmias after myocardial infarction [220] and may have some efficacy in acute supraventricular arrhythmias [310]. It has a half-life of 5–7 hr following oral or intravenous administration, which may be extended when the cardiac output is low [351]. It has been given in a dose of 1–2 mg/kg intravenously to those patients who have not responded satisfactorily to lignocaine. A case report has described ventricular tachycardia and hypotension after the intravenous administration of disopyramide in a patient with a dyskinetic area of myocardium, following a myocardial infarction [392].

Mexiletine

Mexiletine is an antiarrhythmic agent which particularly depresses the maximum rate of depolarization. It has sometimes been used to treat persistent ventricular arrhythmias which have failed to respond to lignocaine or disopyramide. It can be administered intravenously as a loading dose of 100–250 mg given over 4–10 min, and continued as an intravenous infusion. It too can produce hypotension and bradycardia.

Phenytoin and Bretylium Tosylate

Phenytoin and bretylium tosylate have not been used in our anaesthetic experience. Phenytoin is effective in the treatment of digitalis-induced arrhythmias, as a slow intravenous injection of 2 mg/kg. Hypotension, bradycardia and atrioventricular block may complicate its administration.

Propranolol

Propranolol has not found favour during anaesthesia for cardiac surgery, due to its negative inotropic effect. It improves oxygenation of the ischaemic myocardium [313], so that this policy may be reconsidered in future. It is effective in the treatment of supraventricular tachycardias and arrhythmias due to digitalis intoxication, when there is no atrioventricular block. The benefits of its antiarrhythmic action may sometimes outweigh the disadvantages of myocardial depression, as described in a patient with refractory ventricular fibrillation [131]. It is given intravenously in 0·25 mg increments in adults to a total of 2 mg if required. Occasionally propranolol may be indicated before CPB in patients with Fallot's tetralogy if the right to left shunt becomes very great. Its action in depressing myocardial contractility, or increasing systemic vascular resistance may be relevant in this instance.

Digitalis

Digitalis preparations are usually discontinued 48 hr before surgery to reduce the possibility of toxic arrhythmias. They may be related to the digitalis effect of reducing myocardial potassium content [315], and the potassium imbalance induced by diuretics and CPB [418]. Therefore if digitalis is given soon after surgery it is given cautiously and more often for the treatment of supraventricular tachyarrhythmias (not digitalis induced) than for poor ventricular contractility.

Load Reduction

It now seems rational to prevent an increase in left ventricular afterload above normal. Consequently the anaesthetic technique should avoid the circumstances and the use of drugs which increase the systemic resistance adversely. It may be necessary to administer drugs specifically to overcome the hypertension which can occur during [19] or after surgery [438], despite appropriate analgesia. The raised blood pressure may be due to a high systemic vascular resistance or an increase in the velocity of left ventricular contraction. It seems that labile hypertension during surgery may be attributable to fluctuations in contractility especially in patients with coronary artery disease, essential hypertension or aortic regurgitation.

It may also be advisable when the myocardium is failing, to lower the systemic vascular resistance or effect venous unloading of the heart. Due regard must be given to the pulmonary vascular resistance in some congenital and acquired diseases where it is already raised.

The systemic vascular resistance may be elevated due to hypocarbia, pain, hypothermia and heart failure itself. It may be increased during CPB because of some of these factors, or due to awareness, a non-pulsatile flow or surgical stress. Contrary to previous reports, plasma catecholamine levels have not been found to be raised [195].

It is a simple matter to ventilate the patient to produce an arterial $P\text{CO}_2$ within normal limits, and to ensure that sufficient analgesia has been given. A large number of drugs is available to effect load reduction or to depress the hyperdynamic heart. The drugs used for these specific purposes in this Unit include droperidol, pentolinium, nitroprusside, diuretics and halothane.

Droperidol

Droperidol causes peripheral vasodilatation [458] and contributes to the general anaesthetic technique. It is not administered until an intra-arterial means of monitoring the blood pressure is available and it is given in 2·5 mg increments in adults, and 0·1 mg/kg increments in children. The duration of its vascular effect appears to be about 20 min. The total dose is normally limited to 30 mg in adults during anaesthesia, because of the desire to minimize its soporific effect in the postoperative phase. It also reduces pulmonary vascular resistance [276] and may contribute to the management of patients where this is raised.

Pentolinium

Pentolinium, an autonomic ganglion blocker, has been found to be a suitable additional drug in our hands for the control of hypertension during or following surgery. Since it is given after a considerable dose of droperidol it is administered in 0·5 mg increments from a 5 ml syringe containing 5 mg diluted with normal saline. The onset of action is 2–3 min so that a repeat dose is not given before this time. Tachycardia has not been a problem with the small doses required. The ganglion blockade may be advantageous in preventing reflex responses to a fall in carotid sinus and aortic wall pressures. It reduces but does not reverse the hyperglycaemic response to surgery [133]. The fall in serum potassium attributed to its action has not been a problem. It is important to remember that the pupils may become dilated by this drug.

Its use has been commended for the control of blood pressure during coarctation resection [42] and has reduced the need for further hypotensive drugs in the immediate postoperative period. Hypertension and associated abdominal symptoms may, however, be delayed in this condition when other hypotensive agents are more appropriate [138].

Halothane

Halothane with its depression of myocardial contractility, has the merit of rapid and flexible control of blood pressure in patients already treated with droperidol, and who still respond unduly to such stimuli as opening the sternum or manipulation of the ascending aorta prior to bypass. It is also a useful adjunct to the chosen technique of blood pressure control for resection of aortic coarctation in adults, being discontinued prior to removal of the aortic clamps. In the non-failing canine heart, halothane appears to influence the relationship between myocardial oxygen supply and demand in a favourable direction [49] despite its depression of contractility.

Nitroprusside

Nitroprusside specifically lowers systemic resistance by vasodilatation due to its direct action on vessel walls. It can cause cyanide toxicity and the toxic dose in man has not yet been determined [303]. It does not depress the myocardium, although there is no certainty that it does not have a myocardial toxic effect [426]. The oxygen content of coronary sinus blood increases when nitroprusside is administered [370]. This could mean that oxygen supply has improved in relation to demand or that oxygen is not so readily taken up by the myocardium due to toxic or redistribution effects. Chiarello [76] has shown that nitroprusside intensifies myocardial ischaemic injury. Further studies are required to elucidate these points and there are still some reservations regarding its use during cardiac surgery [247].

Nevertheless, because of its effectiveness, rapid onset and recovery it is used for the control of hypertension and to reduce preload and afterload when treating the failing heart. For this therapy in adults it is administered as 50 mg in 500 ml dextrose/saline (100 μg/ml), through a microdrip set (60 drops = 1 ml) at an initial rate of 5–10 drops/min (8–16 μg/min). The minimum monitoring requires central venous and intra-arterial cannulations. Although Stinson [405] found that nitroprusside was associated with the most favourable haemodynamic responses, he advised caution in its use since the relationship between cardiac output and unloading of the heart is variable among individual patients.

Nitroprusside may cause an unfavourable tachycardia and reduction in arterial oxygen tension [386]. This latter effect may be attributed to a reduction in pulmonary vascular resistance [73] which in itself may be advantageous in pulmonary hypertensive heart disease. The application of nitroprusside for its effect on the pulmonary circuit has also been described for the respiratory distress syndrome [3] and it may therefore be useful in the management of a persistent foetal pulmonary circulation or following the Fontan procedure.

Trinitroglycerine

Trinitroglycerine (glyceryl trinitrate) may reduce myocardial oxygen expenditure and therefore relieve angina principally by venous unloading. Consequently it causes a fall in blood pressure in patients with normal cardiac function. Either trinitroglycerine or isosorbide dinitrate (sorbide nitrate) has been recommended sublingually in patients about to undergo coronary artery bypass surgery [439]. It is now commercially available as an intravenous preparation. Previously, it was prepared by dissolving fresh trinitroglycerine tablets (0·5 mg) in saline, sterilizing the solution by millipore filtration, and using as 8 mg in 250 ml. In this form it has been used to limit myocardial oxygen demand during coronary artery surgery [230] and to limit the extent of myocardial infarcts. It seems to be adsorbed by some types of plastic so that infusion from glass syringes and high density polyethylene tubing is recommended [90].

Other Peripheral Vasodilatators

Various other drugs producing peripheral vasodilatation have been used, including chlorpromazine [89], phentolamine [281], phenoxybenzamine [97, 264] and thymoxamine [331], to unload the heart when it has been failing. Other ganglion blockers which have been employed during open heart surgery include hexamethonium [25] and trimetaphan [240]. Trimetaphan increased cardiac output in patients with a high arterial pressure, high left atrial pressure and low cardiac output. Trimetaphan has now been superseded by nitroprusside. When the two were compared, trimetaphan was found to produce an undesired redistribution of cardiac output in favour of skin and muscle [445]. Salbutamol, a beta-2-adrenoceptor agonist caused a fall in systemic vascular resistance and left atrial pressure after cardiac surgery [338]. It produced a substantial rise in heart rate and maximum acceleration of aortic flow, both of which would increase myocardial oxygen consumption.

Diuretics

Frusemide, bumetanide and ethacrynic acid are powerful diuretics and are particularly indicated for the initial treatment of acute pulmonary oedema or congestion and the fluid overload which can be associated with the use of a Ringer's lactate pump prime. Preoperatively they may have been administered for a long time and may cause potassium and chloride depletion, producing a hypochloraemic alkalosis. Hypokalaemia increases the toxicity of digitalis so that close monitoring of serum potassium and appropriate potassium chloride therapy are necessary when these diuretics are given. Occasionally a patient with a failing heart and oliguria may have been treated to such an extent with diuretics that he becomes sodium depleted and develops a hypovolaemic low output state. There is now a more rational trend towards the use of inotropic agents combined with vasodilators, rather than diuretics, in this situation [82]. The intravenous dose of frusemide in an anaesthetic context ranges from 10 to 40 mg in adults and is usually effective despite the much larger doses which may have been given before operation. The effective dose of frusemide has been shown to be less when given by a constant infusion pump [254]. The initial dose of frusemide for infants is 0·5 mg/kg in this Unit.

Mannitol

Mannitol, as a diuretic can rarely be advised in the presence of overload, due to its hyperosmolal effect on plasma volume [298]. It may encourage urine production when other diuretics have failed, and is recommended in the presence of suspected acute renal failure [256].

Mechanical Support

The intra-aortic balloon pump (IABP), one of a number of invasive mechanical devices for assisting the failing circulation, has become a standard facility in cardiac surgical units. The IABP consists of an inflatable balloon catheter which is usually inserted, through a Teflon sleeve attached to the femoral artery, almost as far as the left subclavian artery. The balloon deflates during systole and is inflated by helium during diastole, the mechanism being triggered by the ECG R wave. Thus during systole the resistance to ventricular emptying is suddenly reduced, ventricular work is less, while the systolic blood pressure falls. During diastole the pressure in the proximal aorta is augmented and coronary perfusion, particularly subendocardial perfusion, is enhanced (*Fig. 4.3*). In this way temporary support for the heart and circulation can be provided for several days if necessary, by which time some spontaneous improvement in the myocardium should have occurred. The assist device is usually indicated when the various manoeuvres to produce adequate myocardial contractility have failed at the termination of bypass. It has also been advocated for selected cases of cardiogenic shock following myocardial infarction, and some patients with crescendo angina undergoing investigation by cardiac catheterization prior to surgery [248].

In the operating room the balloon is inserted from necessity before the termination of bypass. The patient can then be weaned off bypass as the IABP assists the circulation. Heparin can be reversed as usual after removal of arterial and venous perfusion cannulas. As the patient improves haemodynamically it may be possible in 24–48 hr to wean him off controlled ventilation despite the presence of the balloon, provided that the criteria of adequate function of the various systems have been met.

The abdominal left ventricular assist device (ALVAD) [323] may have a place for temporary total circulatory support when maximal pharmacological and IABP support have failed. This device has been interposed between the left ventricle and infrarenal abdominal aorta and in spite of the absence of both right and left ventricular function [324] has supported the circulation adequately prior to cardiac and renal transplant.

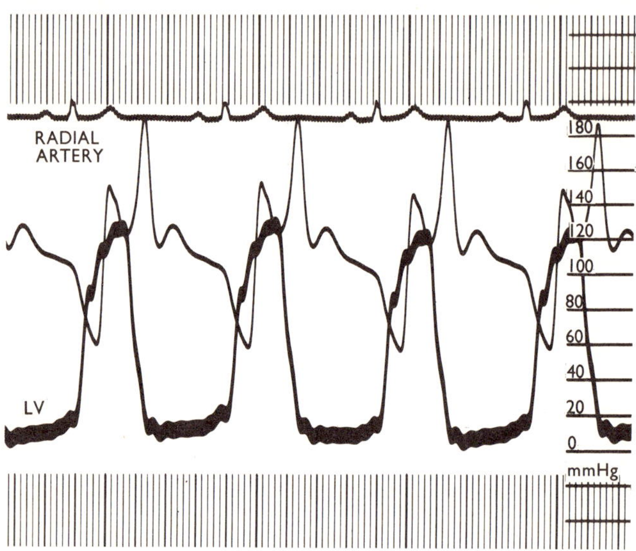

Fig. 4.3. Radial artery and left ventricular pressure in a patient during Intra-aortic Balloon Counter Pulsation. The aortic diastolic pressure exceeds systolic pressure and is sustained. The diastolic pressure time index is large compared with the systolic pressure time index indicating more than adequate subendocardial perfusion.

ANAESTHESIA

In a cardiac surgical unit, patients may require a general anaesthetic in the cardiac catheter laboratory or in the operating room. In the catheter laboratory, the options available to the anaesthetist and the problems he may meet have been reviewed [282]. In the operating room, general anaesthesia is necessary for open heart surgery and for non-bypass operations. These include a variety of palliative procedures [375], ligation of persistent ductus arteriosus, resection of aortic coarctation and the complications of haemorrhage and tamponade. Cardioversion and pacemaker insertion occasionally require general anaesthesia while dental treatment before cardiac surgery may sometimes be undertaken in this way. This review is concerned with anaesthesia for open heart surgery in adults, children and infants. The same considerations of preoperative assessment, precautions and anaesthetic technique apply to anaesthesia for other cardiac operations.

Preoperative Appraisal

It is the normal practice to review the patient's medical history, clinical findings and the results of investigations before surgery is undertaken. The results of various non-invasive and invasive methods of investigation of the heart and circulation are available to the anaesthetist at this time. Medical and surgical problems relevant to the actual conduct of anaesthesia usually become apparent then. The patient's cardiovascular system, with prior medical treatment will usually be as well as the disease allows. In some circumstances, particularly requiring urgent surgery, the patient may still be suffering from left or right heart failure. There may be disturbances of cardiac rhythm, myocardial ischaemia and respiratory, renal or liver dysfunction. Electrolyte imbalance with hypokalaemia and hyponatraemia may be evident. Anaemia, polycythaemia or abnormal coagulation may be manifestations of the heart disease.

Respiratory dysfunction may be secondary to the cardiac condition or due to primary lung disease. The effects of both congenital and acquired heart disease on pulmonary blood volume and water content have been described [251]. The resulting breathlessness and abnormal lung compliance, ventilation, perfusion and oxygenation may not easily be distinguished from lung disease *per se*. Extensive pulmonary function tests are not usually carried out, but it is anticipated that poor preoperative lung function will give rise to some degree of immediate postoperative pulmonary inadequacy, even with improved haemodynamics. Exceptionally, patients with a long history of obstructive airways disease, with a very low forced vital capacity (FVC) and forced expiratory volume (FEV_1) may be regarded as a grave postoperative risk from primary lung disease.

Impaired renal function, with a raised serum creatinine and urea is not uncommon in mitral valve disease particularly due to diminished renal perfusion. This does not demand specific treatment during and after surgery, but requires the established monitoring of renal function at those times. The degree of preoperative renal dysfunction was found to be a consistent predictor of the onset of postoperative renal failure [4].

Impaired liver function is seen in tricuspid valve disease and right ventricular failure. This may have implications regarding the prolongation of action of drugs, coagulation defects and increased postoperative dysfunction, including a high serum bilirubin and associated metabolic disorders [446].

Correction of an abnormal serum potassium, usually hypokalaemia, is desirable before surgery because of the relationship with digitalis toxicity and arrhythmias. Although muscle mass is diminished in chronic low output states [457], there may be a disproportionate deficit of total body potassium even with a normal serum level [318]. Hypochloraemic alkalosis may be associated with hypokalaemia.

Hyponatraemia, a reflection of diminished renal function [123] and the sick cells [142] in heart failure, does not require sodium replacement.

Occasionally a raised serum sodium will be found as a result of zealous diuretic therapy in patients with persistent heart failure. In these patients rehydration and then cardiovascular support may be needed.

There may be anaemia related to infection or previous valve surgery. This is not usually treated by transfusion before anaesthesia. Polycythaemia is found in those congenital heart diseases with large right to left shunts. This can adversely affect the outcome of surgery because of increased viscosity and reduced coagulation factors. Increased viscosity may cause intravascular thrombosis and a state of chronic disseminated intravascular coagulation (DIC) [238]. There may be a reduction in coagulation mechanisms due to this and to the small plasma volume found in severe polycythaemia. Preoperative withdrawal of blood, and administration of heparin to reduce the DIC and loss of clotting factors have been suggested [100]. Adequate hydration and withdrawal of blood together with its replacement by fresh frozen plasma shortly after induction of anaesthesia are also useful manoeuvres.

Open heart surgery in patients with inherited haematological defects has been reviewed [259]. In the 11 patients described, no complications due to the abnormality were evident. Thus thalassaemia minor and the sickle cell trait should give rise to no problems. Our own experience has shown that the management of von Willebrands disease with Koate (human antihaemophilic globulin, Factor VIII) has avoided bleeding problems.

Routine coagulation studies in this Unit include a platelet count, prothrombin ratio and partial thromboplastin time. The incidence of coagulation abnormalities is low. Ellison [126] has described one previously undiagnosed abnormality in 1500 patients who had open heart surgery. However, undetected coagulation defects could give rise to serious problems after bypass, when it is obviously desirable to be forewarned of this possibility.

Drug Therapy

Drug therapy is reviewed before surgery is undertaken.

Digoxin

Digoxin is usually discontinued 24–48 hr before operation to avoid the possibility of digitalis intoxication being precipitated by alterations in electrolyte distribution, especially potassium. Rose [367] was unable to distinguish between digitalis-induced and spontaneously occurring arrhythmias since the serum digitalis level in his patients varied from 0 to 2·8 ng/ml. Hypocalcaemia and hypomagnesaemia were not related to the abnormal rhythms. Digitalis may be required until the morning of operation in patients with atrial fibrillation and a fast ventricular rate.

Beta-adrenoceptor Antagonists

Beta-adrenoceptor antagonists depress myocardial contractility, the response to beta-stimulators, and they delay atrioventricular conduction.

They are almost invariably administered to patients with angina associated with coronary artery disease but are avoided when left ventricular function is compromised. There have been conflicting views on the need to withdraw these drugs before cardiac surgery [137, 226, 239]. There appears to be no contraindication to the continuation of beta-adrenoceptor blockade before operation in patients undergoing aorto-coronary bypass grafts when suitable anaesthetic agents are selected and appropriate blood volume is maintained [288]. The presence of beta-blockade may even be beneficial by improving oxygenation of ischaemic myocardium [313] and providing some myocardial protection [325]. Foëx [145] has pointed out that methoxyflurane, trichlorethylene and enflurane should be avoided, however. He also stressed that hypercapnia or hypoxia during or after operation will depress the heart more, in the presence of beta-blockers. When these drugs are given for the control of essential hypertension, their continuation until surgery provides better stability of the blood pressure during and after anaesthesia, perhaps related in part to diminished renin release [466]. Patients with Fallot's tetralogy who sometimes receive beta-blockers preoperatively [93], usually have the drug withdrawn in view of anticipated reduction in right ventricular function after surgery. When beta-blockers are discontinued, a gradual withdrawal over 48 hr is regarded as optimal [226]. This avoids the risks of severe angina and myocardial infarction associated with sudden withdrawal in patients with coronary artery disease [12, 306].

There would seem to be benefits in continuing antihypertensive drugs until the time of surgery [342]. The facility to monitor and manipulate the cardiovascular system during heart surgery should ensure that their presence has no adverse effects. Patients may for unassociated reasons be taking steroids before operation and these are managed in conventional fashion.

Numerous drugs alter the number, stickiness or ability of platelets to aggregate. It is therefore desirable to discontinue drugs known to produce these effects, so that platelet function after bypass is not impaired from this cause. It has been suggested that clofibrate should be discontinued 2 weeks before cardiac surgery.

Premedication

A preoperative visit to the patient establishes an important rapport with him, when the nature of the pre- and postoperative events can be described to him. It also enables an assessment of any problems associated with the proposed technique of anaesthesia and monitoring to be made.

A large range of drugs is available to relieve the anxiety of patients before heart surgery, and to provide sedation. The difficulties of evaluating these drugs have been described [146]. A night sedative such as nitrazepam is sometimes desired by patients, while some benefit by taking diazepam or chlordiazepoxide during the day. The personal management of the patient by doctors, nurses and fellow patients probably makes a greater contribution towards allaying anxiety than the prescribed drugs.

Lyons [274] compared no premedication in cardiac surgical patients with a premedication of either diazepam or pentobarbitone with morphine and hyoscine. He found that the latter combination did not cause cardiovascular or respiratory depression, and the patients were calm and sedated. Adults in this Unit are usually given papaveretum 10 mg and hyoscine 0·4 mg intramuscularly 1 hr before induction of anaesthesia. The more anxious, usually younger adults, receive pentobarbitone 100 mg by mouth on the night before operation. Particularly ill or old patients may receive less than the usual dose of premedication and for emergency surgery no premedication is given at all if the cardiovascular state is precarious. Children of more than 6 months receive papaveretum 0·5 mg and hyoscine 0·01 mg/kg intramuscularly to a maximum of 10 mg and 0·2 mg respectively, 1 hr before anaesthesia. Infants are given atropine 0·1–0·2 mg by intramuscular injection.

Anaesthetic Agents

A wide variety of drugs has been used with success to provide the anaesthesia for cardiac surgery. There is no evidence, based on the results of surgery, that one technique is superior to another. It would seem vital however that the anaesthetist appreciates fully the haemodynamics of the patient's disease and the way in which this may be altered by his choice of drugs and mechanical support.

Thiopentone

Thiopentone in the widest field of anaesthesia is the intravenous induction agent of choice [122]. Despite the introduction of methohexitone, propanidid, Althesin (alphaxalone/alphadolone acetate), etomidate, hydroxybutyrate, ketamine and diazepam, thiopentone still seems to have a lower incidence of adverse reactions. The well-recognized depression of the cardiovascular system by thiopentone may be a serious danger to patients with cardiac disease so that it is used with great caution. Because the circulation time may be slow, the effects of even 25 mg thiopentone on the blood pressure may not be evident for two or three minutes. Unless great patience is exercised, there is a tendency to give more thiopentone which may produce profound hypotension. The appropriate dose of this drug must therefore be guided as much by the observed blood pressure trend, as the loss of patient consciousness. When methohexitone and Althesin were compared with thiopentone in cardiac surgical patients, the blood pressure fell to a similar degree [273]. For this reason many anaesthetists have looked to other induction methods, using nitrous oxide and oxygen alone, morphine, neuroleptanalgesia, ketamine or diazepam.

Nitrous Oxide

Nitrous oxide with muscle relaxants has been the mainstay of anaesthesia for heart surgery for decades [169]. It is a weak anaesthetic and therefore unsuitable as the sole agent for induction. It is used principally to supplement a variety of narcotics. Employed in this way it does limit the percentage of oxygen which can be administered. However, it must be very rare that more than 50 per cent oxygen is required to provide a safe arterial oxygen content. In fact, when the 'virtual shunt' [41] is more than 50 per cent there is very little increase in arterial oxygen tension with high inspired oxygen concentrations, and a marginal increase in oxygen content. The mere correction of hypoxia by increasing the inspired concentration of oxygen is a simplistic approach and other methods of improving oxygen delivery must be employed [467]. Nitrous oxide does not cause noticeable haemodynamic changes in the systemic circulation [409, 425] or in a small series, the pulmonary circulation [106]. Dottori found that tracheal intubation with muscle relaxants and this agent alone produced a transient increase of 31 per cent in the mean systemic pressure and 78 per cent in the mean pulmonary artery pressure.

The detrimental effects of nitrous oxide might be considered in three particular respects. It does cause some degree of myocardial depression and increase in pulmonary vascular resistance when the high dose morphine or fentanyl technique is used [246, 409]. It causes expansion of gas within the body, in particular air bubbles inadvertently introduced into the patient by the bubble oxygenator, as a result of opening the heart chambers, or from intravenous drips and injection sites by the anaesthetist [286]. It interferes with vitamin B12 metabolism even with less than 6 hr exposure [15] although recovery occurs when nitrous oxide is discontinued.

Morphine

Profound morphine narcosis has its advocates [269] but this technique has not been widely adopted in the United Kingdom. The dose of morphine for anaesthetizing cardiac surgical patients was as high as 8–10 mg/kg [180, 289], but because of disadvantages the total dose was reduced to 1–2 mg/kg [268]. The administration is at a rate of 5 mg/min, either as a bolus or by infusion [400]. It may produce a fall in blood pressure, due to changes in peripheral resistance and venous capacitance [188], is a comparatively slow induction method and does not produce certain unconsciousness. The addition of hyoscine 0·01–0·02 mg/kg during the course of surgery, will eliminate the problem of awareness [43] while physostigmine up to 0·07 mg/kg will reverse the effect of hyoscine at the completion of surgery [297]. The addition of nitrous oxide increases cardiovascular depression [468]. Surgical stimulation still produces a blood pressure rise despite adequate narcosis [19] and this if untreated causes an unwanted increase in myocardial oxygen demand. Residual respiratory depressant effects of morphine require intermittent positive pressure ventilation, often overnight, which may be regarded as a disadvantage. Romagnola [366] was able to extubate patients having aorto-coronary bypass surgery at 15·7 hr after morphine and 6·4 hr on average, after a fentanyl technique. The antidiuretic hormone response to surgery is suppressed by morphine in a dose of 2 mg/kg [334].

Neuroleptanalgesia

Neuroleptanalgesia (NLA) uses a combination of droperidol with fentanyl or phenoperidine to produce intense analgesia and a degree of peripheral vasodilation. This combination also induces anaesthesia slowly, with the possibility of a fall in blood pressure requiring treatment. The side effect of muscle rigidity should not be a problem when muscle relaxants are given. Morgan [312] used conventional doses of neuroleptics to induce anaesthesia for major surgery including heart surgery. He gave 5–20 mg of droperidol to produce drowsiness, followed by fentanyl 0·1–0·8 mg slowly while 50–70 per cent nitrous oxide was being administered by facemask. This produced a fall in systolic blood pressure of more than 40 mmHg in 3 per cent of patients having open heart surgery, and falls of 20–40 mmHg in 19 per cent. In the absence of preinduction hypertension or a hyperdynamic circulation, this might be regarded as undesirable.

Perhaps NLA can be regarded more favourably for maintenance of anaesthesia. A mean of 0·1 mg of fentanyl per hr was given by Morgan for this purpose, while Manners [287] used phenoperidine 4–20 mg given incrementally in the course of cardiac operations. The use of droperidol in the latter instance was confined to limiting the systolic pressure to less than 140 mmHg.

Järnberg [218] reported that central haemodynamics were preserved using NLA in non-cardiac patients but renal perfusion was reduced. Postoperatively this became normal and it was concluded that the technique was acceptable for the poor-risk patient. Santesson [378] found that NLA had a direct metabolic depressant effect since the fall in cardiac output associated with it related to a diminished tissue oxygen demand. However, the stimulus of surgery increased left ventricular stroke work above control values. In contrast, Stoelting [408] found that the addition of droperidol or nitrous oxide to large doses of fentanyl decreased myocardial contractility and cardiovascular dynamics. The depressant effect of large doses of fentanyl on cardiac output and blood pressure in dogs can be partially reversed with diazepam 0·5 mg/kg, and completely antagonized with pancuronium 0·1 mg/kg [265].

The use of fentanyl 0·005 mg/kg to maintain analgesia has been compared with morphine 0·5 mg/kg [112]. There seemed to be no advantage in using morphine rather than fentanyl.

Recent studies have shown that there is no difference in the duration of action of equianalgesic doses of morphine and fentanyl in respect of respiratory depression [358] or analgesia [199]. Delayed respiratory depression after fentanyl has been described [9] so that early extubation after large doses may be hazardous.

Ketamine

Ketamine has been recommended as the anaesthetic of choice for the poor-risk patient [88]. However, the sympathetic stimulation and effect on myocardial oxygen balance may not be beneficial [382, 434]. The patient in severe heart failure with depleted myocardial noradrenaline may respond adversely by the direct myocardial depressant effect [102]. More control of the poor-risk patient may therefore be achieved with specific induction agents and additional exogeneous catecholamines if necessary.

Ketamine would not seem to be the best choice when there is muscular obstruction to ventricular outflow, in Fallot's tetralogy or hypertrophic cardiomyopathy for instance. Nor would it seem suitable for patients with pulmonary hypertension [419] although Gassner [152] concluded that changes in pulmonary haemodynamics were due to an increased cardiac output, not pulmonary vasoconstriction.

Nevertheless, ketamine is used for paediatric and adult cardiac anaesthesia. The cardiovascular effects are less in children and are minimal by intramuscular injection. Radnay [349] gave children ketamine 5 mg/kg intramuscularly on the operating room table followed by an additional 2·5 mg/kg if necessary. A premedication of pentobarbitone 3–4 mg/kg, morphine 0·2 mg/kg and atropine 0·01 mg/kg had preceded this induction. Anaesthesia was maintained with 50 per cent nitrous oxide and oxygen, and relaxation was provided with pancuronium. Additional intravenous supplements of ketamine amounting to 6·1 $\mu g\,kg^{-1}\,min^{-1}$ were given. Levin [260] reported that a ketamine–pancuronium technique did not prove to be superior to halothane, nitrous oxide and curare for cardiovascular surgery in infants. In adults, ketamine has been given using an infusion pump and supplemented with nitrous oxide, pancuronium and increments of diazepam [182]. A 0·1 per cent solution of ketamine was administered by Holter infusion pump or microdrip set throughout the operation and CPB. Jackson [213] showed that when diazepam preceded ketamine in adults undergoing open heart surgery, there was no change of mean blood pressure when ketamine was given.

Diazepam

Diazepam has been advocated as an induction agent in patients with little cardiovascular reserve [236], because of its benign effects on the heart and circulation [96, 113]. Significant cardiovascular depression may occur however, and it must still be administered with some care even to patients without heart disease [219]. Stanley [398] described a modest fall in cardiac output when as little as 5 mg diazepam was given to patients undergoing open heart surgery who were anaesthetized with morphine. A comparison of diazepam as an induction agent with thiopentone and methohexitone showed its limitations particularly with regard to delay in onset of action and in recovery time [59]. It causes significant respiratory depression [96], and the prolonged effect of sedation may be regarded as a disadvantage in the early postoperative period.

Eisenberg [124] described an anaesthetic technique which could be applied to cardiac patients using a combination of diazepam and morphine. After a premedication of diazepam 5–20 mg and atropine 0·4–0·6 mg intramuscularly, anaesthesia was induced by morphine 1–2 mg and diazepam 2·5 mg every 30 sec into a fast-running intravenous drip, while giving 70 per cent nitrous oxide by facemask. A total of 5–20 mg diazepam was given in this way. The patients were then intubated using suxamethonium and relaxation was continued with Tubarine (tubocurarine chloride). Additional morphine was given as required. A blood pressure fall of 10–15 per cent was reported, while emergence from anaesthesia was rapid.

A different combination of diazepam–pentazocine has been described for an unselected series of 320 open heart operations [181]. Anaesthesia was induced with increments of diazepam to a total of 0·3–0·4 mg/kg and pentazocine 1·5–3 mg/kg infused over 15 min. This was followed by 50 per cent nitrous oxide with oxygen, incremental doses of diazepam 5 mg and pentazocine 10–20 mg and muscle relaxation with Tubarine or pancuronium. Three patients recalled the defibrillation procedure. The rise in systemic vascular resistance which may occur with pentazocine [11] is undesirable in patients with coronary artery disease or a failing left ventricle.

Volatile Anaesthetics

Volatile anaesthetics are sometimes used for both induction and maintenance of anaesthesia for cardiac surgery. As induction agents they are probably used principally for infants in some centres. To maintain anaesthesia they are often combined with nitrous oxide and oxygen, or with oxygen alone when added to the oxygenator. Halothane, enflurane, methoxyflurane and trichlorethylene have all had their advocates, while cyclopropane is still available as an induction agent. Ether has been used particularly for the specific technique of profound hypothermia with surface cooling in infants.

Both halothane and enflurane produce myocardial depression [300, 397], enflurane more than any other volatile anaesthetic [71]. Both should therefore be used with even more caution, if at all, as induction agents in infants with congestive heart failure [160] or obstruction to cardiac output. Halothane increases the sensitivity of the myocardium to catecholamines much more than enflurane. The effect of halothane in reducing pulmonary vascular resistance seems to be equivocal [206, 266]. The reduction of systemic vascular resistance with enflurane during open heart surgery was found to persist for only 10 min [231].

The merit of either of these agents may be related to a reduction in myocardial oxygen consumption associated with a fall in blood pressure and cardiac output as described for halothane [49]. They may be used to produce an easily reversible control of a hyperdynamic circulation with high myocardial oxygen demand as seen in patients with coronary artery disease, and sometimes aortic valve disease. They may also contribute to the control of hypertension in aortic coarctation. The benefit of rapid recovery from these agents may lead to their increased use if prolonged postoperative mechanical ventilation is not required [223]. These agents are still given to produce anaesthesia during bypass, by addition to the oxygenator gas supply. Methods of scavenging to prevent their pollution of the operating room have been described [17, 304, 317]. The place of halothane, because of an association with hepatic necrosis, is still controversial [210, 388, 412] and its substitution by enflurane uncertain [343].

Methoxyflurane is no longer desirable because of its nephrotoxic effects. Ether is generally unsatisfactory due to its flammability. Its popularity for the profound hypothermia technique has been related to an absence of myocardial irritability and absence of vasoconstriction [294, 469]. When halothane was used instead of ether, the safe period of circulatory occlusion was shorter [381]. It was postulated that this was due to a higher brain oxygen consumption than when ether was used [212].

Muscle Relaxants

Pancuronium* has now largely replaced other non-depolarizing muscle relaxants during anaesthesia for cardiac surgery. It was compared with tubocurarine, gallamine and alcuronium in cardiac surgical patients during induction of anaesthesia and laryngeal intubation [273]. Pancuronium produced a greater rise in heart rate but less fall in mean blood pressure before intubation than tubocurarine and alcuronium. Its myocardial stimulant effect [385] may be regarded as disadvantageous in patients with hypertension or coronary artery disease [395], since the blood pressure may rise well above preinduction levels after laryngeal intubation. The choice of tubocurarine for these patients is equivocal. It may be preferable to control the cardiovascular reactivity by continuing beta-blockade than to use tubocurarine which could cause an uncontrolled hypotensive episode during induction. The safe use of tubocurarine in the presence of beta-blockade has not yet been established, while pancuronium can be given without hazard [288]. Tubocurarine would seem to be a more suitable choice for adult patients undergoing resection of coarctation, however.

Fazadinium, like gallamine, produces a marked tachycardia which in general is considered undesirable in patients with cardiac disease. These two drugs might be considered when there is a bradycardia in patients taking beta-blockers. Dimethylcurare, were it available in the United

**See* important note added in proof, p. 260.

Kingdom, might be a suitable relaxant for open heart surgery since it does not cause changes in heart rate and has a long duration of action [407].

Suxamethonium is often mentioned as a means of rapid intubation before cardiac surgery. It may be ineffective when the circulation time is prolonged and has adverse effects on cardiac rhythm in the presence of digitalis. Before pancuronium was available, Gilston [155] described the use of suxamethonium mixed with tubocurarine to avoid the possibility of the patient coughing on the endotracheal tube as the effect of suxamethonium diminished and before the non-depolarizing relaxant had taken effect. There seem to be few indications now to employ suxamethonium for tracheal intubation before cardiac surgery. There is usually no reason why controlled ventilation for two or three minutes with a facemask cannot be carried out until a non-depolarizing muscle relaxant has become effective.

Anaesthetic Technique

Whichever technique of anaesthesia is selected, preparation before arrival of the sedated patient in the anaesthetic room is required. It must be assumed that all patients requiring heart surgery are liable to serious disturbances of the cardiovascular system. It is mandatory to be prepared for such eventualities, by having the necessary equipment, apparatus and drugs ready from the outset. These include the ECG oscilloscope, defibrillator with external and internal paddles, routine drugs, disposable equipment and infusion sets.

Drugs drawn up and immediately available in this Unit are

Calcium gluconate 1 g in 10 ml and

Adrenaline 10 mg in 500 ml of 4 per cent dextrose and 1/5 N saline in a microdrop drip set, so that 3 drops contain 1 μg.

Induction

Adults are anaesthetized by the following technique in the Wessex Unit. Children weighing more than 10 kg are managed in a similar way, with drug dosages adjusted according to weight (Table 4.5). Orthopnoeic patients are supported by pillows, as required. ECG monitoring is established from the outset. A butterfly needle or 21G Venflon is inserted into the left hands and 1–2 mg phenoperidine, administered. Left radial artery cannulation is then performed to provide a continuous display of blood pressure throughout induction of anaesthesia and during surgery. Anaesthetic induction consists of a further 2–3 mg phenoperidine in all but the smallest and most frail adults followed by pancuronium 8 mg and thiopentone 25–50 mg initially. Further increments of thiopentone are guided by the state of patients' wakefulness and the displayed blood pressure. Induction may be slow when the cardiac output is low or there is a left to right shunt. Respiration is gently assisted, then controlled, using a face-

Table 4.5. A Guide to the Dose of Drugs Used During Anaesthesia in Infants and Small Children

Guide only to anaesthetic drugs in infants and children.

Name: . . . . Weight:. . . . . kg

		per kg
4 mg/2 ml	Pancuronium	0·1 mg
100 mg/2 ml	Suxamethonium	0·5 mg
15 mg/1·5 ml	Tubocurarine	0·5 mg
0·6 mg/ml	Atropine	0·02 mg
0·5 mg/ml	Neostigmine	0·08 mg
10 mg/2 ml	Droperidol	0·1 mg
2 g/10 ml	Glucose	2·5 ml
20 units/ml	Insulin	0·2 units
10 mg/ml	Heparin	3 mg
100 mg/10 ml	Protamine	6 mg
0·5 mM/ml	Sodium bicarbonate	2 ml
1 g/10 ml	Calcium gluconate	0·1 ml
1 mg/10 ml	Adrenaline	0 02 ml (2 μg)
4 μg/ml	Isoprenaline	0·05 ml (0·2 μg)
100 mg/500 ml	Dopamine drip	
2 mg/500 ml	Adrenaline drip	
1 mg/500 ml	Isoprenaline drip	
20 mg/2 ml	Frusemide	0·5 mg
13 mM/5 ml	Potassium chloride	0·2 mM slowly in 15 min
100 mg/10 ml	Lignocaine	1 mg
50 mg/5 ml	Disopyramide	1 mg
0·5 mg/2 ml	Digoxin, *total dose*	0·9 mg/m^2
8 mg/2 ml	Dexamethasone	0·2 mg
500 mg/7 ml	Methylprednisolone	30 mg

mask and a mixture of 6 l nitrous oxide and 3 l oxygen for the majority of patients. Fifty per cent oxygen is given in the presence of cyanotic heart disease and for those patients showing signs of a low cardiac output or pulmonary congestion.

Intubation is carried out after about 3 min, without topical anaesthetic spray of larynx and trachea, using a cuffed disposable Portex oroendotracheal tube. Inflation of both lungs is confirmed. It is particularly easy to overlook accidental endobronchial intubation in children. Occasionally it may seem desirable to avoid muscle paralysis to facilitate intubation. In these particular instances such as late cardiac tamponade [301], induction can easily be accomplished with nitrous oxide and oxygen, a narcotic or diazepam in small doses and limited topical anaesthesia to the larynx. Spontaneous respiration can then continue until the chest is about to be opened. The additional effect of muscle relaxation and IPPV before this may immediately reduce venous return and cause a further fall in cardiac output. The effect of IPPV in causing a reversal to or increase of right to left intracardiac shunts, especially when the chest has been opened, has been explored by Strong [411]. This usually merely demands the establishment of bypass without undue delay, rather than administration of beta-blockers [93] or alpha-stimulators [441].

Nasopharyngeal and oesophageal thermometers are inserted. A 12 g or 14 g cannula is placed in a vein in the right hand or arm, and attached via a drip extension to an infusion of compound sodium lactate injection. Cannulation of the internal jugular vein is then performed, to provide the means of measuring central venous pressure and a route for the administration of catecholamines. The contraindications and precautions regarding this technique are observed at this point. If the patient requires catecholamine support before induction of anaesthesia or the need is anticipated before controlled ventilation is established, an intravenous catheter can be inserted into an antecubital vein. All intravenous and arterial lines are secured and the arms are protected at the sides of the trunk.

The bladder is catheterized and a urimeter attached beneath the head of the operating table.

Mechanical IPPV is continued with 67 per cent nitrous oxide and oxygen, to achieve an arterial $P\text{co}_2$ within the normal range. A variety of sophisticated ventilators [8] meet most of the essential and desirable features described by Loh [267]. Although simpler patient ventilators can be used for the majority of patients, the facilities for humidification, a wide range in inspiratory and expiratory times and the application of PEEP may not always be met.

Before the operation proceeds it is again necessary to check the performance of ventilator, humidifier and ventilator alarms, with the patient now attached. It is also the moment to be sure that intravenous drips, central venous catheters and arterial cannula are functioning satisfactorily.

Before Bypass

Nitrous oxide analgesia is supplemented with incremental doses of phenoperidine 1–2 mg to a total of 2–10 mg except in the most fragile patients. Fentanyl has been used when it was anticipated that patients would be sufficiently stable soon after a short operation, to be extubated. This group included many children and young adults with relatively uncomplicated congenital heart disease. The recent evidence that equianalgesic doses of phenoperidine and fentanyl have the same duration of action [199, 358] suggests that such a policy is unnecessary.

Pancuronium is given in 2 mg increments in adults if required, but is not usually needed before bypass. For adults pancuronium 4 mg and phenoperidine 2 mg are added to the oxygenator prime.

Droperidol is given in increments to a total of 20 mg to control a systolic blood pressure in excess of 140 mmHg. This is followed if necessary by pentolinium in 0·5 mg increments in a solution containing 1 mg/ml. Halothane may also be used to provide additional flexibility of control. Uncommonly, blood volume expansion or catecholamine support is required before bypass. Manipulation of the heart is most likely to produce transient hypotension or arrhythmias. Serious haemorrhage is possible when the sternum is opened in patients who have had previous heart surgery. All preparations are therefore made for this eventuality.

Blood samples are taken for clotting control and for blood gas, acid–base, PCV and serum electrolyte estimations. The blood sugar is also measured in neonates and in particularly ill children and adults.

The St Thomas's Hospital Cardioplegia Injection 20 ml is added to 1 l of Ringer's solution. This infusate is kept in melting ice in the operating room until required together with 1 l bags of Hartmann's solution. Drip extension tubing is passed from the table and connected to drip sets in the suspended Ringer's and Hartmann's solutions. The bag of cardioplegia solution is pressurized, using a pressure infusor, after air has been flushed from the system.

Heparin is given in a dose of 90 mg/m^2, into the central venous catheter, after confirming the correct catheter position. A half dose of heparin is given at 1 hr, and one-fourth of the initial dose at each following hour until bypass is terminated.

Bypass

Nitrous oxide is discontinued as bypass commences, and the oxygen monitor turned off. Urine volume is noted at this time. The venous pressure should fall while the arterial pressure trend is noted. There should be no movement of the diaphragm.

CPB is described as total when the superior and inferior venae cavae are snared, when ventricular fibrillation occurs while on bypass, or when the aorta is cross-clamped. In the first instance coronary sinus blood or shunted blood may still be traversing the lungs, but nevertheless at this stage mechanical ventilation is discontinued. It is customary to give a low flow of oxygen through the manual circuit with escape via a spill valve. Recent evidence suggests that there may be no advantage over allowing the lungs to collapse [399].

Cardioplegia solution is now given through a cannula or catheter inserted into the ascending aorta proximal to a clamp, or in the presence of aortic regurgitation, through separate coronary cannulas after the aorta has been cross-clamped and opened. The solution is delivered over a

3–5 min period, and care is taken that the cannula does not trip or damage the aortic valve. There have been some comments that excess pressure in the proximal aorta during infusion might contribute to subsequent myocardial oedema, and therefore monitoring of this pressure has been proposed [140]. The possibility of bubbles evolving in the cold solution as it perfuses the warm heart may not be unimportant. It is conceivable that bubbles in the coronary circulation at this stage could cause uneven distribution of the cardioplegia solution.

In adults, the infusate returns to the oxygenator after emerging from the coronary sinus. This addition to the total perfusate includes potassium and magnesium, and will reduce the PCV somewhat. If the cavae have been snared, the right atrium is opened before the cardioplegic solution is given, to prevent distension of the heart. In infants and children the solution is always discarded in this way.

During the period of hypothermic cardioplegic arrest, cold Hartmann's solution is trickled into the pericardial cavity so that the heart lies in a cold pool. This solution when aspirated is discarded, and not returned to the oxygenator.

Pancuronium 2 mg and phenoperidine 2 mg are given to adult patients after each 1 hr of bypass. Thiopentone, Althesin, and other intravenous induction agents or volatile anaesthetics have been employed, to avoid the real risk of awareness during bypass [46]. If the mean arterial pressure exceeds 90 mmHg, an additional 2 mg of phenoperidine may be given, followed by increments of droperidol. A high arterial pressure despite these measures is unusual. It could be caused by the position of the aorta cannula in relation to the left subclavian artery. If it is not due to this or other mechanical causes and is not relieved by increased analgesia and modest alpha-blockade, the flow from the heart–lung machine may be reduced somewhat.

A low mean radial artery pressure during bypass may also be caused by mechanical factors, or by a low systemic resistance if the usual pump output of $2{\cdot}4\ l/m^2$ has been achieved. An increased flow from the pump after the addition of more fluid to the oxygenator will increase the pressure when the resistance is low. Although central nervous system dysfunction has been attributed to hypotension during bypass [430], we rely on increasing the flow rate rather than giving peripheral vasoconstrictors in this event. The effect of hypotension on coronary flow during bypass in dogs was investigated by Simmonds [417]. He found that subendocardial perfusion improved when methoxamine, an alpha-adrenergic agonist, was given.This has no relevance during cardioplegic myocardial preservation.

Blood samples from the oxygenator are analysed half-hourly for blood gases, acid–base balance, PCV and serum potassium. Potassium chloride 1 g is added to the perfusate if the serum level is less than 4·5 mM/l. Urine output usually exceeds a rate of 0·5–1 ml kg^{-1} hr^{-1}, but is encouraged with 10–20 mg frusemide if it is less than optimal after 30 min of bypass. In anticipation of the post-bypass phase, 2 units of fresh frozen plasma are thawed for use in adults and 1 unit for children.

Gentle manual ventilation with oxygen is recommenced when the final heart cavity (e.g. aorta, right ventricle, or right atrium) is nearly closed, or when weaning from CPB commences. Mechanical ventilation is then continued. It is possible to overlook the need for IPPV at this stage and a special effort needs to be made to avoid this elementary and dangerous omission. At this point various surgical manoeuvres are carried out to remove air from the left side of the heart and aorta, to avoid right coronary artery or cerebral air emboli particularly [421]. An effective heart beat may not be restored immediately without the need to defibrillate the heart, or cardiovert it from an unacceptable atrial or nodal rhythm. Electrical defibrillation is usually effective provided that the heart has rewarmed, acid–base and potassium levels are normal, myocardial preservation has been adequate and coronary perfusion has been effectively restored. If defibrillation is not achieved and these factors have been corrected, the anaesthetist's contribution to the problem usually entails the administration of lignocaine 1 mg/kg intravenously, or if this is ineffective, disopyramide 1 mg/kg given slowly. In the presence of a slow heart rate appropriate management may include ventricular or atrial pacing, or the use of chronotropic drugs.

The restoration of an effective filling pressure is guided by the central venous or left atrial pressures, as the venous drainage from the patient is gradually reduced and the perfusion from the heart–lung machine to the patient diminished. When the venous line is finally clamped, a single 10 ml bolus of 10 per cent calcium gluconate is given if the systolic blood pressure is barely approaching 90–100 mmHg. If the venous pressures are high, blood pressure low and heart contractility sluggish, an appropriate catecholamine is administered during weaning from bypass, and continued afterwards if necessary. The need for mechanical circulatory support, or further surgery, is usually evident within minutes.

After Bypass

Mechanical ventilation is continued. Fifty per cent nitrous oxide is added after 5 min if the cardiovascular performance seems adequate and there is no clinical evidence suggesting that an air embolus has occurred. Nitrous oxide can usually be increased to 60 per cent subsequently without detriment to the cardiovascular system.

An appropriate filling pressure is maintained by transfusion from the oxygenator initially, followed by fresh frozen plasma and blood. Kaplan [229] concluded from clotting studies alone that the routine use of fresh frozen plasma and platelets in cardiac surgery was not justified. However, we still administer fresh frozen plasma on the assumption that additional labile clotting factors will be beneficial, that the plasma oncotic pressure may be reduced, and as an alternative volume expander to blood at this stage. The blood is ACD- or CPD-preserved. Because it is less than 4 days old and is rarely given in large quantities, it is not generally administered through a 20–40 μm filter. Blood filters have been evaluated by Cullen [92] and Marshall [292, 293] and their use reviewed by Walker [443]. We have not found a practical application of the various Cell Saver or auto-transfusion systems as yet. Several methods of obtaining fresh autologous blood so that it may be given after bypass have been described [173, 255]. Pliam [336] and Sherman [389] did not find that bank-blood requirements were reduced by giving autologous blood. Our blood usage in 100 consecutive patients is shown in *Fig. 4.4*. This compares with 2·6

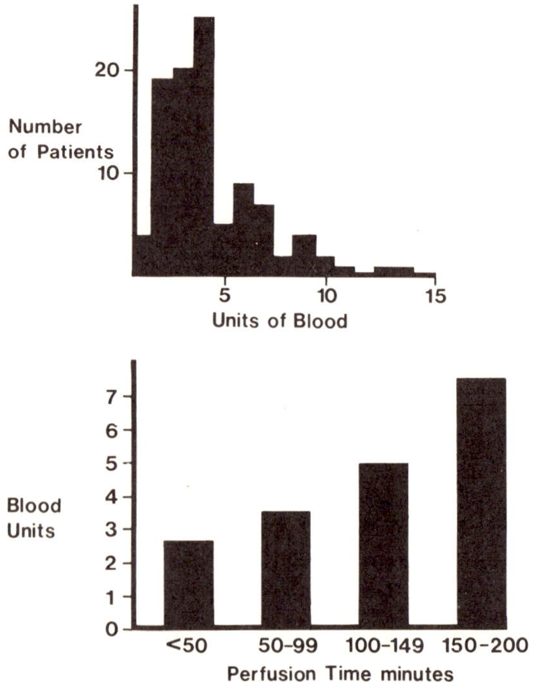

Fig. 4.4. Total blood usage in 100 consecutive adult patients undergoing cardio-pulmonary bypass in the Wessex Unit. The majority of patients require 2–4 units of blood. Blood usage increased with perfusion time.

units/patient reported by Tector [423] and 4·8 units/patient by Cohn [83] using autologous transfusion.

Protamine administration, to reverse the effects of heparin, is commenced when venous and arterial perfusion cannulas are removed. Protamine 2 mg for each mg of heparin the patient received before bypass is given over a period of 15 min. Myocardial depression due to protamine

[291] may require volume and catecholamine support, and a reduction in the rate of protamine administration. About 15 min after protamine has been given, blood samples are taken for a thrombin time, blood gas, acid–base and serum potassium estimations.

Although fibrinolysis is usual during open heart surgery [168], we do not routinely employ aminocaproic acid or tranexamic acid to inhibit plasminogen activator activity, or Trasylol (aprotinin), an antiplasmin. McClure [275] has suggested that aminocaproic acid should be considered for use in patients with cyanotic congenital heart disease who are expected to have a long period of CPB. He administered 75 mg of epsilon-amino-caproic acid per kg in the first hour, and 15 mg kg^{-1} hr^{-1} for 24 hr in this group of patients. The corresponding dose of tranexamic acid would be 15 mg/kg every 6–8 hr.

If bleeding is more than expected it is necessary to consider giving additional protamine, more fresh frozen plasma, and ensuring a continuing supply of blood, preferably fresh. It is customary to carry out a platelet count and give a platelet transfusion if indicated. Heavy bleeding entails the exercise of all the accepted practices for the management of massive transfusions [305]. The Gorman Rupp blood warmer is a particularly convenient piece of equipment. It has a bubble trap, so does not require the additional microfilter suggested for this purpose by Watson [448]. The proposal to increase the temperature of blood warmers to 46 °C is based on tenuous evidence [436]. It may occasionally be necessary to re-establish CPB to control severe haemorrhage from some inaccessible site, or because of acute severe heart failure. The patient must be given a standard dose of heparin again. It is prudent to repeat the thrombin time, to confirm the incoagubility of the perfusate.

The control of ventricular ectopic beats after bypass commonly entails the administration of potassium and occasionally lignocaine or disopyramide. One gram of potassium chloride is given over 10 min in adults, if the serum potassium is found to be less than 4·5 mM/l.

Dexamethasone 8 mg intravenously is still given in the operating room or recovery room if an episode occurs which may be responsible for a period of persistent cerebral hypoxia or ischaemia. The rationale for this is based on the presumption that the ensuing brain oedema will be reduced by steroids [149]. Experimentally this steroid effect has been shown to be better with pretreatment in doses of dexamethasone of 1 mg/kg initially and 1 mg/kg every 6 hr [237]. Reulen [356] has reviewed the formation of vasogenic brain oedema and the merits of steroids, hyperventilation and diuretic agents.

Profound Hypothermia Technique in Infants

Anaesthesia for infants weighing less than 10 kg, using the Kyoto technique of surface cooling, followed by extracorporeal cooling, differs in some details from the general approach in children and adults.

Premedication may consist of atropine alone.

Drugs are prepared for anaesthesia and resuscitation (Table 4.5) and the ECG is attached to the patient.

Anaesthetic induction is by nitrous oxide and oxygen with a low percentage of halothane.

Orotracheal intubation is carried out following the administration of pancuronium, when halothane is discontinued.

Anaesthesia is maintained with nitrous oxide and oxygen.

Carbon dioxide 2–5 per cent is added when the nasopharyngeal temperature reaches 30 °C, when nitrous oxide is discontinued.

Although a high arterial Po_2 is desirable because of the increased oxygen reserve when the circulation is arrested, its adverse effects could have clinical consequences. Betts [44] has found that there is a danger of retrolental fibroplasia if the arterial Po_2 exceeds 13 kPa for more than 2 hr in premature infants weighing less than 2·5 kg or of less than 38 weeks maturity.

Droperidol may be given to promote vasodilatation.

Venous and arterial cannulas are inserted after induction of anaesthesia, to monitor central venous and arterial pressures, and to provide an infusion line. Thermometers are placed in oesophagus and nose, and the bladder is catheterized. As soon as the patient has been anaesthetized, he is cooled by a circulating blanket beneath him, using a Gorman Rupp Aquamatic K thermia. When the intravascular cannulas have been placed, crushed ice in small plastic bags is packed around the patient's trunk, limbs and head, avoiding the genital area. A further circulating blanket is then placed on top of the patient and the whole enclosed in a space blanket, eliminating as much air space as possible. Cooling proceeds rapidly. It is a simple matter to plot the patient's temperature at 10 min intervals to project it to the estimated time of the target temperature, since the rate of cooling is almost uniform (*Fig. 4.5*). It is necessary to ensure complete paralysis and vasodilàtation to promote cooling. Neonates are surface cooled to an oesophageal temperature of 25 °C while surgery in older children usually commences at 26 °C. Ice bags are removed at a temperature 1–2 °C higher than the target but cooling from the underblanket continues as the patient is prepared for bypass.

Blood samples are taken during cooling, for clotting control, blood gas and acid–base balance, serum potassium and blood glucose levels.

If the venous pressure is low or blood pressure falls during cooling, Hartmann's solution 5–10 ml/kg is infused, but no other cardiovascular support is given. The slower sinus rhythm seen below 30 °C is not treated. Glucose is routinely given after anaesthetic induction, as 2·5 ml/kg of a 20 per cent solution. The patient is heparinized with 3 mg/kg.

Some features of perfusion are relevant to the anaesthetist. One litre of fresh heparinized blood is used to prime the heart–lung machine, and usually requires the addition of sodium bicarbonate 10 mM.

A base deficit, a plasma potassium of less than 4 mM/l or plasma glucose of less than 10 mM/l in the priming fluid are corrected.

The patient is perfused at a rate of 100 ml/kg for 5–10 min to complete the cooling process. A high oxygen reserve at this time is desirable. However, a high Po_2 in the oxygenator blood could theoretically be harmful because of its toxic effects and the possibility of bubble formation as the blood warms towards the patient's temperature. At a nasopharyngeal temperature of 18–20 °C the perfusion is stopped and blood drained into the oxygenator.

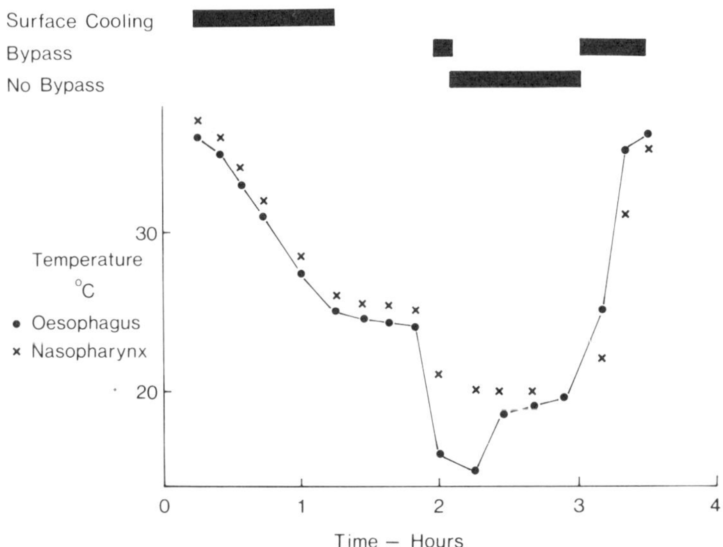

Fig. 4.5. Temperature changes in a 5 kg infant undergoing total correction of Fallot's tetralogy, using the Kyoto profound hypothermia technique. The duration of bypass is short. The period of no circulation is less than 1 hr, at a nasopharyngeal temperature of 20 °C.

After the cardiac correction, rewarming is not commenced as soon as bypass is re-established, but only when the tissue oxygen debt has been made good. Rewarming is then achieved with bypass and a circulating blanket at a rate of 1 °C/min.

Blood gas analysis when the temperature reaches 30 °C does not usually show an important non-respiratory acidaemia. If it does, sodium bicarbonate is given. Perfusion is terminated in the normal manner.

After bypass, filling pressures of the ventricles are sustained with fresh frozen plasma, 10–20 ml/kg, platelet concentrates 5–10 ml/kg and packed red cells. Supporting drugs, most commonly calcium, dopamine and frusemide, are given as indicated.

Transfer to Recovery Room

A nasogastric tube is passed, before leaving the operating room. The transfer of patients to the recovery room or intensive care unit entails the disconnection from monitoring and ventilator equipment. If the distance from operating room to recovery room is not very short, it is necessary to provide ECG and pressure monitoring, and resuscitation apparatus *en route*. Continued controlled ventilation can be provided in various ways, the simplest being the use of oxygen with a reservoir bag and valve mount.

POSTOPERATIVE CARE

A survey of anaesthesia for cardiac surgery cannot be complete without some comments about postoperative patient care. Although the role of the anaesthetist undoubtedly varies according to local custom, it is probable that in almost all units he will take some part in postoperative respiratory management. In addition he may have an involvement, or at least an interest in the closely related state of the heart and circulation. He may contribute to fluid and electrolyte management and surveillance of the nutritional status of the patient. There may of course be other immediate postoperative problems of kidney or liver dysfunction, cerebral damage or infections.

The instrumentation of the postoperative intensive care area may be sophisticated, with computerized programmes of care [361] and some degree of automation regarding cardiovascular support or respiratory monitoring [432]. In simpler terms, written protocols of management for the various systems of the body are often available to provide the safe routine care of cardiac patients postoperatively. The same principles of staffing, facilities and coordination apply to this area as to any general intensive care unit, with the focus more particularly on the heart and circulation.

Cardiovascular Monitoring and Support

Cardiovascular monitoring and support in the Recovery Room follow well-established methods [316], some principles of which have already been outlined. The main circulatory problems are a low cardiac output, hypotension or hypertension, arrhythmias or conduction defects, continued bleeding and cardiac tamponade. Maintenance of suitable right and left atrial pressures, with the use of drugs to increase myocardial contractility, alter vascular resistance and control arrhythmias are the mainstays of treatment. Hypertension is not uncommon during emergence from anaesthesia and is treated by relief from pain and ventricular load reduction. Hypertension beyond the first few hours may require such drugs as methyldopa, hydrallazine, or beta-blockers. Bleeding due to coagulation defects or surgical causes can be a problem. In the absence of abnormal coagulation, re-exploration of the chest may be required. The development of cardiac tamponade can be an early or late complication, and can present an anaesthetic challenge.

Controlled Ventilation

Controlled ventilation is frequently continued into the immediate postoperative period, except in the least complicated and shortest open heart procedures. The incidence of continued IPPV postoperatively has been variously reported as 100 per cent [163, 296], 40 per cent [420], and 0 per cent [184] for periods of 4–48 hr. To some extent the need for IPPV is related to the anaesthetic technique. The respiratory depression associated with profound morphine narcosis persisted for many hours postoperatively, while the effect of fentanyl appeared to be shorter [366]. There is no place for the use of doxapram or naloxone to shorten the period of narcotic respiratory depression, due to their adverse haemodynamic effects [101, 141]. When a ketamine drip was used in the place of narcotics or volatile anaesthetics, postoperative IPPV was not required in a reported series of 200 patients [184].

The advantages of continuing IPPV after open heart surgery include the elimination of residual anaesthesia before the resumption of spontaneous respiration, a safe airway and appropriate control of arterial blood gases. The patient can be given complete relief from pain, he can rest and can be given periodic deep breaths. If he has not completely rewarmed in the operating room, this can be achieved in the presence of residual anaesthesia, without shivering and an increase in oxygen consumption and cardiac output [35]. The work of spontaneous breathing, increased after cardiac surgery [465] can be eliminated. If the patient is in a low cardiac output state due to myocardial failure, a reduction in ventricular filling pressure caused by the raised intrathoracic pressure of IPPV can be beneficial [84]. If circulatory problems arise, there are no delays in re-establishing an airway and controlled ventilation.

The disadvantages of continuing IPPV include the possible need for more staff and equipment. There are many recognized dangers of mechanically ventilating patients, not the least of which are accidental disconnection from the machine or displacement and obstruction of the airway. Larger quantities of drugs may be given to control spontaneous respiration and toleration of the endotracheal tube. There is a possibility of producing hypocapnia, alkalaemia and a fall in serum potassium, with its attendant risk of ventricular arrhythmias in the presence of digitalis. The haemodynamic effects of IPPV and hypocapnia could adversely affect cardiac output and tissue perfusion [16, 189]. The fact that pulmonary vascular resistance is increased may be particularly relevant following the Fontan procedure [77].

After surgery, IPPV may be terminated in the operating room, within a few hours or after elective ventilation overnight. Occasionally it is necessary to continue IPPV for an extended period due to functional considerations of the cardiovascular, respiratory or renal systems. In the Wessex Unit it is our usual policy to omit the reversal of non-depolarizing relaxants at the end of surgery, and to leave the oroendotracheal tube in place. Some centres prefer to replace it in infants and children by a nasotracheal tube at this stage [32], but unless it is very evident that infants especially will require IPPV for more than 24 hr, this is not our practice. The patient is therefore manually ventilated while being taken to the recovery room, with a secure airway and ventilation, and time is not spent unnecessarily in the operating room to establish safe spontaneous respiration. The majority of children, and many adults, including those undergoing coronary artery bypass grafts, single and double valve replacements can now be extubated on the day of operation.

Ventilation is controlled in this Unit using a Manley Pulmovent for adults and for children over 10 kg. A Baby Bird is used for patients who are smaller than this. Milner [308] has reviewed a number of ventilators suitable for infants. The initial ventilator settings are based on the post-perfusion variables, which usually include a large tidal volume and low respiratory rate [464] and postperfusion blood gas analysis. They are subsequently adjusted to provide an arterial $P\text{o}_2$ of 10–15 kPa and $P\text{co}_2$ of 4·5–5·5 kPa if possible. Auscultation of the chest and a chest X-ray at this stage are necessary to confirm air entry into both lungs. An unexpected pneumothorax or haemothorax will thus be detected. The precise position of the endotracheal tube will also be confirmed and the venous catheters and nasogastric tube identified on X-ray.

Positive-end Expiratory Pressure

PEEP is rarely applied to adults in this Unit since an arterial $S\text{o}_2$ of 85–90 per cent can almost always be achieved in our experience with a $FI\text{o}_2$ of 0·5 or less. There is also a reluctance to use it routinely after cardiac surgery in young children as in other centres [335]. Whether it is preferable to increase $FI\text{o}_2$ to 0·4–0·5 rather than increasing functional residual capacity (FRC) by the application of PEEP is as yet undecided. More consideration would be given to the application of PEEP if a high $FI\text{o}_2$ was required for more than 24 hr to prevent undue hypoxaemia. PEEP may decrease or increase cardiac output, as well as increase arterial $P\text{o}_2$ [84]. Clearly the best PEEP should not merely increase arterial $P\text{o}_2$ but should contribute towards oxygen flux. Best PEEP in patients with acute respiratory failure coincided with the best lung and chest wall compliance [413], but this has not yet been confirmed after cardiac surgery. PEEP can readily be provided by a threshold resistor on the Pulmovent and similar ventilators.

Continuous Positive Airway Pressure

Continuous positive airway pressure (CPAP), which is applied during all phases of spontaneous respiration, is a useful manoeuvre when intubated patients are being weaned from IPPV [91]. It particularly prevents the otherwise inevitable reduction in FRC and fall in arterial Po_2 in patients with low pulmonary compliance [170, 183]. Its principal application after cardiac surgery seems to be in a minority of small children who require extended IPPV progressing to intermittent mandatory ventilation.

Intermittent Mandatory Ventilation
Intermittent mandatory ventilation (IMV) is an aid to weaning patients from ventilatory support [107]. It allows the patient to breath spontaneously while still being mechanically ventilated at a reduced rate. The need for drugs to diminish respiratory drive has been less since its introduction. The criteria for a ventilator circuit for IMV, and a simple modification of a Manley ventilator have now been published [252]. The application of CPAP to an IMV circuit of this type requires important further modifications. For the majority of those patients in the Wessex Unit who are ventilated overnight, termination of IPPV has not been a problem. The IMV facility is simply included in the circuit to diminish the need for respiratory depressants.

Patient Control During IPPV
Initially residual anaesthetic effects enable many patients to tolerate an endotracheal tube and controlled ventilation. Subsequently drugs with respiratory depressant, sedative and analgesic properties are required, in preference to muscle relaxants. The drugs commonly used in this Unit are papaveretum 1–2·5 mg increments and diazepam 2·5 mg increments, in adults given intravenously. Most of the non-volatile anaesthetic agents already described have also been used for the same purpose. Nitrous oxide was originally employed in this way for tetanus management but its dangers over a prolonged period were soon evident. Its use in some cardiac units has no doubt now been reconsidered in view of the known effects after only a few hours [15]. Any drugs with a significant depressant effect on the cardiovascular system are obviously best avoided when selecting the means of settling patients on ventilators. A prolonged action is also undesirable so that the use of lorazepam would seem to be limited. Even repeated doses of diazepam may cause undue drowsiness.

Termination of Controlled Ventilation
Termination of controlled ventilation after cardiac surgery is undertaken according to a number of criteria [207]. Thus the cardiovascular system should be secure, with a mean arterial pressure of 70 mmHg, left atrial pressure less than 20 mmHg and stable heart rate and rhythm. There should be minimal bleeding, the extremities should be warm and well perfused, and urine output should be 0·5–1 ml kg^{-1} hr^{-1}. The patient may still at this stage require a little catecholamine support and assistance from the IABP device. These do not contraindicate the discontinuation of IPPV,

provided that the various criteria have been met. If the cardiovascular system is not secure, discontinuation of IPPV may result not in an increase in oxygen transport [21], but in an exacerbation of left or right heart failure and a paradoxical decrease in cardiac output [36]. This may be due to a redistribution of blood volume as the mean intrathoracic pressure falls [157, 429] causing an increase in ventricular preload and afterload, both detrimental to the failing heart. There is a danger of pulmonary congestion [244] with its clinical signs and deteriorating blood gas exchange. Right heart failure may not be so evident but should be suspected if there is increasing agitation, restlessness or arrhythmias [249].

In the respiratory system there should be few wheezes and crackles on auscultation of the lungs, arterial Po_2 should be at least 8 kPa with an FIo_2 of 0·4, whilst the tidal volume and inflation pressure in relation to arterial Pco_2 should not be grossly abnormal. The problem of identifying respiratory variables during IPPV which relate to the patient's ability to breathe spontaneously and adequately has not been resolved. Delooz [98] found that successful spontaneous breathing was characterized by an increase in cardiac output, arterial pressure and mixed venous Po_2. The group unable to tolerate prolonged voluntary ventilation showed no change in oxygen availability. Hilberman [192] examined more than 50 potential predictors of postoperative respiratory inadequacy. A vital capacity of more than 15 ml/kg or maximum inspiratory force of more than 28 cm water were the most useful prognostic measurements that spontaneous breathing would be adequate. Blood gas analysis and passive pulmonary mechanics were poor predictors.

Acute renal failure may be a reason for delaying extubation. Respiratory insufficiency related to renal failure is due to a variety of causes [394] including effusions, pulmonary infection, water and salt overload, and peritoneal dialysis.

Finally, when termination of ventilation is considered, the patient should have no residual effects of muscle relaxants, and should not have received recent heavy sedation. He should be alert and cooperative with no gross neurological deficit.

There is no need to wean patients gradually from IPPV if the various criteria are met within 24 hr. Only when patients have been ventilated beyond this period does it seem necessary sometimes to hesitate to remove the endotracheal tube. If in doubt it seems wise to leave the tube, and occasionally a trial of spontaneous respiration through it will resolve the situation. This may not be easily tolerated especially by adults. It may then be preferable to remove the tube and reintubate within a few hours if necessary.

Following Extubation

Following extubation careful continuing clinical observation, cardiovascular assessment and blood gas analysis are required. Patients are most comfortable in a head-up position, which has been found to neither decrease cardiac output, nor improve oxygenation [348]. A further period of IPPV may sometimes be needed if there is serious right or left heart failure, or further complications of the cardiovascular, respiratory or central nervous systems. Blood gas analysis may be misleadingly normal when the signs of respiratory distress are present and IPPV is indicated [156]. Gilston has devised a clinical scoring system for adult respiratory distress. A tick chart is in use in the Wessex Unit to observe infants and children after extubation (Table 4.6).

Table 4.6. A Tick Chart as an Aid to the Assessment of Infants Following Heart Surgery, When Breathing Spontaneously. The Observations are Made Every 15 Min

Spontaneous respiration	*Time*
Expiratory grunting	
Flared nostrils	
Subcostal retraction	
Respiratory rate	
Anxious	
Restless	
Drowsy	
Limp limbs	
Cold periphery	
Cyanosis	
Urine volume	

Oxygen Therapy and Physiotherapy

Oxygen therapy and physiotherapy are applied after extubation when the problems of lung collapse, pulmonary congestion and pulmonary oedema commonly arise [132]. The objectives are maintenance of arterial Po_2 and So_2 at a safe level, proper expansion of the lungs and encouragement to cough.

In general, adults and children in this Unit receive 40 per cent oxygen through a venturi nebulizer and facemask at an oxygen flow of more than 6 l/min. If the arterial Po_2 exceeds 10 kPa oxygen is discontinued. An arterial Po_2 exceeding 8 kPa or saturation of 90 per cent breathing air, is accepted. Occasionally arterial Po_2 of 7–8 kPa is well tolerated by patients who are alert, active and taking normal meals, and does not appear to be detrimental. A lower Po_2 is inevitable in some infants undergoing palliative shunts. The infrequent patient suffering from chronic respiratory disease and a raised preoperative arterial Pco_2 is given oxygen by 24 per cent or 28 per cent Ventimask, and a Po_2 below 8 kPa may also be accepted. It has not been found necessary to vary FIo_2 widely in an attempt to produce an optimum $Pa,_{O_2}$ within a narrow range [41] but the isoshunt diagram can be useful to quantify respiratory progress.

A headbox is used for babies after extubation. This is provided with 40 per cent oxygen from a venturi nebulizer. Additional humidity is added from an ultrasonic nebulizer if the endotracheal tube has been in place for some time. The danger of excess water intake with this type of humidification [167] has not been apparent. This is probably related to the fact that insensible water loss is increased in infants nursed under an overhead radiant heat shield [459, 461]. In addition urine osmolality is routinely monitored as one guide to fluid balance and administration [87, 227].

Pain Relief

Pain relief postoperatively while the patient continues to be mechanically ventilated, presents no problem. Complete relief as well as amnesia can be achieved with small intravenous doses of narcotics and diazepam, in addition to residual anaesthetic agents, without detriment to the cardiovascular system. Relief of pain when the patient is breathing unassisted may not always get the attention it deserves [105]. The plethora of new analgesics over the last 20 years is a reminder that the right drug has still not been found [119]. The transition from parenteral to oral analgesics may be difficult to bridge. An effervescent tablet of soluble aspirin 500 mg with papaveretum 10 mg has been commended, giving 1–2 tablets every 4–6 hr in adults [118]. A confident and caring medical and nursing staff contribute a great deal to the relief of the anxieties, aches and pains soon after cardiac surgery.

Fluids and Electrolytes

Various methods for prescribing water and electrolyte intake are based on the patients' surface area or weight. Using surface area, a total of 750 ml/m^2 on day 0, 1000 ml/m^2 on day 1 and 1250 ml/m^2 on day 3 is commonly given. On a weight basis, patients in the Wessex Unit are prescribed 3 ml kg^{-1} hr^{-1} if less than 20 kg, 2 ml kg^{-1} hr^{-1} if 20–30 kg and 1 ml kg^{-1} hr^{-1} if more than 30 kg, by all routes. This volume may be varied especially in infants, or in adults after the immediate postoperative period according to frequent assessment. An account is always taken of fluid intake in the operating room, urine output, temperature, the effects of added humidification and radiant heater, as well as laboratory investigations. Patients over 10 kg receive a solution of 4 per cent dextrose in one-fifth normal saline. Babies of 10 kg or less receive 10 per cent dextrose to which 1 g sodium chloride is added to 500 ml. In this latter group, the flushing fluid of the arterial and venous cannulas by an Intraflo [391] amounts to 6 ml/hr. This is a considerable proportion of total intake, so that 10 per cent dextrose with added sodium is also used. Additional intravenous glucose may be required if regular blood sugar estimates fall below about 2 mM/l.

As nasogastric or oral feeds are introduced, intravenous glucose is gradually reduced.

Potassium Chloride

Potassium chloride 1 g in 500 ml is added to the intravenous water and electrolyte solution, unless the serum potassium exceeds 5 mM/l. Potassium chloride is also administered into the 30 ml reservoir chamber of a central venous drip, or as a bolus over 15–30 min, if the serum potassium is less than 4·5 mM/l adults or less than 4 mM/l in children. Thirteen mM of potassium chloride is given to adults, and 0·2 mM/kg to children. The serum potassium is then estimated and the dose repeated if indicated.

Calcium

Calcium may sporadically be administered as a bolus for its inotropic action in children and adults. In infants it is given in 1 hourly increments as 10 per cent calcium gluconate (0·1 ml/kg) unless intravenous nutrition has been established, when it is included in the infusion.

Magnesium

Magnesium administration as a routine after open heart surgery has been described. It has been regarded as the treatment of choice for neonatal tetany [431] and may therefore have a place in the management of infants with congenital heart disease in the first few days of life. The dose suggested is 0·2 ml/kg intramuscularly of a 50 per cent solution of magnesium sulphate. Magnesium is only given regularly to patients in the Wessex Unit when parenteral nutrition has been instituted.

Renal Insufficiency

Renal insufficiency in the postoperative period, as a result of surgery, has a variable incidence depending to some extent on the assiduity of the investigator [4]. Oliguria may occur during or following surgery, it may be delayed for 12–24 hr, or may develop subsequently. It may proceed to a polyuric phase within one or two days, or may persist and require continued management for days or weeks. Renal insufficiency may, however only be manifest as a polyuria with poor renal concentration and a serum creatinine exceeding 140 μg/l. The management of renal failure requires its early recognition, and consideration of the heterogeneous factors influencing its development as well as treatment of incipient and established ARF [256]. Chesney [75] has summarized its management in infants after cardiac surgery.

The effect of diuretics on central haemodynamics and renal function has been investigated in non-cardiac patients undergoing abdominal surgery [216, 217]. Frusemide decreased cardiac output, increased systemic vascular resistance and decreased glomerular filtration rate.

Mannitol increased cardiac output, decreased systemic vascular resistance and maintained glomerular filtration rate. It was concluded that in patients without increased preload or left ventricular insufficiency mannitol would be the diuretic of choice in the treatment of postoperative oliguria.

Liver Failure

Liver failure is now a rare event following heart surgery, but preoperative liver dysfunction may worsen postoperatively [321]. The management of liver failure follows conventional lines [446] and like renal failure, requires some modification of the nutritional regime.

Neurological Problems

Neurological problems after cardiac surgery may be related to preoperative disease and deficits, operative events, particularly emboli and reduced cerebral perfusion, and postoperative complications relating to a low cardiac output or prosthetic valves. Evidence of brain damage may not be immediate. Brunberg [60] has described a delayed onset as a complication of deep hypothermia with total circulatory arrest. The anaesthetist's contribution to the management of the brain-damaged patient includes prompt recognition and treatment of cerebral oedema, and proper care of the airway, ventilation and tracheobronchial secretions. It is helpful to ascertain that the patient is awake on return to the recovery room, and that he is able to move all limbs.

Gastrointestinal Bleeding

The minority of patients who are seriously ill after cardiac surgery are susceptible to the development of gastrointestinal bleeding as seen in many stress situations [121]. Antacids are frequently given in the hope that the occurrence of acute gastric erosions will be diminished. Some antacids contain a considerable amount of sodium, and if given 4-hourly could provide an intake in excess of 40 mM in 24 hr [30]. The substitution of cimetidine for some antacids may therefore be appropriate, and may reduce the incidence of gastrointestinal haemorrhage as it has done in fulminant hepatic failure [278]. The reduction of gastric acidity may not be beneficial however, since it may cause the stomach to become a reservoir of bacterial growth. This may be responsible for gastric erosions [58] and respiratory infection [22].

Nutrition

The nutrition of patients after cardiac surgery is deficient by Intensive Care standards [283, 442]. Preoperative malnutrition is associated with poorer surgical results but postoperative parenteral nutrition has not reversed this relationship [6]. Further studies are required [47]. On general principles it would seem reasonable to nourish patients after this major surgery if it can be achieved easily, safely and inexpensively.

It is uncommon for patients after heart surgery to be unable to accept an oral diet with oral supplements. Sometimes food must be given by the nasogastric route (Table 4.7) if the patient has an extended period of mechanical ventilation, or does not take food by mouth because of inanition or swallowing difficulties. The parenteral route is only indicated when there is failure of absorption by the gastrointestinal tract. The presence of artificial valves must increase the hazards of intravenous feeding and catheter sepsis. There is a natural reluctance to commence

Table 4.7. The Wessex Tube Feed for Nasogastric Administration. The Constituents Can be Varied According to Nutritional Assessment

Food	*Quantity*	*Calories*	*Nitrogen (g)*	*Sodium (mM)*	*Potassium (mM)*
Milk ml	1000	660	5·3	21	40
Eggs	3	330	4·5	10	7
Caloreen g	200	800			
Prosparol g	100	450			
Yoghourt ml	200	115	1·4	6	8
Potassium chloride g	2				26
Water as required					
Iron					
Vitamins					
Total		2355	11·2	37	81

intravenous nutrition early for this reason. Patients most likely to require this form of therapy also require mechanical ventilation, have an associated poor cardiovascular performance, are prone to sepsis, and may be suffering from cardiac cachexia. The food available by the various routes after cardiac surgery and in intensive therapy units has been described, together with associated metabolic problems [14, 284].

Even when patients are able to take food by mouth, they may take very little nourishment [283]. Therefore a supplement to the normal hospital diet may be helpful in achieving a desirable nutritional intake. Many formulations are available for nasogastric feeding from liquified hospital diets, feeds based on milk, eggs, caloreen and fat emulsions, convenience foods such as Clinifeed and Isocal to various elemental diets [200, 285]. The use of a small-bore tube [302] requires that feeds are homogeneous and fluid enough to be administered by drip feed.

There are many commercial intravenous sources of calories and nitrogen. Each preparation may have advantages and disadvantages. On the rare occasions when parenteral nutrition is required, the Wessex Unit relies on 20 per cent glucose, intralipid and vamin glucose, with additional vitamins (multivitamin infusion, or Solivito and Vitlipid) and minerals (Addam electrolyte solution or Ped-El and potassium phosphate). Ellis [125] has summarized the general management and prevention of hazards, and Baum [34] and Panter-Brick [329] have given practical guides for infant feeding.

Proper surveillance of food intake by the nasogastric or intravenous route, and measurement of nutritional states are no less important in cardiac patients than in the circumstances of general intensive care. The perils of parenteral nutrition are equally important and sinister after cardiac surgery. A strict routine of care of intravenous catheters dedicated to the infusion of nutriments is essential. Some hospitals have now instituted hyperalimentation units with especially trained nurses to rationalize the use of intravenous food and minimize the risks of infection [5].

REFERENCES

1. Abbott T. R. (1972) The use of glucagon following open heart surgery in children. *Br. J. Anaesth.* **44,** 854.
2. Abbott T. R. (1977) Oxygen uptake following deep hypothermia. *Anaesthesia* **32,** 524.
3. Abbott T. R., Rees G. J., Dickinson D. et al. (1978) Sodium nitroprusside in idiopathic respiratory distress syndrome. *Br. Med. J.* **1,** 1113.
4. Abel R. M., Buckley M. J., Austen W. G. et al. (1976) Acute postoperative renal failure in cardiac surgical patients. *J. Surg. Res.* **20,** 341.
5. Abel R. M., Fischer J. E., Buckley M. J. et al. (1974) Hyperalimentation in cardiac surgery. A review of sixty four patients. *J. Thorac. Cardiovasc. Surg.* **67,** 294.
6. Abel R. M., Fischer J. E., Buckley M. J. et al. (1976) Malnutrition in cardiac surgical patients. Results of a prospective randomized evaluation of early postoperative parenteral nutrition. *Arch. Surg.* **111,** 45.
7. Abele J. E. (1963) The physical background to freezing point osmometry and its medical–biological applications. *Am. J. Med. Electronics* **2,** 32.
8. Adams A. P. (1976) Anaesthetic ventilators and associated breathing circuits. *Br. J. Clin. Equip.* **1,** 133.
9. Adams A. P. and Pybus D. A. (1978) Delayed respiratory depression after use of fentanyl during anaesthesia. *Br. Med. J.* **1,** 278.
10. Adler D. and Bryan-Brown C. W. (1975) Use of the axillary artery for intravascular monitoring. *Crit. Care Med.* **1,** 148.
11. Alderman E. L., Barry W. H., Graham A. F. et al. (1972) Hemodynamic effects of morphine and pentazocine differ in cardiac patients. *N. Engl. J. Med.* **287,** 623.
12. Alderman E. L., Coltart D. J., Wettach G. E. et al. (1974) Coronary artery syndromes after sudden propranolol withdrawal. *Ann. Intern. Med.* **81,** 625.
13. Allen E. V. (1929) Thromboangiitis obliterans. Methods of diagnosis of chronic occlusive arterial disease lesions distal to the wrist with illustrative cases. *Am. J. Med. Sci.* **178,** 237.
14. Allison S. P. (1977) Metabolic aspects of intensive care. *Br. J. Anaesth.* **49,** 689.
15. Amess J. A. L., Rees G. M., Burman J. F. et al. (1978) Megaloblastic haemopoiesis in patients receiving nitrous oxide. *Lancet* **2,** 339.
16. Andersen M. N. and Kuchiba K. (1967) Depression of cardiac output with mechanical ventilation: comparative studies of intermittent positive, positive negative and assisted ventilation. *J. Thorac. Cardiovasc. Surg.* **54,** 182.
17. Annis J. T., Carlson D. A. and Simmons D. H. (1976) Scavenging system for the Harvey blood oxygenator. *Anesthesiology* **45,** 359.

18. Aps C., Bell J. A., Jenkins B. S. et al. (1976) Logical approach to lignocaine therapy. *Br. Med. J.* **1**, 13.
19. Arens J. F., Benbow B. P., Ochsner J. L. et al. (1972) Morphine anesthesia for aorto–coronary bypass procedures. *Anesth. Analg. (Cleve.)* **51**, 901.
20. Armstrong R. F., St. Andrew D., Cohen S. L. et al. (1978) Continuous monitoring of mixed venous oxygen tension (PVo_2) in cardiorespiratory disorders. *Lancet* **1**, 632.
21. Askitopoulou H., Sykes M. K. and Young C. (1978) Cardiorespiratory effects of increased airway pressure during controlled and spontaneous breathing after cardiac surgery. *Br. J. Anaesth.* **50**, 1203.
22. Atherton S. T. and White D. J. (1978) Stomach as source of bacteria colonising respiratory tract during artificial ventilation. *Lancet* **2**, 968.
23. Azzoli S. G., Shahinian T. K. and Cha Chung J. A. (1972) Correlation among mean central venous pressure, mean pulmonary wedge pressure and cardiac output after acute haemorrhage and replacement with Ringers lactate solution in the dog. *Am. J. Surg.* **123**, 385.
24. Babka R., Colby C., El-Etr A. et al. (1977) Monitoring of intraoperative heparinization and blood loss following cardiopulmonary bypass surgery. *J. Thorac. Cardiovasc. Surg.* **73**, 780.
25. Balchum O. J., Gensini G. and Blount S. G. J. (1957) The effect of hexamethonium upon the pulmonary vascular resistance in mitral stenosis. *J. Lab. Clin. Med.* **50**, 186.
26. Barash P. G., Glanz S., Katz J. D. et al. (1978) Ventricular function of children during halothane anesthesia. An echocardiographic evaluation. *Anesthesiology* **49**, 79.
27. Barnes R. W., Foster E. J. Janssen G. A. et al. (1976) Safety of brachial artery catheters as monitors in the intensive care unit – prospective evaluation with the Doppler ultrasonic velocity detector. *Anesthesiology* **44**, 260.
28. Barratt-Boyes B. G. (1976) The technique of intracardiac repair in infancy using deep hypothermia with circulatory arrest and limited cardiopulmonary bypass. In: Ionescu M. I. and Wooler G. H. (ed.), *Current Techniques in Extracorporeal Circulation.* London, Butterworth, p. 197.
29. Barrer M. J. and Ellison N. (1977) Platelet function. *Anesthesiology* **46**, 202.
30. Barry R. E. and Ford J. (1978) Sodium content and neutralising capacity of some commonly used antacids. *Br. Med. J.* **1**, 413.
31. Bartlett R. H. and Gazzaniga A. B. (1976) Physiology and pathophysiology of extracorporeal circulation. In: Ionescu M. I. and Wooler G. H. (ed.), *Current Techniques in Extracorporeal Circulation.* London, Butterworth, p. 7.
32. Battersby E. F., Hatch D. J. and Towey R. M. (1977) The effects of prolonged naso-endotracheal intubation in children. A study in infants and young children after cardiopulmonary bypass. *Anaesthesia* **32**, 154.
33. Baum D., Dillard D. H. and Porte D. (1968) Inhibition of insulin release in infants undergoing deep hypothermic cardiovascular surgery. *N. Engl. J. Med.* **279**, 1309.
34. Baum J. D., Aynsley-Green A., Brown R. et al. (1974) Total intravenous feeding for infants and children. *Clin. Trials J.* (Suppl. 1), 140.
35. Bay J., Nunn J. F. and Prys-Roberts C. (1968) Factors influencing arterial Po_2 during recovery from anaesthesia. *Br. J. Anaesth.* **40**, 398.
36. Beach T., Millen E. and Grenvik A. (1973) Hemodynamic response to discontinuance of mechanical ventilation. *Crit. Care Med.* **1**, 85.
37. Beattie H. W., Evans G., Garnett E. S. et al. (1972) Sustained hypovolaemia and extracellular fluid volume expansion following cardiopulmonary bypass. *Surgery* **71**, 891.
38. Becker R. M., Smith M. R. and Dobel A. R. C. (1974) Effect of platelet inhibition on platelet phenomena in cardiopulmonary bypass in pigs. *Ann. Surg.* **179**, 52.

39. Bedford R. F. (1977) Radial artery function following percutaneous cannulation with 18 and 20 gauge catheters. *Anesthesiology* **47**, 37.
40. Bell H., Stubbs D. and Pugh D. (1971) Reliability of central venous pressure as an indicator of left atrial pressure. *Chest* **59**, 169.
41. Benatar S. R., Hewlett A. M. and Nunn J. F. (1973) The use of isoshunt lines for control of oxygen therapy. *Br. J. Anaesth.* **45**, 711.
42. Bennett E. J. and Dalal F. Y. (1974) Hypotensive anaesthesia for coarctation. A method of prevention of postoperative hypertension. *Anaesthesia* **29**, 269.
43. Bennett G. M., Loeser E. A. and Stanley T. H. (1977) Cardiovascular effects of scopolamine during morphine–oxygen and morphine–nitrous oxide–oxygen anesthesia in man. *Anesthesiology* **46**, 225.
44. Betts E. K., Downes J. J., Schaffer D. B. et al. (1977) Retrolental fibroplasia and oxygen administration during general anaesthesia. *Anesthesiology* **47**, 518.
45. Bevan D. R. (1978) Osmometry: 3. Clinical applications. *Anaesthesia* **33**, 809.
46. Blacher R. S. (1975) On awakening paralyzed during surgery: a syndrome of traumatic neurosis. *JAMA* **234**, 67.
47. Blackburn G. L., Gibbons G. W., Bothe A. et al. (1977) Nutritional support in cardiac cachexia. *J. Thorac. Cardiovasc. Surg.* **73**, 489.
48. Blackburn J. P. (1978) What is new in blood-gas analysis? *Br. J. Anaesth.* **50**, 51.
49. Bland J. H. L. and Lowenstein E. (1976) Halothane-induced decrease in experimental myocardial ischaemia in the non-failing canine heart. *Anesthesiology* **45**, 287.
50. Boyd A. D., Tremblay R. E., Spencer F. C. et al. (1959) Estimation of cardiac output soon after intracardiac surgery with cardiopulmonary bypass. *Ann. Surg.* **150**, 613.
51. Bradley R. D. and Branthwaite M. A. (1970) Circulatory effects of potassium, glucose and insulin following open heart surgery. *Thorax* **25**, 716.
52. Branthwaite M. A. (1974) Cerebral blood flow and metabolism during open heart surgery. *Thorax* **29**, 633.
53. Braunwald E. (1972) Myocardial function – 1972. *Anesth. Analg. (Cleve.)* **51**, 489.
54. Braunwald E. (1974) Regulation of the circulation (Part I). *N. Engl. J. Med.* **290**, 1124.
55. Braunwald E. (1974) Regulation of the circulation (Part II). *N. Engl. J. Med.* **290**, 1420.
56. Brazier J., Cooper N. and Buckberg G. D. (1974) The adequacy of subendocardial oxygen delivery: the interaction of determinants of flow, arterial oxygen content and myocardial oxygen need. *Circulation* **49**, 968.
57. Brock, Lord (1975) Observations on peripheral and central temperatures with particular reference to the occurrence of vasoconstriction. *Br. J. Surg.* **62**, 589.
58. Brooks D. K. (1978) Stomach as reservoir for respiratory pathogens. *Lancet* **2**, 1147.
59. Brown S. S. and Dundee J. W. (1968) Clinical studies of induction agents XXV: diazepam. *Br. J. Anaesth.* **40**, 108.
60. Brunberg J. A., Doty D. B. and Reilly E. L. (1974) Choreoathetosis in infants following cardiac surgery with deep hypothermia and circulatory arrest. *J. Pediatr.* **84**, 232.
61. Bryce-Smith R. (1972) Complications. In: Hewer C. I. (ed.), *Recent Advances in Anaesthesia and Analgesia,* 11th ed. Edinburgh, Churchill Livingstone, p. 246.
62. Buchbinder N. and Ganz W. (1976) Hemodynamic monitoring: invasive techniques. *Anesthesiology* **45**, 147.
63. Buckberg G. D. and Ross G. (1972) Effects of isoproterenol on coronary blood flow, its distribution, and myocardial performance. *Surg. Forum* **23**, 197.
64. Büky B. (1970) Effect of magnesium on ventricular fibrillation due to hypothermia. *Br. J. Anaesth.* **42**, 886.

65. Bull B. S., Korpman R. A., Huse W. M. et al. (1975) Heparin therapy during extracorporeal circulation. 1. Problems inherent in existing heparin protocols. *J. Thorac. Cardiovasc. Surg.* **69**, 674.
66. Bull M. H., Huse W. M. and Bull B. S. (1975) Evaluation of tests to monitor heparin therapy during extracorporeal circulation. *Anesthesiology* **43**, 346.
67. Bunker J. P., Bendixen H. H. and Murphy A. J. (1962) Hemodynamic effects on intravenously administered sodium citrate. *N. Engl. J. Med.* **266**, 372.
68. Bunker J. P., Stetson J. B., Coe R. C. et al. (1955) Citrate intoxication. *JAMA* **157**, 1361.
69. Byrick R. J., Finlayson D. C. and Noble W. H. (1977) Pulmonary arterial pressure increases during cardiopulmonary bypass, a potential cause of pulmonary oedema. *Anesthesiology* **46**, 433.
70. Calverley R. K., Jenkins L. C. and Griffiths J. (1973) A clinical study of serum magnesium concentrations during anaesthesia and cardiopulmonary bypass. *Can. Anaesth. Soc. J.* **20**, 499.
71. Calverley R. K., Smith N. T., Prys-Roberts C. et al. (1975) Cardiovascular effects of prolonged enflurane anesthesia in man. Abstracts of Scientific Papers, American Society of Anesthesiologists Annual Meeting, p. 57.
72. Chapman J. M. and Davies J. R. (1978) Dopamine dosage. *Br. Med. J.* **2**, 437.
73. Chatterjee K., Parmley W. W., Ganz W. et al. (1973) Hemodynamic and metabolic responses to vasodilator therapy in acute myocardial infarction. *Circulation* **48**, 1183.
74. Chauve A., Castro A. and Fontan F. (1977) Effect of dopamine in cardiac patients after open heart surgery. *Proc. R. Soc. Med.* **70** (Suppl. 2), 50.
75. Chesney R. W., Kaplan B. S., Freedom R. M. et al. (1975) Acute renal failure: an important complication of cardiac surgery in infants. *J. Pediatr.* **87**, 381.
76. Chiarello M., Gold H. K., Leinbach R. C. et al. (1976) Comparison between the effects of nitroprusside and nitroglycerin on ischaemic injury during acute myocardial infarction. *Circulation* **54**, 766.
77. Choussat A., Fontan F. and Besse P. (1978) Selection criteria for Fontan's procedure. In: Anderson R. H. and Shinebourne E. A. (ed.), *Paediatric Cardiology*, 1977. Edinburgh, Churchill Livingstone, p. 559.
78. Clements A. J. (1976) Anaesthesia for open heart surgery. *Int. Anesthesiol. Clin.* **14**, 63.
79. Coffin L. H., Ankeney J. L. and Beheler E. M. (1966) Experimental study and clinical use of epinephrine for treatment of low cardiac output syndrome. *Circulation* **33** (Suppl. 1), 78.
80. Cohen R. D. and Simpson R. (1975) Lactate metabolism. *Anesthesiology* **45**, 661.
81. Cohn J. N. and Franciosa J. A. (1977) Drug therapy: vasodilator therapy of cardiac failure (Part I). *N. Engl. J. Med.* **297**, 27.
82. Cohn J. N. and Franciosa J. A. (1978) Selection of vasodilator, inotropic or combined therapy for the management of heart failure. *Am. J. Med.* **65**, 181.
83. Cohn L. H., Fosberg A. M., Anderson W. P. et al. (1975) The effects of phlebotomy, hemodilution and autologous transfusion on systemic oxygenation and whole blood utilization in open heart surgery. *Chest* **68**, 283.
84. Colgan F. J., Nichols F. A. and Deweese J. A. (1974) Positive end expiratory pressure, oxygen transport and the low output state. *Anesth. Analg. (Cleve.)* **53**, 538.
85. Colvin M. P., Curran J. P., Jarvis D. et al. (1977) Femoral artery pressure monitoring. Use of the Seldinger technique. *Anaesthesia* **32**, 451.
86. Cooley D. A., Beall A. C. Jr and Grondin P. (1962) Open heart operations with disposable oxygenators, 5% dextrose and normothermia. *Surgery* **52**, 713.
87. Coran A. G., Das J. B. and Eraklis A. J. (1971) Use of osmometry in the preoperative and postoperative management of the newborn. *J. Pediatr. Surg.* **6**, 529.

88. Corssen G., Allarde R., Brosch F. et al. (1970) Ketamine as the sole anesthetic in open heart surgery. A preliminary report. *Anesth. Analg. (Cleve.)* **49**, 1025.
89. Corssen G., Chodoff P., Domino E. F. et al. (1965) Neuroleptanalgesia and anaesthesia for open heart surgery: pharmacologic rationale and clinical experience. *J. Thorac. Cardiovasc. Surg.* **49**, 901.
90. Cossum P. A., Roberts M. S., Galbraith A. J. et al. (1978) Loss of nitroglycerin from intravenous infusion sets. *Lancet* **2**, 349.
91. Crew A. D., Varkonyi P. I., Gardner L. G. et al. (1974) Continuous positive airway pressure breathing in the postoperative management of the cardiac infant. *Thorax* **29**, 437.
92. Cullen D. J. and Ferrara L. (1974) Comparative evaluation of blood filters. *Anesthesiology* **41**, 568.
93. Cumming G. R. (1970) Propranolol in tetralogy of Fallot. *Circulation* **41**, 13.
94. Cutler E. C., Levine S. A. and Beck C. S. (1924) The surgical treatment of mitral stenosis. *Arch. Surg.* **9**, 689.
95. Daenen W., de Leval M. and Stark J. (1977) Dopamine in open-heart surgery for congenital heart disease. *Proc. R. Soc. Med.* **70** (Suppl. 2), 48.
96. Dalen J. E., Evans G. L., Banas J. S. et al. (1969) The hemodynamic and respiratory effects of diazepam (Valium) *Anesthesiology* **30**, 259.
97. Deitzman R. H., Ersek R., Lillehei C. W. et al. (1969) Low output syndrome: recognition and treatment. *J. Thorac. Cardiovasc. Surg.* **57**, 138.
98. Delooz H. H. (1976) Factors influencing successful discontinuance of mechanical ventilation after open heart surgery: a clinical study of 41 patients. *Crit. Care Med.* **4**, 265.
99. Denlinger J. K., Nahrwold M. L., Gibbs P. S. et al. (1976) Hypocalcaemia during rapid blood transfusion in anaesthetized man. *Br. J. Anaesth.* **48**, 995.
100. Dennis L. H., Stewart J. L. and Conrad M. E. (1967) Heparin treatment of haemorrhagic diathesis in cyanotic congenital heart disease. *Lancet* **1**, 1088.
101. Desmonts J. M., Bohm G. and Couderc E. (1978) Hemodynamic responses to low doses of naloxone after narcotic nitrous oxide anaesthesia. *Anesthesiology* **49**, 12.
102. Diaz F. A., Bianco J. A., Bello A. et al. (1976) Effect of ketamine on canine cardiovascular function. *Br. J. Anaesth.* **48**, 941.
103. Dietzman R. H., Lunseth J. B. and Goot B. (1975) The use of methylprednisolone during cardiopulmonary bypass: a review of 427 cases. *J. Thorac. Cardiovasc. Surg.* **69**, 870.
104. Dillard D. H., Mohri H. and Merindino K. A. (1971) Correction of heart disease in infancy utilising deep hypothermia and total circulatory arrest. *J. Thorac. Cardiovasc. Surg.* **61**, 64.
105. Donald I. (1976) At the receiving end: a doctor's personal recollections of second-time cardiac valve replacement. *Scott. Med. J.* **21**, 49.
106. Dottori O., Korsgren M., Löf B. A. et al. (1976) The haemodynamic effects of unsupplemented nitrous oxide–oxygen relaxant anaesthesia in cardiac patients. *Acta Anaesthesiol. Scand.* **20**, 195.
107. Downes J. B., Klein E. F., Desautels D. et al. (1973) Intermittent mandatory ventilation. A new approach to weaning patients from mechanical ventilators. *Chest* **64**, 331.
108. Drew C. E. and Anderson I. M. (1959) Profound hypothermia in cardiac surgery; report of three cases. *Lancet* **1**, 748.
109. Drop L. J. and Laver M. B. (1975) Low plasma ionized calcium and response to calcium therapy in critically ill man. *Anesthesiology* **43**, 300.
110. Duarte C. G. (1968) Effects of ethacrynic acid and furosemide on urinary calcium, phosphate and magnesium. *Metabolism* **17**, 867.
111. Dubois M., Savege T. M., O'Carroll T. M. et al. (1978) General anaesthesia and changes on the cerebral function monitor. *Anaesthesia* **33**, 157.

112. Dubois-Primo J. (1975) Comparison between fentanyl and morphine for use in analgesic anaesthesia during open heart surgery. *Acta Anaesthesiol. Belg.* **26**, 5.
113. Dundee J. W. and Keilty S. R. (1969) Diazepam. In: Clarke R. S. J. (ed.), *The Newer Intravenous Anaesthetics. Int. Anesthesiol. Clin.* 7, 91.
114. Dyckner T. and Wester P. O. (1978) Intracellular potassium after magnesium infusion. *Br. Med. J.* **1**, 822.
115. Edie R. N., Jaubert S. N. and Malm J. R. (1976) The use of haemodilution and non-haemic prime for cardiopulmonary bypass. In: Ionescu M. I. and Wooler G. H. (ed.), *Current Techniques in Extracorporeal Circulation.* London, Butterworth, p. 117.
116. Editorial (1977) Potassium in heart failure. *Br. Med. J.* **2**, 469.
117. Editorial (1977) Disopyramide for cardiac arrhythmias. *Lancet* **2**, 912.
118. Editorial (1976) Postoperative pain. *Br. Med. J.* **2**, 664.
119. Editorial (1978) Postoperative pain. *Br. Med. J.* **2**, 517.
120. Editorial (1978) Swan Ganz catheters. *Lancet* **2**, 357.
121. Editorial (1978) Gastrointestinal bleeding in acute respiratory failure. *Br. Med. J.* **1**, 531.
122. Editorial (1978) Adverse reactions to intravenous induction agents. *Br. Med. J.* **2**, 648.
123. Editorial (1978) Hyponatraemia. *Lancet* **1**, 642.
124. Eisenberg L. and Kwan A. M. (1971) Neuroleptanaesthesia with diazepam morphine in poor risk surgical patients. *Can. Anaesth. Soc. J.* **18**, 465.
125. Ellis B. W. de L., Stansbridge R., Fielding L. P. et al. (1976) A rational approach to parenteral nutrition. *Br. Med. J.* **1**, 1388.
126. Ellison N. (1977) Diagnosis and management of bleeding disorders. *Anesthesiology* **47**, 171.
127. Ellison N., Beatty C. P., Blake D. R. et al. (1974) Heparin rebound. Studies in patients and volunteers. *J. Thorac. Cardiovasc. Surg.* **67**, 723.
128. English D. C. W., Frew R. M. and Piggott J. J. (1969) Percutaneous catheterization of the internal jugular vein. *Anaesthesia* **24**, 521.
129. English T. A. H. (1978) *Soc. Thorac. Surg. Engl.*, Leeds, Sept. 1978. (Unpublished.)
130. English T. A. H., Digerness S. and Kirklin J. W. (1971) Changes in colloid osmotic pressure during and shortly after open intracardiac operation. *J. Thorac. Cardiovasc. Surg.* **61**, 338.
131. Entress A. and Doshi D. M. (1978) Use of propranolol to control ventricular tachycardia upon termination of cardiopulmonary bypass. *Anesthesiology* **49**, 56.
132. Estafanous F. G. (1975) Respiratory care following open heart surgery. *Surg. Clin. North Am.* **55**, 1229.
133. Fahmy N. R. and Battit G. E. (1975) Effects of pentolinium on blood sugar and serum potassium concentrations during anaesthesia and surgery. *Br. J. Anaesth.* **47**, 1309.
134. Farman J. V. (1976) A new central venous catheter. *Lancet* **1**, 780.
135. Farman J. V. (1978) Which venous catheter? *Br. J. Clin. Equip.* **3**, 210.
136. Farnsworth A. E., Angerpointner T. A., Lewis G. J. R. et al. (1977) A monitor for the continuous assessment of left ventricular performance after open heart operations. *Ann. Thorac. Surg.* **23**, 169.
137. Faulkner S. L., Hopkins J. T., Boerth R. C. et al. (1973) Time required for complete recovery from chronic propranolol therapy. *N. Engl. J. Med.* **289**, 607.
138. Fisher A. and Benedict C. R. (1977) Adult coarctation of the aorta: anaesthesia and postoperative management. *Anaesthesia* **32**, 533.
139. Fisher M. L., Defelice C. E. and Parisi A. F. (1975) Assessing left ventricular pressure with flow directed (Swan-Ganz) catheter. Detection of sudden changes in patients with left ventricular dysfunction. *Chest* **68**, 542.

140. Fisk R. L., Gelfand E. T. and Callaghan J. C. (1977) Hypothermic coronary perfusion for intraoperative cardioplegia. *Ann. Thorac. Surg.* **23,** 58.

141. Flacke J. W., Flacke W. E. and Williams G. D. (1977) Acute pulmonary oedema following naloxone reversal of high dose morphine anesthesia. *Anesthesiology* **47,** 376.

142. Flear C. T. G. and Singh C. M. (1973) Hyponatraemia and sick cells. *Br. J. Anaesth.* **45,** 976.

143. Flemma R. J. and Singh H. M. (1977) Intraoperative preservation of left ventricular function: past, present and future directions. *Adv. Cardiol.* **20,** 81.

144. Fluck D. C., Bescos L. L. and Gilkes R. R. (1973) Effect on blood volume of maintaining a high central venous pressure after major aortic surgery. *Thorax* **28,** 762.

145. Foëx P. (1978) Preoperative assessment of patients with cardiac disease. *Br. J. Anaesth.* **50,** 15.

146. Forrest W. H., Brown C. R. and Brown B. W. (1977) Subjective responses to six common preoperative medications. *Anesthesiology* **47,** 241.

147. Forrester J. S., Diamond G., McHugh T. J. et al. (1971) Filling pressures in the right and left sides of the heart in acute myocardial infarction. *N. Engl. J. Med.* **285,** 190.

148. Forrester J. S., Ganz W., Diamond G. et al. (1972) Thermodilution cardiac output determination with a single flow-directed catheter. *Am. Heart J.* **83,** 306.

149. French L. A. and Galichich J. H. (1964) The use of steroids for control of cerebral oedema. *Clin. Neurosurg.* **10,** 212.

150. Fry J. L. and Proctor H. J. (1977) Effects of hypoxia acidosis and peripheral vascular resistance on endocardial viability ratio. *Surg. Gynecol. Obstet.* **144,** 850.

151. Fuhrman G. J., Fuhrman F. A. and Field J. (1950) Metabolism of rat heart slices, with special reference to effects of temperature and anoxia. *Am. J. Physiol.* **163,** 642.

152. Gassner S., Cohen M. and Aygen M. (1974) The effect of ketamine on pulmonary artery pressure. An experimental and clinical study. *Anaesthesia* **29,** 141.

153. Gautam H. P. (1969) Improved cardiac performance with potassium glucose and insulin. *Lancet* **1,** 1315.

154. Gibbon J. H. (1954) Application of a mechanical heart and lung apparatus to cardiac surgery. *Minn. Med.* **37,** 171.

155. Gilston A. (1971) Anaesthesia for cardiac surgery. *Br. J. Anaesth.* **43,** 217.

156. Gilston A. (1976) A clinical scoring system for adult respiratory distress. Preliminary report of its use in heart diseases. *Anaesthesia* **31,** 448.

157. Gilston A. (1976) Venous hypertension after mechanical ventilation. *Anaesthesia* **31,** 513.

158. Gilston A. and Resnekov L. (1971) *Cardiorespiratory Resuscitation.* Philadelphia, F. A. Davis Company, p. 43.

159. Glick G., Parmley W. W. and Wechsler A. S. (1968) Glucagon. Its enhancement of cardiac performance in the cat and dog and persistence of its inotropic action despite beta-receptor blockade with propranolol. *Circ. Res.* **22,** 789.

160. Glover W. J. (1977) Management of cardiac surgery in the neonate. *Br. J. Anaesth.* **49,** 59.

161. Gnanadurai T. V., Branthwaite J. F., Colbeck J. F. et al. (1978) Lysosomal enzyme release from lungs after cardiopulmonary bypass. *Anaesthesia* **33,** 227.

162. Godfrey S. and Costeloe K. (1976) Clinical use of an indwelling umbilical artery electrode. *Lancet* **1,** 311.

163. Goenen M., Norlander O., Carlens P. et al. (1972) Circulation ventilation and fluid balance in patients during and immediately after heart valve replacement. *Scand. J. Thorac. Cardiovasc. Surg.* **6,** 6.

164. Goldberg L. I. (1978) Dopamine and dobutamine. *Br. Med. J.* **2,** 1163.
165. Goodman L. S. and Gilman A. (1975) *The Pharmacological Basis of Therapeutics,* 5th ed. New York, Macmillan Publishing Co., p. 369.
166. Gordon B. L. and Carleton R. A. (1969) *Clinical Cardiopulmonary Physiology,* 3rd ed. New York, Grune and Stratton.
167. Graff T. D. and Benson D. W. (1969) Systemic and pulmonary changes with inhaled humid atmospheres. *Anesthesiology* **30,** 199.
168. Gralnick H. R. and Fischer R. D. (1971) The hemostatic response to open heart operations. *J. Thorac. Cardiovasc. Surg.* **61,** 909.
169. Gray T. C. and Riding J. E. (1957) Anaesthesia for mitral valvotomy. *Anaesthesia* **12,** 129.
170. Gregory G. A., Edmunds L. H., Kitterman J. A. et al. (1975) Continuous positive airway pressure and pulmonary and circulatory function after cardiac surgery in infants less than three months of age. *Anesthesiology* **43,** 426.
171. Griepp R. B., Stinson E. B. and Shumway N. E. (1973) Profound local hypothermia for myocardial protection during open heart surgery. *J. Thorac. Cardiovasc. Surg.* **66,** 731.
172. Guyton A. C. and Jones C. E. (1973) Central venous pressure: physiological significance and clinical implications. *Am. Heart J.* **86,** 431.
173. Hallowell P., Bland J. H. L., Buckley M. J. et al. (1972) Transfusion of fresh autologous blood in open heart surgery. *J. Thorac. Cardiovasc. Surg.* **64,** 941.
174. Hanisharo P. K. and Weil M. H. (1972) Reliability of central venous pressure as a measure of changes in left sided intracardiac pressure. *Chest* **62,** 479.
175. Hardaway R. M. (1971) The problem of acute severe trauma and shock. *Surg. Gynec. Obstet.* **133,** 799.
176. Harris E. A. (1973) Metabolic aspects of profound hypothermia. In: Barratt-Boyes B. G., Neutze J. M. and Harris E. A. (ed.), *Heart Disease in Infancy. Diagnosis and Surgical Treatment.* Edinburgh and London, Churchill Livingstone.
177. Harris E. A., Seelye E. R. and Barratt-Boyes B. G. (1974) On the availability of oxygen to the body during cardiopulmonary bypass in man. *Br. J. Anaesth.* **46,** 425.
178. Harrison D. C. (1975) Practical guidelines for the use of lidocaine: prevention and treatment of cardiac arrhythmias. *JAMA* **233,** 1202.
179. Harrison G. G. (1978) Death attributable to anaesthesia. *Br. J. Anaesth.* **50,** 1041.
180. Hasbrook J. D. (1970) Morphine anaesthesia for open heart surgery. *Ann. Thorac. Surg.* **10,** 364.
181. Hatano S., Keane D., Wade M. A. et al. (1974) Diazepam–pentazocine anaesthesia for cardiovascular surgery. *Can. Anaesth. Soc. J.* **21,** 586.
182. Hatano S., Sadove M. S., Keane D. M. et al. (1976) Diazepam–ketamine anaesthesia for open heart surgery. 'Micro-mini' drip administration technique. *Anaesthesist* **25,** 457.
183. Hatch D. J., Taylor B. W., Glover W. J. et al. (1973) Continuous positive airway pressure after open heart operations in infancy. *Lancet* **2,** 469.
184. Hazrati S. (1977) Maintaining spontaneous respiration in the postoperative phase of cardiac surgery. *Int. Surg.* **62,** 199.
185. Hearse D. J., Stewart D. A. and Braimbridge M. V. (1975) Hypothermia arrest and potassium arrest: metabolic and myocardial protection during elective cardiac arrest. *Circ. Res.* **36,** 481.
186. Hearse D. J., Stewart D. A. and Braimbridge M. V. (1976) Cellular protection during myocardial ischaemia: the development and characterization of a procedure for the induction of reversible ischaemic arrest. *Circulation* **54,** 193.
187. Hennessy V. L. Jr, Hicks R. E., Niewiarowski S. et al. (1977) Function of human platelets during extracorporeal circulation. *Am. J. Physiol.* **232,** 622.

188. Henney R. P., Vasko J. S., Brawley R. K. et al. (1966) The effects of morphine on the resistance and capacitance vessels of the peripheral circulation. *Am. Heart J.* **72**, 242.
189. Hewitt P. B., Chamberlain J. H. and Seed R. F. (1973) The effect of carbon dioxide on cardiac output in patients undergoing mechanical ventilation following open heart surgery. *Br. J. Anaesth.* **45**, 1035.
190. Hicks R. E., Dutton R. C., Ries C. A. et al. (1973) Production and fate of platelet aggregate emboli during venovenous perfusion. *Surg. Forum* **24**, 250.
191. Hikasa Y., Shirotani H., Satomura K. et al. (1967) Open heart surgery in infants with an aid of hypothermia anaesthesia. *Arch. Jpn Chir.* **36**, 495.
192. Hilberman M., Kamm B., Lamy M. et al. (1976) An analysis of potential physiological predictors of respiratory adequacy following cardiac surgery. *J. Thorac. Cardiovasc. Surg.* **71**, 711.
193. Hill D. G., Sonksen P. H. and Braimbridge M. V. (1974) Levels of plasma insulin and glucose after open-heart surgery. *J. Thorac. Cardiovasc. Surg.* **67**, 712.
194. Hill J. D., Osborn J. J., Swank R. L. et al. (1970) Experience using a new dacron filter during extracorporeal circulation. *Arch. Surg.* **101**, 649.
195. Hine I. P., Wood W. G., Mainwaring-Burton R. W. et al. (1976) The adrenergic response to surgery involving cardiopulmonary bypass, as measured by plasma and urinary catecholamine concentrations. *Br. J. Anaesth.* **48**, 355.
196. Hobelmann C. F. Jr, Smith D. E., Virgilio R. W. et al. (1974) Left atrial and pulmonary artery wedge pressure difference with positive end expiratory pressure. *Surg. Forum* **25**, 232.
197. Hoffman J. I. E. and Buckberg G. D. (1975) Pathophysiology of subendocardial ischaemia. *Br. Med. J.* **1**, 76.
198. Holloway E. L., Stinson E. B., Derby G. C. et al. (1975) Action of drugs in patients early after cardiac surgery. I. Comparison of isoproterenol and dopamine. *Am. J. Cardiol.* **35**, 656.
199. Holmes C. McK. (1976) Supplementation of general anaesthesia with narcotic analgesics. *Br. J. Anaesth.* **48**, 907.
200. Holmes J. T. (1975) Parenteral feeding and elemental diets. *Br. J. Hosp. Med.* **13**, 747.
201. Horecky J. and Siska K. (1972) Colloid osmotic and dispersion stability of hemodilutional perfusion during open heart surgery. *Abstr. 7th Conf. Europ. Soc. Microcirc.*, Aberdeen.
202. Horton R. and Biglieri E. G. (1962) Effect of aldosterone on the metabolism of magnesium. *J. Clin. Endocrinol. Metab.* **22**, 1187.
203. Howland W. S., Schweitzer O., Ragasa J. et al. (1976) Colloid oncotic pressure and levels of albumin and total protein during major surgical procedures. *Surg. Gynec. Obstet.* **143**, 592.
204. Huch A., Seiler D., Meinzer K. et al. (1977) Transcutaneous $P\text{co}_2$ measurement with a miniaturised electrode. *Lancet* **1**, 982.
205. Huch R., Lübbers D. W. and Huch A. (1974) Reliability of transcutaneous monitoring of arterial $P\text{o}_2$ in newborn infants. *Arch. Dis. Child.* **49**, 213.
206. Hughes J. M. (1977) Pulmonary circulation and fluid balance. *Int. Rev. Physiol.* **14**, 135.
207. Humphries J. O., Gott V. L. and Benson D. W. (1973) Care of the patient undergoing valvular heart surgery. *Prog. Cardiovasc. Dis.* **25**, 449–489.
208. Hurley E. J., Lower R. R., Dong E. Jr et al. (1964) Clinical experience with local hypothermia in elective cardiac arrest. *J. Thorac. Cardiovasc. Surg.* **47**, 51.
209. Hussum B. and Palm T. (1978) Arterial dominance in the hand. *Br. J. Anaesth.* **50**, 913.
210. Inman W. H. W. and Mushin W. W. (1978) Jaundice after repeated exposure to halothane: a further analysis of reports to the Committee on Safety of Medicines. *Br. Med. J.* **2**, 1455.

211. Ionescu M. I. and Wooler G. H. (ed.) (1976) *Current Techniques in Extracorporeal Circulation.* London Butterworth.
212. Ishitoya T., Sato S., Dibenedetto G. et al. (1977) Oxygen consumption during surface induced deep hypothermia under halothane anesthesia. *Ann. Thorac. Surg.* **23,** 52.
213. Jackson A. P. F., Dhadphale P. R., Callaghan M. L. et al. (1978) Haemodynamic studies during induction of anaesthesia for open-heart surgery using diazepam and ketamine. *Br. J. Anaesth.* **50,** 375.
214. Jakubowski H. D. and Taube H. D. (1975) Plasma renin activity in surgical patients. In: Arias A. (ed.), *Recent Progress in Anesthesiology and Resuscitation,* Amsterdam, Excerpta Medica, p. 359.
215. Janssen P. J. (1976) Anesthesia for corrective open heart surgery of congenital defects beyond infancy. *Int. Anesthesiol. Clin.* **14,** 205.
216. Järnberg P. O. (1978) Acute effect of furosemide and mannitol on renal function in the early postoperative period. *Acta Anaesthesiol. Scand.* **22,** 173.
217. Järnberg P. O. (1978) Acute effects of furosemide and mannitol on central haemodynamics in the early postoperative period. *Acta Anaesthesiol. Scand.* **22,** 184.
218. Järnberg P. O., Santesson J. and Eklund J. (1978) Renal function during neurolept anaesthesia. *Acta Anaesthesiol. Scand.* **22,** 167.
219. Jenkinson J. L., Macrae W. R., Scott D. B. et al. (1974) Haemodynamic effects of diazepam used as a sedative for oral surgery. *Br. J. Anaesth.* **46,** 294.
220. Jennings G., Jones M. S., Besterman E. M. et al. (1976) Oral disopyramide in prophylaxis of arrhythmias following myocardial infarction. *Lancet* **1,** 51.
221. Jewell B. R. (1977) A re-examination of the influence of muscle length on myocardial performance. *Circ. Res.* **40,** 221.
222. Jewitt D., Birkhead J., Mitchell A. et al. (1974) Clinical cardiovascular pharmacology of dobutamine, a selective inotropic catecholamine. *Lancet* **2,** 263.
223. Jobes D. R. (1975) Anesthesia for cardiac surgery. *Surg. Clin. North Am.* **55,** 893.
224. Johnston A. E., Radde I. C., Steward D. J. et al. (1974) Acid base and electrolyte changes in infants undergoing profound hypothermia for surgical correction of congenital heart defects. *Can. Anaesth. Soc. J.* **21,** 23.
225. Johnstone R. E. and Greenhow D. E. (1973) Catheterization of the dorsalis pedis artery. *Anesthesiology* **39,** 654.
226. Jones E. L., Kaplan J. A., Dorney E. R. et al. (1976) Propranolol therapy in patients undergoing myocardial revascularization. *Am. J. Cardiol.* **38,** 696.
227. Jones R. W. A., Rochefort M. J. and Baum J. D. (1976) Increased insensible water loss in newborn infants nursed under radiant heaters. *Br. Med. J.* **2,** 1347.
228. Jynge P., Hearse D. J. and Braimbridge M. V. (1977) Myocardial protection during ischaemic cardiac arrest: a possible hazard with calcium-free cardioplegia infusates. *J. Thorac. Cardiovasc. Surg.* **73,** 848.
229. Kaplan J. A., Cannarella C., Jones E. L. et al. (1977) Autologous blood transfusion during cardiac surgery. *J. Thorac. Cardiovasc. Surg.* **74,** 4.
230. Kaplan J. A., Dunbar R. W. and Jones E. L. (1976) Nitroglycerin infusion during coronary artery surgery. *Anesthesiology* **45,** 14.
231. Karliczek G., Hempelmann G. and Piepenbrock S. (1974) Hemodynamic changes of enflurane (Ethrane) in open cardiac surgery. *Acta Anaesthesiol. Belg.* **2,** 276.
232. Khan R. M. A., Hodge J. S. and Bassett H. F. M. (1973) Magnesium in open heart surgery. *J. Thorac. Cardiovasc. Surg.* **66,** 185.
233. Kirklin J. W. and Theye R. A. (1973) Cardiac performance after open intracardiac surgery. *Circulation* **28,** 1061.
234. Kirklin J. W. (1976) Symposium on monitoring. *Anesthesiology* **45,** 113.

235. Kirsch U., Rodewald G. and Kalmar P. (1972) Induced ischaemic arrest clinical experience with cardioplegia in open heart surgery. *J. Thorac. Cardiovasc. Surg.* **63**, 121.
236. Knapp R. B. and Dubow H. S. (1970) Diazepam as an induction agent for patients with cardiopulmonary disease. *South. Med. J.* **63**, 1451.
237. Kobrine A. I. and Kempe L. G. (1973) Studies in head injury II. Effect of dexamethasone on traumatic brain swelling. *Surg. Neurol.* **1**, 38.
238. Komp D. M. and Sparrow A. W. (1970) Polycythemia in cyanotic heart disease – a study of altered coagulation. *J. Pediatr.* **76**, 231.
239. Kopriva C. J., Brown A. C. D. and Pappas G. (1978) Hemodynamics during general anaesthesia in patients receiving propranolol. *Anesthesiology* **48**, 28.
240. Kouchoukos N. T., Sheppard L. C. and Kirklin J. W. (1972) Effect of alterations in arterial pressure on cardiac performance early after the open intracardiac operations. *J. Thorac. Cardiovasc. Surg.* **64**, 563.
241. Krauss X. H., Verdouw P. D., Hugenholtz P. G. et al. (1975) On line monitoring of mixed venous oxygen saturation after cardiothoracic surgery. *Thorax* **30**, 636.
242. Krohn B. G., Urquhart R. R. and Magidson O. (1968) Metabolic alkalosis following heart surgery. *J. Thorac. Cardiovasc. Surg.* **56**, 732.
243. Kubicek W. G., Kottke F. J., Ramos M. V. et al. (1974) The Minnesota impedance cardiograph – theory and application. *Biomed. Eng.* **9**, 410.
244. Laaksonen V. O., Arola M. K., Inberg M. V. et al. (1977) Effect of different respirator adjustments on central haemodynamics in open heart surgery patients. *Acta Anaesthesiol. Scand.* **21**, 200.
245. Lancet (1978) Resources for bypass surgery. **2**, 587.
246. Lappas D. G., Buckley M. J., Laver M. B. et al. (1975) Left ventricular performance and pulmonary circulation following addition of nitrous oxide to morphine during coronary artery surgery. *Anesthesiology* **43**, 61.
247. Lappas D. G., Lowenstein E., Waller J. et al. (1976) Hemodynamic effects of nitroprusside infusion during coronary artery operation in man. *Circulation* **54** (Suppl. 3), 4.
248. Lappas D. G., Powell W. M. J. and Daggett W. M. (1977) Cardiac dysfunction in the perioperative period. *Anesthesiology* **47**, 117.
249. Laver M. B. (1975) Anesthesia for open heart surgery: its contribution to the care of the critically ill. *Bull. N.Y. Acad. Med.* **51**, 930.
250. Laver M. B. (1976) A time to measure. *Anesthesiology* **45**, 114.
251. Laver M. B., Hallowell P. and Goldblatt A. (1970) Pulmonary dysfunction secondary to heart disease. *Anesthesiology* **33**, 161.
252. Lawler P. G. P. and Nunn J. F. (1977) Intermittent mandatory ventilation. A discussion and a description of necessary modifications to a Brompton Manley Ventilator. *Anaesthesia* **32**, 138.
253. Laws H. L., Kirklin M. K., Diethelm A. G. et al. (1978) Training and use of surgeons assistants. *Surgery* **83**, 445.
254. Lawson D. H., Gray J. M. B., Henry D. A. et al. (1978) Continuous infusion of frusemide in refractory oedema. *Br. Med. J.* **2**, 476.
255. Lawson N. W., Ochsner J. L., Mills N. L. et al. (1974) Use of hemodilution and fresh autologous blood in open heart surgery. *Anesth. Analg.* (*Cleve.*) **53**, 672.
256. Lee H. A. (1977) The management of acute renal failure. *Br. J. Anaesth.* **49**, 697.
257. Leier C. V., Webel J. and Bush C. A. (1977) The cardiovascular effects of the continuous infusion of dobutamine in patients with severe cardiac failure. *Circulation* **56**, 468.
258. de Leval M. R., Hill J. D. and Mielke C. H. (1976) Haematological aspects of extra corporeal circulation. In: Ionescu M. I. and Wooler G. H. (ed.), *Current Techniques in Extracorporeal Circulation.* London, Butterworth, p. 312.

259. de Leval M. R., Taswell H. F., Bowie E. J. W. et al. (1974) Open heart surgery in patients with inherited hemoglobinopathies, red cell dyscrasias and coagulopathies. *Arch. Surg.* **109**, 618.
260. Levin R. M., Seleny F. L. and Streczyn M. V. (1975) Ketamine pancuronium narcotic technique for cardiovascular surgery in infants – a comparative study. *Anesth. Analg. (Cleve.)* **54**, 800.
261. Libby P., Maroko P. R., Bloor C. M. et al. (1972) Hydrocortisone induced reduction in infarct size following experimental acute coronary occlusion. (Abstr.) *Circulation* **46** (Suppl. II), 14.
262. Libby P., Maroko P. R., Bloor C. M. et al. (1973) Reduction of experimental myocardial infarction size by corticosteroid administration. *J. Clin. Invest.* **52**, 599.
263. Lilleaason P. (1977) Moderate and extreme haemodilution in open heart surgery. *Scand. J. Thorac. Cardiovasc. Surg.* **11**, 97.
264. Lillehei R. C., Lillehei C. W., Grismer J. T. et al. (1963) Plasma catecholamines in open heart surgery; the prevention of their pernicious effects by pretreatment with dibenzline. *Surg. Forum* **13**, 269.
265. Liu W. S., Bidwai A. V., Stanley T. H. et al. (1976) The cardiovascular effects of diazepam and of diazepam and pancuronium during fentanyl and oxygen anaesthesia. *Can. Anaesth. Soc. J.* **23**, 395.
266. Loh L., Sykes M. K. and Chakrabarti M. K. (1977) The effect of halothane and ether on the pulmonary circulation in the innervated perfused cat lung. *Br. J. Anaesth.* **49**, 309.
267. Loh L., Sykes M. K. and Chakrabarti M. K. (1978) The assessment of ventilator performance. *Br. J. Anaesth.* **50**, 63.
268. Lowenstein E. (1971) Morphine 'anaesthesia'. A perspective. *Anesthesiology* **35**, 563.
269. Lowenstein E., Hallowell P., Levine F. H. et al. (1969) Cardiovascular response to large doses of intravenous morphine in man. *N. Engl. J. Med.* **281**, 1389.
270. Lowenstein E., Little J. W. and Lo H. H. (1971) Prevention of cerebral embolisation from flushing radial artery cannulae. *New Engl. J. Med.* **285**, 1414.
271. Lozman J., Powers S. R. Jr, Older T. et al. (1974) Correlation of pulmonary wedge and left atrial pressures. A study in patients receiving positive end expiratory pressure ventilation. *Arch. Surg.* **109**, 270.
272. Lubbers J., Ten Hof J. P., Van der Veen P. H. et al. (1974) Microgas emboli in a pump oxygenator during open heart surgery. *Arch. Chir. Neerl.* **26**, 41.
273. Lyons S. M. and Clarke R. S. J. (1972) A comparison of different drugs for anaesthesia in cardiac surgical patients. *Br. J. Anaesth.* **44**, 575.
274. Lyons S. M., Clarke R. S. J. and Vulgaraki K. (1975) The premedication of cardiac surgical patients. A clinical comparison of four regimes. *Anaesthesia* **30**, 459.
275. McClure P. D. and Izsak J. (1974) The use of epsilon-aminocaproic acid to reduce bleeding during cardiac bypass in children with congenital heart disease. *Anesthesiology* **40**, 604.
276. Macdonald H. R., Braid D. P., Stead B. R. et al. (1966) Clinical and circulatory effects of neuroleptanalgesia with dehydrobenzperidol and phenoperidine. *Br. Heart J.* **28**, 654.
277. McDonald R. H., Taylor R. R. and Cingolani H. E. (1966) Measurement of myocardial developed tension and its relation to oxygen consumption. *Am. J. Physiol.* **211**, 667.
278. MacDougall B. R. D., Bailey R. J. and Williams R. (1977) H_2-receptor antagonists and antacids in the prevention of acute gastrointestinal haemorrhage in fulminant hepatic failure. *Lancet* **1**, 617.
279. McKenna R., Bachmann F., Whittaker B. et al. (1975) The hemostatic mechanism after open heart surgery. *J. Thorac. Cardiovasc. Surg.* **70**, 298.

280. Majid P. A., Meeran M. K. M., Sharma B. et al. (1972) Insulin and glucose in the treatment of heart failure. *Lancet* **2**, 937.
281. Majid P. A., Sharma B. and Taylor S. H. (1971) Phentolamine for vasodilator treatment of severe heart failure. *Lancet* **2**, 719.
282. Manners J. M. (1971) Anaesthesia for diagnostic procedures in cardiac disease. *Br. J. Anaesth.* **43**, 276.
283. Manners J. M. (1974) Nutrition after cardiac surgery. *Anaesthesia* **29**, 675.
284. Manners J. M. (1976) Diet as therapy after cardiac surgery. *Drug Therapy*, May, p. 200.
285. Manners J. M. (1976) A new tube feed. Aminutrin and Calonutrin. *Anaesthesia* **31**, 441.
286. Manners J. M. (1977) Air embolism during anaesthesia. *Anaesthesia* **32**, 670.
287. Manners J. M., Monro J. L. and Ross J. K. (1977) Pulmonary hypertension in mitral valve disease: 56 surgical patients reviewed. *Thorax* **32**, 691.
288. Manners J. M. and Walters F. J. M. (1979) Beta-adrenoceptor blockade and anaesthesia. *Anaesthesia* **34**, 3.
289. Mannheimer W. H. (1971) The use of morphine and intravenous alcohol in the anaesthetic management of open heart surgery. *South. Med. J.* **64**, 1125.
290. Mansberger A. R., Boyd D. R., Cowley R. A. et al. (1969) Refractometry and osmometry in clinical surgery. *Ann. Surg.* **169**, 672.
291. Marin-Neto J. A., Sykes M. K., Marin J. L. B. et al. (1978) Myocardial depressant effects of protamine sulphate. *Br. J. Anaesth.* **50**, 1079.
292. Marshall B. E., Wurzel H. A., Ellison N. et al. (1975) Microaggregate formation in stored blood. III. Comparison of Bentley, Fenwall, Pall and Swank micropore filters. *Circulation* **2**, 249.
293. Marshall B. E., Wurzel H. A., Neufeld G. R. et al. (1976) Effect of Intercept micropore filtration of blood on microaggregates and other constituents. *Anesthesiology* **44**, 525.
294. Matsumoto A., Sato S., Kondo J. et al. (1977) Open heart surgery by means of deep hypothermia with surface cooling for the age group under one year. *Cardiovasc. Surg.* **18**, 163.
295. Matthews H. R., Meade J. B. and Evans C. C. (1974) Significance of prolonged peripheral vasoconstriction after open heart surgery. *Thorax* **29**, 343.
296. Maung T. and Kyll D. T. (1972) The role of the respirator in the management of patients after cardiac surgery. *Med. J. Aust.* **1**, 175.
297. May A. E., Machin J. R. and Wyatt R. (1978) Physostigmine in open heart surgery. Reversal of hyoscine supplementation of morphine oxygen–air-relaxant technique. *Anaesthesia* **33**, 547.
298. Mazze R. I. (1977) Critical care of the patient with acute renal failure. *Anesthesiology* **47**, 138.
299. Mentzer R. M., Alegre C. A. and Nolan S. P. (1976) The effects of dopamine and isoproterenol on the pulmonary circulation. *J. Thorac. Cardiovasc. Surg.* **71**, 807.
300. Merin R. G., Kumazawa T. and Luka N. L. (1976) Enflurane depresses myocardial function perfusion and metabolism in the dog. *Anesthesiology* **45**, 501.
301. Merrill W., Donahoo J. S., Brawley R. K. et al. (1976) Late cardiac tamponade: a potentially lethal complication of open-heart surgery. *J. Thorac. Cardiovasc. Surg.* **72**, 929.
302. Metz G., Dilawari J. and Kellock T. D. (1978) Simple technique for naso enteric feeding. *Lancet* **2**, 454.
303. Michenfelder J. D. (1977) Cyanide release from sodium nitroprusside in the dog. *Anesthesiology* **46**, 196.
304. Miller J. D. (1976) A device for the removal of waste anaesthetic gases from the extracorporeal oxygenator. *Anesthesiology* **44**, 181.
305. Miller R. D. (1973) Complications of massive blood transfusions. *Anesthesiology* **39**, 82.

306. Miller R. R., Olson H. G., Amsterdam E. A. et al. (1975) Propranolol withdrawal rebound phenomenon. Exacerbation of coronary events after abrupt cessation of antianginal therapy *N. Engl. J. Med.* **293**, 416.
307. Millington P. A., Hsiao H. and Proctor H. J. (1976) Design and preliminary evaluation of an endocardial viability ratio (EVR) monitor. In: Martin J. (ed.), *San Diego Symposium for Biochemical Engineering.* New York, Academic Press.
308. Milner A. D., Robertson N. C. R. and Hale P. (1977) Neonatal intensive therapy equipment. *Br. J. Clin. Equip.* **2**, 169.
309. Minty B. D. and Barrett A. M. (1978) Accuracy of an automated blood gas analyser operated by untrained staff. *Br. J. Anaesth.* **50**, 1031.
310. Mitzgala H. F. and Huvelle P. R. (1976) Acute termination of cardiac arrhythmias with intravenous disopyramide. *J. Int. Med. Res.* **4** (Suppl. 1), 82.
311. Monro J. L., Mollo S., Brookbank S. et al. (1978) The cost of cardiac surgery. *Br. Med. J.* **1**, 1684.
312. Morgan M., Lumley J. and Gillies I. D. S. (1974) Neuroleptanaesthesia for major surgery. Experience with 500 cases. *Br. J. Anaesth.* **46**, 288.
313. Mueller H. and Ayres S. M. (1976) Propranolol in acute myocardial infarction in man: effects on haemodynamics and myocardial oxygenation. *Postgrad. Med. J.* **52** (Suppl. 4), 141.
314. Mueller H., Ayres S. M., Giannelli S. et al. (1972) Effect of isoproterenol 1-norepinephrine and intra-aortic counterpulsation on hemodynamics and myocardial metabolism in shock following acute myocardial infarction. *Circulation* **45**, 335.
315. Muller P. (1965) Ouabain effects on cardiac contraction, action potential and cellular potassium. *Circ. Res.* **17**, 46.
316. Mundth E. D. and Austen W. G. (1968) Postoperative intensive care in the cardiac surgical patient. *Prog. Cardiovasc. Dis.* **11**, 229.
317. Muravchik S. (1977) Scavenging enflurane from extracorporeal pump oxygenator. *Anesthesiology* **47**, 468.
318. Nagant de Deuxchaisnes C., Collet R. A., Busset R. et al. (1961) Exchangeable potassium in wasting amyotrophy, heart disease and cirrhosis of the liver. *Lancet* **1**, 681.
319. Nelson R. R., Gobel F. L., Jorgensen C. R. et al. (1974) Hemodynamic predictors of myocardial oxygen consumption during static and dynamic exercise. *Circulation* **50**, 1179.
320. Neville W. E., Faber L. P. and Peacock H. (1964) Total prime of the disc oxygenator with Ringer's lactate solution for cardiopulmonary bypass. *Dis. Chest* **45**, 320.
321. Nielson M. S. and Manners J. M. (1979) Valve replacement in carcinoid syndrome: anaesthetic management for tricuspid and pulmonary valve surgery. *Anaesthesia* **34**, 494.
322. Norman J. (1978) An assessment of acid–base balance. *Br. J. Anaesth.* **50**, 45.
323. Norman J. C., Cooley D. A. and Igo S. R. (1977) Prognostic indices for survival during postcardiotomy intra-aortic balloon pumping. *J. Thorac. Cardiovasc. Surg.* **74**, 709.
324. Norman J. C., Cooley D. A., Kahan B. D. et al. (1978) Total support of the circulation of a patient with postcardiotomy stone-heart syndrome by a partial artificial heart (ALVAD) for 5 days followed by heart and kidney transplantation. *Lancet* **1**, 1125.
325. Norris R. M., Clarke E. D., Samuel N. L. et al. (1978) Protective effect of propranolol in threatened myocardial infarction. *Lancet* **2**, 907.
326. Nunn J. F. and Freeman J. (1964) Problems of oxygenation and oxygen transport during haemorrhage. *Anaesthesia* **19**, 206.

327. Orloff J. and Blake W. D. (1951) Effects of concentrated salt-poor albumin on metabolism and excretion of water and electrolytes in dogs. *Am. J. Physiol.* **164**, 167.
328. Pace N. L. (1977) A critique of flow directed pulmonary artery catheterization. *Anesthesiology* **47**, 455.
329. Panter-Brick M., Wagget J. and Dale G. (1977) *Intravenous Nutrition in Paediatrics.* Dorchester, Dorset Press.
330. Parr G. V. S., Blackstone E. H. and Kirklin J. W. (1975) Cardiac performance and mortality after intracardiac surgery in infants and young children. *Circulation* **51**, 867.
331. Pearson D. T. (1972) The use of isoprenaline and alpha-adrenergic blockade in open heart surgery. *Resuscitation* **1**, 149.
332. Petrie J. C., Galloway D. B., Jeffers T. A. et al. (1976) Adverse reactions to beta-blocking drugs; a review. *Postgrad. Med. J.* **52** (Suppl. 4), 63.
333. de Peyer E., Rouge J. C., Sizonenko P. C. et al. (1977) Evolution du magnesium sanguin et urinaire pendant et après la circulation extra-corporelle en chirurgie cardiaque de l'enfant. *Ann. Anesthesiol. Fr.* **18**, 205.
334. Philbin D. M. and Coggins C. H. (1978) Plasma antidiuretic hormone levels in cardiac surgical patients during morphine and halothane anaesthesia. *Anesthesiology* **49**, 95.
335. Pick M. J., Hatch D. J. and Kerr A. A. (1976) The effect of positive end expiratory pressure on lung mechanics and arterial oxygenation after open heart surgery in young children. *Br. J. Anaesth.* **48**, 983.
336. Pliam M. B., McGoon D. C. and Tarhan S. (1975) Failure of transfusion of autologous whole blood to reduce banked blood requirements in open heart surgical patients. *J. Thorac. Cardiovasc. Surg.* **70**, 338.
337. Pombo J. F., Troy B. L. and Russell R. O. Jr (1971) Left ventricular volume and ejection fraction by echocardiography. *Circulation* **43**, 480.
338. Poole-Wilson P. A., Lewis G., Angerpointer T. et al. (1977) Haemodynamic effects of salbutamol and nitroprusside after cardiac surgery. *Br. Heart J.* **39**, 721.
339. Prescott L. F., Adjepon-Yamoah K. K. and Talbot R. G. (1976) Impaired lignocaine metabolism in patients with myocardial infarction and cardiac failure. *Br. Med. J.* **1**, 939.
340. Prince S. R., Sullivan R. L. and Hackel A. (1976) Percutaneous catheterization of the internal jugular vein in infants and children. *Anesthesiology* **44**, 170.
341. Prior P. E., Maynard D. E. and Brierley J. B. (1978) E.E.G. monitoring for the control of anaesthesia produced by the infusion of althesin in primates. *Br. J. Anaesth.* **50**, 993.
342. Prys-Roberts C. (1976) Medical problems of surgical patients. *Ann. R. Coll. Surg. Engl.* **58**, 465.
343. Prys-Roberts C. (1977) New wine in old bottles. *Br. J. Anaesth.* **49**, 845.
344. Prys-Roberts C. (1978) Cardiovascular monitoring. In: *Monitoring in Anesthesia.* New York, J. Wiley and Sons, p. 53.
345. Prys-Roberts C., Green L. T. and Meloche R. et al. (1971) Studies of anaesthesia in relation to hypertension. II. Haemodynamic consequences of induction and endotracheal intubation. *Br. J. Anaesth.* **43**, 531.
346. Purschke R., Brucke P. and Schulte H. D. (1974) Studies on the reliability of determining stroke-volume from the aortic-pressure contour. *Anaesthesist* **23**, 525.
347. Qvist J., Pontoppidan H. and Wilson R. S. (1975) Hemodynamic response to mechanical ventilation with PEEP: the effect of hypervolaemia. *Anesthesiology* **42**, 45.
348. Rabow F. I., Dwane P. and Don H. (1972) The effect of posture on gas exchange following cardiac surgery. *Can. Anaesth. Soc. J.* **19**, 647.

349. Radnay P. A., Hollinger I. and Santi A. (1976) Ketamine for pediatric cardiac anesthesia. *Anaesthesist* **25**, 259.
350. Radzivil G. G., Mikheeva E. V. and Kutasova I. V. (1975) Izmenenie Kontsentratsii obshchego magniia V krovi bol'nykh perenesshikh operatsiiu s iskusstvennym krovoobrashcheniem. *Kardiologiia* **15**, 118.
351. Rangno R. E., Warnica W., Ogilvie R. I. et al. (1976) Correlation of disopyramide pharmacokinetics with efficacy in ventricular tachyarrhythmias. *J. Int. Med. Res.* **4** (Suppl. 1), 54.
352. Rao T. L. K., Wong A. Y. and Salem M. R. (1977) A new approach to catheterization of the internal jugular vein. *Anesthesiology* **46**, 362.
353. Rathod R., Jacobs H. K., Kramer N. E. et al. (1978) Echocardiographic assessment of ventricular performance following induction with two anaesthetics. *Anesthesiology* **49**, 86.
354. Reidemeister J. C., Heberer G. and Bretschneider H. J. (1967) Induced cardiac arrest by sodium and calcium depletion and application of procaine. *Int. Surg.* **47**, 536.
355. Reul G. J., Romagholi A., Sandiford F. M. et al. (1974) Protective effect of propranolol on the hypertrophied heart during cardiopulmonary bypass. *J. Thorac. Cardiovasc. Surg.* **68**, 283.
356. Reulen H. J. (1976) Vasogenic brain oedema. *Br. J. Anaesth.* **48**, 741.
357. Richardson A. E. and Bereen F. J. (1977) Effect of piracetam on level of consciousness after neurosurgery. *Lancet* **2**, 1110.
358. Rigg J. R. A. and Goldsmith C. H. (1976) Recovery of ventilatory response to carbon dioxide after thiopentone, morphine and fentanyl in man. *Can. Anaesth. Soc. J.* **23**, 370.
359. Rithalia S. V. S. and Tinker J. (1978) Automatic infusion devices. *Br. J. Clin. Equip.* **3**, 163.
360. Roberts R., DeMello V. and Sobel B. E. (1976) Deleterious effects of methylprednisolone in patients with myocardial infarction. *Circulation* **53** (Suppl. I), 204.
361. Robicsek F., Reichertz P. L., Masters T. N. et al. (1975) Computers in cardiology: computerized intensive care of postoperative cardiac surgical patients. *Long Beach Calif. I.E.E.E. Comput. Soc.*, 83.
362. Roche J. K. and Stengle J. M. (1973) Open heart surgery and the demand for blood. *JAMA* **225**, 1516.
363. Roe B. B. (1973) Physiologic changes occurring after open heart surgery. *Surg. Annu.* **5**, 299.
364. Roe B. B., Hutchinson J. C., Fishman W. H. et al. (1977) Myocardial protection with cold, ischaemic, potassium-induced cardioplegia. *J. Thorac. Cardiovasc. Surg.* **73**, 366.
365. Roe C. F., Goldberg M. J., Blair C. S. et al. (1966) The influence of body temperature on early postoperative oxygen consumption. *Surgery* **60**, 85.
366. Romagnoli A. (1973) Duration of action of fentanyl. *Anesthesiology* **39**, 568.
367. Rose M. R., Glassman E. and Spencer F. C. (1975) Arrhythmias following cardiac surgery: relation to serum digoxin level. *Am. Heart J.* **89**, 288.
368. Ross J. K., Diwell A. E., Marsh J. et al. (1978) Wessex cardiac surgery follow up survey: the quality of life after operation. *Thorax* **33**, 3.
369. Ross J. K., Monro J. L., Manners J. M. et al. (1976) Cardiac surgery in Wessex: review of 1000 consecutive open-heart procedures. *Br. Med. J.* **2**, 1485.
370. Rowe G. G. and Henderson R. H. (1974) Systemic and coronary hemodynamic effects of sodium nitroprusside. *Am. Heart J.* **87**, 83.
371. Rowe M. I. and Marchildon M. B. (1976) Physiological considerations in the newborn surgical patient. *Surg. Clin. North Am.* **56**, 245.
372. Rubin L. R. and Bongiovi J. (1970) Central venous pressure. An unreliable guide to fluid therapy in burns. *Arch. Surg.* **100**, 269.

373. Russell W. J. (1974) *Central Venous Pressure: Its Clinical Use and Role in Cardiovascular Dynamics.* London, Butterworth.
374. Rygg I. H. and Valentin N. (1976) The Rygg-Kyvsgaard pump–oxygenator: In: Ionescu M. I. and Wooler G. H. (ed.), *Current Techniques in Extracorporeal Circulation.* London, Butterworth, p. 139.
375. Sade R. M. and Castaneda A. R. (1976) Recent advances in cardiac surgery in the young infants. *Surg. Clin. North Am.* **56,** 451.
376. Sade R. M., Cosgrove D. M. and Castanada A. R. (1977) *Infant and Child Care in Heart Surgery.* Chicago, Year Book Medical Publishers Inc., p. 44.
377. Saidman L. J. and Ty Smith H. (1978) *Monitoring in Anesthesia.* New York, J. Wiley & Sons.
378. Santesson J., Järnberg P. O. and Amer S. (1978) The effect of surgical stress on haemodynamics during neurolept anaesthesia. *Acta Anaesthesiol. Scand.* **22,** 123.
379. Sarin C. L., Yalav E., Clement A. J. et al. (1970) The necessity for measurement of left atrial pressure after cardiac surgery. *Thorax* **25,** 185.
380. Sarnoff S. J., Braunwald E., Welch G. H. Jr. et al. (1958) Hemodynamic determinants of oxygen consumption of the heart with special reference to the tension–time index. *Am. J. Physiol.* **192,** 148.
381. Sato S., Vanini V., Mohri H. et al. (1974) A comparative study of the effect of carbon dioxide and perfusion rewarming on limited circulatory occlusion during surface hypothermia under halothane and ether anesthesia. *Ann. Surg.* **180,** 192.
382. Savege T. M., Colvin M. P., Weaver E. J. M. et al. (1976) A comparison of some cardiorespiratory effects of althesin and ketamine when used for induction of anaesthesia in patients with cardiac disease. *Br. J. Anaesth.* **48,** 1071.
383. Schaer H. (1976) Effects on ionized calcium of a correction of acidosis with alkalinizing agents. *Br. J. Anaesth.* **48,** 327.
384. Schwartz B. (1977) A safer IV catheter. *Anesthesiology* **47,** 234.
385. Seed R. F. and Chamberlain J. H. (1977) Myocardial stimulation by pancuronium bromide. *Br. J. Anaesth.* **49,** 401.
386. Seltzer J. L., Doto J. B. and Jacoby J. (1976) Decreased arterial oxygenation during sodium nitroprusside administration for intraoperative hypertension. *Anesth. Analg. (Cleve.)* **55,** 880.
387. Sheppard L. C. and Kouchoukos N. T. (1976) Computers as monitors. *Anesthesiology* **45,** 250.
388. Sherlock S. (1978) Halothane hepatitis. *Lancet* **2,** 364.
389. Sherman M. M., Dobnik D. B., Dennis R. C. et al. (1976) Autologous blood transfusion during cardiopulmonary bypass. *Chest* **70,** 592.
390. Shils M. E. (1969) Experimental human magnesium depletion. *Medicine* **48,** 61.
391. Shinebourne E. and Pfitzner J. (1973) Continuous flushing device for indwelling arterial and venous cannulae. *Brit. J. Hosp. Med.* **9** (Equip. Suppl.), 64.
392. Siklos P., Chalmers T. M. and Evans D. W. (1978) Ventricular tachycardia after disopyramide. *Lancet* **1,** 98.
393. Smith A. L. (1977) Barbiturate protection in cerebral hypoxia. *Anesthesiology* **47,** 285.
394. Smith B. H. (1973) Anaesthetic problems of renal transplantation. *Proc. R. Soc. Med.* **66,** 42.
395. Smith G. (1976) The coronary circulation and anaesthesia. *Br. J. Anaesth.* **48,** 933.
396. Smith G. H. and Chandra K. (1972) Haemodynamic effects of glucagon after mitral valve replacement. *Thorax* **27,** 591.
397. Sonntag H., Donath U., Millebrand W. et al. (1978) Left ventricular function in conscious man and during halothane anaesthesia. *Anesthesiology* **48,** 320.

398. Stanley T. H., Bennett G. M., Loeser E. A. et al. (1976) Effects of diazepam and droperidol on cardiovascular dynamics during morphine anesthesia. *Anesthesiology* **44**, 255.
399. Stanley T. H., Liu W. S. and Gentry S. (1977) Effects of ventilatory techniques during cardiopulmonary bypass on post-bypass and postoperative pulmonary compliance and shunt. *Anesthesiology* **46**, 391.
400. Stanski D. R., Greenblatt D. J., Lappas D. G. et al. (1976) Kinetics of high dose intravenous morphine in cardiac surgery patients. *Clin. Pharmacol. Ther.* **19**, 752.
401. Stein L., Beraud J. J., Cavanilles J. et al. (1974) Pulmonary oedema during fluid infusion in the absence of heart failure. *JAMA* **299**, 65.
402. Stein L., Beraud J. J., Morissette M. et al. (1975) Pulmonary oedema during volume infusion. *Circulation* **52**, 483.
403. Stephenson L. W., Blackstone E. H. and Kouchoukos N. T. (1976) Dopamine vs epinephrine in patients following cardiac surgery: randomized study. *Surg. Forum* **27**, 272.
404. Stevenson J. G., Stone E. F., Dillard D. H. et al. (1974) Intellectual development of children subjected to prolonged circulatory arrest during hypothermic open heart surgery in infancy. *Circulation* **50** (Suppl. II), 54.
405. Stinson E. B., Holloway E. L., Derby G. et al. (1975) Comparative hemodynamic responses to chlorpromazine, nitroprusside, nitroglycerin and trimetephan immediately after open-heart operations. *Circulation* **51** (Suppl. I), 26.
406. Stinson E. B., Holloway E. L., Derby G. C. et al. (1977) Control of myocardial performance early after open-heart operations by vasodilator treatment. *J. Thorac. Cardiovasc. Surg.* **73**, 523.
407. Stoelting R. K. (1974) Hemodynamic effects of dimethyltubocurarine during nitrous oxide–halothane anesthesia. *Anesth. Analg. (Cleve.)* **53**, 513.
408. Stoelting R. K., Gibbs P. S., Creasser C. W. et al. (1975) Hemodynamic and ventilatory responses to fentanyl, fentanyl-droperidol, and nitrous oxide in patients with acquired valvular heart disease. *Anesthesiology* **42**, 319.
409. Stoelting R. K., Reis R. R. and Longnecker D. E. (1972) Hemodynamic responses to nitrous oxide–halothane in patients with valvular heart disease. *Anesthesiology* **37**, 430.
410. Stoner J. D., Bolen J. L. and Harrison D. C. (1977) Comparison of dobutamine and dopamine in treatment of severe heart failure. *Br. Heart J.* **39**, 536.
411. Strong M. J., Keats A. S. and Cooley D. A. (1967) Arterial gas tensions under anaesthesia in tetralogy of Fallot. *Br. J. Anaesth.* **39**, 472.
412. Strunin L. (1978) Halothane hepatitis. *Lancet* **2**, 468.
413. Suter P. M., Fairley H. B. and Isenberg M. D. (1975) Optimum end expiratory airway pressure in patients with acute pulmonary failure. *N. Engl. J. Med.* **292**, 284.
414. Swaminathan R., Morgan D. B., Ionescu M. et al. (1978) Hypophosphataemia and its consequences in patients following heart surgery. *Anaesthesia* **33**, 601.
415. Swan H. J. C., Ganz W., Forrester J. et al. (1970) Catheterization of the heart in man with use of a flow-directed balloon-tipped catheter. *N. Engl. J. Med.* **283**, 447.
416. Sykes M. K. (1963) Venous pressure as a clinical indication of adequacy of transfusion. *Ann. R. Coll. Surg. Engl.* **33**, 185.
417. Symmonds J. B., Kleinmann L. H. and Wechsler A. S. (1977) Effects of methoxamine on the coronary circulation during cardiopulmonary bypass. *J. Thorac. Cardiovasc. Surg.* **74**, 577.
418. Taggart P. and Slater J. D. H. (1970) The possible significance of ionic gradient changes associated with cardiopulmonary bypass surgery. *Clin. Sci.* **38**, 260.
419. Takahashi K., Shima T., Koga Y. et al. (1971) The effects of ketamine hydrochloride on the pulmonary hemodynamics in dogs. *Jpn J. Anesthesiol.* **20**, 842.

420. Tarhan S. and Moffitt E. A. (1972) Anesthesia and supportive care during and after cardiac surgery. *Ann. Thorac. Surg.* **11,** 64.
421. Tarhan S., White R. D. and Moffitt E. A. (1977) Anesthesia and postoperative care for cardiac operations. *Ann. Thorac. Surg.* **23,** 173.
422. Taylor K. M. (1978) Injury and wound sepsis. Hypothalamic and wound changes in relation to injury. *Ann. R. Coll. Surg. Engl.* **60,** 229.
423. Tector A. J., Gabriel R. P., Mateicka W. E. et al. (1976) Reduction of blood usage in open heart surgery. *Chest* **70,** 454.
424. Thomas D. J. B. and Alberti K. G. M. M. (1978) Hyperglycaemic effects of Hartmann's solution during surgery in patients with maturity onset diabetes. *Br. J. Anaesth.* **50,** 185.
425. Thornton J. A., Fleming J. S., Goldberg A. D. et al. (1973) Cardiovascular effects of 50% nitrous oxide and 50% oxygen mixture. *Anaesthesia* **28,** 484.
426. Tinker J. H. and Michenfelder J. D. (1976) Sodium nitroprusside: pharmacology, toxicology and therapeutics. *Anesthesiology* **45,** 350.
427. Tinker J. L., Tarhan S., White R. D. et al. (1976) Dobutamine for inotropic support during emergence from cardiopulmonary bypass. *Anesthesiology* **44,** 281.
428. Toyama M. and Reis R. L. (1975) Effects of myocardial ischaemia on ventricular compliance. *J. Thorac. Cardiovasc. Surg.* **70,** 458.
429. Trichet B., Falke K., Togut A. et al. (1975) The effect of pre-existing pulmonary vascular disease on the response to mechanical ventilation with PEEP following open heart surgery. *Anesthesiology* **42,** 56.
430. Tufo H. M., Ostfeld A. M. and Shekelle T. (1970) Central nervous system dysfunction following open heart surgery. *JAMA* **212,** 1333.
431. Turner T. L., Cockburn F. and Forfar J. O. (1977) Magnesium therapy in neonatal tetany. *Lancet* **1,** 283.
432. Turney S. Z., McCluggage C., Blumenfeld W. et al. (1972) Automatic respiratory gas monitoring. *Ann. Thorac. Surg.* **14,** 159.
433. Tuttle R. R., Pollock G. D., Todd G. et al. (1977) The effect of dobutamine on cardiac oxygen balance, regional blood flow and infarction severity after coronary artery narrowing in dogs. *Circ. Res.* **41,** 357.
434. Tweed W. A., Minuck M. and Mymin D. (1972) Circulatory responses to ketamine anesthesia. *Anesthesiology* **37,** 613.
435. Tyers G. F. O., Williams E. H., Hughes H. C. et al. (1977) Effect of perfusate temperature on myocardial protection from ischaemia. *J. Thorac. Cardiovasc. Surg.* **73,** 766.
436. Van der Walt J. H. and Russell W. J. (1978) Effect of heating on the osmotic fragility of stored blood. *Br. J. Anaesth.* **50,** 815.
437. Vaughan Williams E. M. (1970) Classification of anti-arrhythmic drugs. In: Sandue E. (ed.), *Symposia on Cardiac Arrhythmias.* Sweden, AB Astra, p. 449.
438. Viljoen J. F., Estafanous F. G. and Tarazi R. C. (1976) Acute hypertension immediately after coronary artery surgery. *J. Thorac. Cardiovasc. Surg.* **71,** 548.
439. Viljoen J. F. and Gindi M. Y. (1971) Anesthesia for coronary artery surgery. *Surg. Clin. North Am.* **51,** 1081.
440. Virgilio R. W., Smith D. E., Rice C. L. et al. (1976) Effect of colloid osmotic pressure and pulmonary capillary wedge pressure on intrapulmonary shunt. *Surg. Forum* **27,** 168.
441. Voegelpoel L., Schrire V., Nellen M. et al. (1960) The use of phenylephrine in the differentiation of Fallot's tetralogy from pulmonary stenosis with intact ventricular septum. *Am. Heart J.* **59,** 489.
442. Walesby R. K., Goode A. W. and Bentall H. H. (1978) Nutritional status of patients undergoing valve replacement by open heart surgery. *Lancet* **1,** 76.
443. Walker A. K. Y. (1978) Blood microfiltration: a review. *Anaesthesia* **33,** 35.

444. Walston A. II. and Kendall M. E. (1973) Comparison of pulmonary wedge and left atrial pressure in man. *Am. Heart J.* **86**, 159.
445. Wang H. H., Liu L. M. P. and Katz R. L. (1977) A comparison of the cardiovascular effects of sodium nitroprusside and trimetaphan. *Anesthesiology* **46**, 40.
446. Ward M. E., Trewby P. N., Williams R. et al. (1977) Acute liver failure. Experience in a special unit. *Anaesthesia* **32**, 228.
447. Ware S. and Osborne J. P. (1976) Postoperative hypoglycaemia in small children. *Br. Med. J.* **2**, 499.
448. Watson B. G., Pearson D. T. and Williams W. (1977) Prevention of venous blood gas embolism with blood microfilters. *Anaesthesia* **32**, 174.
449. Weil M. H., Shubin H. and Rosoff L. (1965) Fluid repletion in circulatory shock. *JAMA* **192**, 669.
450. Weiskopf R. B. and Severinghaus J. W. (1972) Lack of effect of high altitude on hemoglobin oxygen affinity. *J. Appl. Physiol.* **33**, 276.
451. Westhorpe R. N., Varghese Z., Petrie A. et al. (1978) Changes in ionized calcium and other plasma constituents associated with cardiopulmonary bypass. *Br. J. Anaesth.* **50**, 951.
452. Wexler L. F. and Pohost G. M. (1976) Hemodynamic monitoring: noninvasive technique. *Anesthesiology* **45**, 156.
453. Wheeldon D. R., Bethune D. W., Gill R. D. et al. (1976) A simple cooling circuit for topical cardiac hypothermia. *Thorax* **31**, 565.
454. Whitby J. D. and Dunkin L. J. (1969) Temperature differences in the oesophagus. The effect of intubation and ventilation. *Br. J. Anaesth.* **41**, 615.
455. Whitby J. D. and Dunkin L. J. (1971) Cerebral, oesophageal and nasopharyngeal temperatures. *Br. J. Anaesth.* **43**, 673.
456. White R. D., Goldsmith R. S., Rodriguel R. et al. (1976) Plasma ionic calcium levels following injection of chloride, gluconate and gluceptate salts of calcium. *J. Thorac. Cardiovasc. Surg.* **71**, 609.
457. White R. J., Chamberlain D. A., Hamer J. et al. (1969) Potassium depletion in severe heart disease. *Br. Med. J.* **2**, 606.
458. Whitwam J. G. and Russell W. J. (1971) The acute cardiovascular changes and adrenergic blockade by droperidol in man. *Br. J. Anaesth.* **43**, 581.
459. Wil P. Y. K. and Hodgman J. E. (1974) Insensible water loss in preterm infants: changes with postnatal development and non-ionizing radiant energy. *Pediatrics* **54**, 704.
460. Williams J. F., Childress R. H., Chip J. N. et al. (1969) Hemodynamic effects of glucagon in patients with heart disease. *Circulation* **39**, 38.
461. Williams P. R., and Oh W. (1974) Effects of radiant warmer on insensible water loss in newborn infants. *Am. J. Dis. Child.* **128**, 511.
462. Williams S. E. (1976) Hydrogen ion infusion for treating severe metabolic alkalosis. *Br. Med. J.* **1**, 1189.
463. Wilson R. S. (1976) Monitoring the lung: mechanics and volume. *Anesthesiology* **45**, 135.
464. Wilson R. S. and Rie M. A. (1975) Management of mechanical ventilation. *Surg. Clin. North Am.* **55**, 591.
465. Wilson R. S., Sullivan S. F., Malm J. R. et al. (1973) The oxygen cost of breathing following anesthesia and cardiac surgery. *Anesthesiology* **39**, 387.
466. Wilton A. and Joshi P. I. S. (1977) Adrenergic receptors and renin release. *Lancet* **1**, 698.
467. Winter P. M. and Smith G. (1972) The toxicity of oxygen. *Anesthesiology* **37**, 210.
468. Wong K. C., Martin W. E., Hornbein T. F. et al. (1973) The cardiovascular effects of morphine sulphate with oxygen and with nitrous oxide in man. *Anesthesiology* **38**, 542.

469. Wong K. C., Mohri H., Dillard D. et al. (1974) Deep hypothermia and diethyl ether anaesthesia for open heart surgery in infants: a clinical report of 8 years experience. *Anesth. Analg.* (*Cleve.*) **53**, 765.
470. Woods H. F., Ash G., Weston M. J. et al. (1978) Prostacyclin can replace heparin in haemodialysis in dogs. *Lancet* **2**, 1075.
471. Wright G., Sanderson J. M. and Furness A. (1978) Pulsatile pumps for open heart surgery. *Lancet* **1**, 217.
472. Yates A. (1978) Dopamine and dobutamine. *Br. Med. J.* **1**, 1622.
473. Zapol W. M., Snider M. T. and Schneider R. C. (1977) Extracorporeal membrane oxygenation for acute respiratory failure. *Anesthesiology* **46**, 272.
474. Zimmer S. and Maule B. H. (1978) The Swan Ganz catheter: use in an intensive care unit – an initial impression. *Anaesthesia* **33**, 199.
475. Zorab J. S. M. (1969) Continuous display of the arterial pressure. A simple manometric technique. *Anaesthesia* **24**, 431.

Note Added in Proof (*see* p. 219)

There have been some recent doubts about the suitability of pancuronium for patients in atrial fibrillation particularly [i]. This is due to its action of increasing atrioventricular conduction [ii].

REFERENCES

i. Pratila M. G. and Pratilas V. (1977) A case of tachydysrhythmia: refractory to propranolol and responsive to neostigmine. *Anaesthesia* **32**, 1017.
ii. Rozelle B. C., Geha D. G., Raessler K. L. et al. (1975) The effect of pancuronium bromide on atrio-ventricular conduction in halothane anesthetized dogs. Abstracts of Scientific Papers, American Society of Anesthesiologists Annual Meeting, p. 151.

Index